Intraocular Lens (IOL) Power Calculation

Gede Pardianto
Editor

Intraocular Lens (IOL) Power Calculation

A Practical Guide

Springer

Editor
Gede Pardianto
Department of Ophthalmology and Vision Sciences
Universitas Prima Indonesia
Medan, Indonesia

Sabang Merauke Eye Center (SMEC)
Medan, Indonesia

Prima Vision Eye Hospital
Medan, Indonesia

Star Premiere Eye Center (SPEC)
Medan, Indonesia

ISBN 978-981-92-1222-4 ISBN 978-981-92-1223-1 (eBook)
https://doi.org/10.1007/978-981-92-1223-1

This Springer imprint is published by the registered company Springer Nature Singapore Pte Ltd.
The registered company address is: 152 Beach Road, #21-01/04 Gateway East, Singapore 189721, Singapore

In loving memory of our beloved teacher and mentor: Vidyapati Widiarto Mangunkusumo, MD, PhD (1945–2026). A profound educator, a brilliant mind, a soul of great wisdom, and a lifelong inspiration to us all.

Foreword

Intraocular Lens (IOL) Power Calculation: A Practical Guide, edited by Gede Pardianto, MD, PhD, represents a landmark achievement in ophthalmic education and clinical practice. The subject of intraocular lens (IOL) power calculation has long stood at the intersection of precise science and refined surgical art, demanding from clinicians not only a command of formulas and biometry but also the judgment to individualize refractive outcomes for every patient. This book addresses that demanding balance with clarity, authority, and remarkable breadth.

The volume unfolds systematically, beginning with the historical development of IOLs and the foundations of calculation methods, before advancing into the multi-faceted challenges encountered in daily surgical practice. Each chapter illuminates its theme with depth and relevance: pediatric cataracts, eyes with prior keratoplasty, eyes altered by previous refractive surgery, vitrectomized and uveitic eyes, as well as the nuances of simultaneous vision and also phakic IOLs. Equally important is the attention devoted to emerging technologies such as femtosecond laser-assisted cataract surgery, advanced optical biometry, and toric IOL calculation. By integrating these innovations with insights from high-volume surgical settings and outreach programs, the text succeeds in bridging the most advanced techniques with the global realities of ophthalmic care.

What distinguishes this book is the consistency and authority of its contributors. Internationally recognized experts distill complex knowledge into accessible guidance, creating a text that is at once scholarly and eminently practical. The breadth of the audience addressed is notable: from surgeons seeking to refine their outcomes, to residents and fellows establishing the foundations of their training, to researchers, optometrists, and ophthalmic nurses who contribute to the continuum of care. Each will find in these pages a synthesis of evidence, experience, and vision that elevates the understanding of IOL power calculation.

Through the editorial leadership of Dr. Pardianto and the collective expertise of the contributing authors, this book has achieved a rare accomplishment: it not only documents the current state of knowledge but also sets a standard for the future. Its enduring value will lie in guiding clinicians to achieve refractive excellence while reminding the ophthalmic community of the profound impact that precise lens power calculation exerts on the quality of life for patients worldwide.

Ruhr University Bochum, Knappschaft Kliniken
Bochum, Germany

H. Burkhard Dick

Preface

In the rapidly evolving field of modern cataract surgery, the significance of accurate intraocular lens (IOL) power calculation cannot be overstated. As cataract surgery continues to be one of the most significant discoveries of mankind and the most commonly performed procedures worldwide, the demand for excellent visual outcomes has been greater. This book, *Intraocular Lens (IOL) Power Calculation: A Practical Guide*, is born out of a necessity to bridge the gap between theoretical knowledge and practical application in IOL power calculations.

Over the years, I have witnessed firsthand the profound impact that accurate IOL power calculation can have on patient satisfaction and the overall success of the surgery. Despite advancements in surgical techniques and technology, many practitioners still grapple with the complexities of IOL calculations, leading to suboptimal results. This guide aims to demystify the process, providing a comprehensive yet accessible resource for ophthalmologists at all levels of experience.

Within these pages, you will find a wealth of practical insights, detailed methodologies, and essential tools that can enhance your understanding and execution of IOL power calculations. From foundational principles to innovative approaches, this book encompasses a diverse range of strategies tailored to meet the needs of various practice settings, whether in urban hospitals or rural clinics and mass charity settings.

I encourage you to approach this guide with an open mind and a willingness to explore new techniques and perspectives. By embracing the knowledge shared in this book, you can elevate your practice and, ultimately, improve the quality of care you provide to your highly valuable patients.

This book is dedicated as a tribute to our beloved teacher, Dr. Vidyapati Widiarto Mangunkusumo, a great cataract surgeon whose immense contributions have touched the lives of millions.

I extend my heartfelt gratitude to my mentors, colleagues, and the countless patients who have inspired my journey in ophthalmology. It is my hope that this book serves as a valuable resource and legacy in humanity, empowering you to achieve remarkable outcomes in your very finest cataract surgeries.

Welcome to a journey of discovery and excellence in IOL power calculation.

Medan, Indonesia Gede Pardianto

Intraocular Lens (IOL) Power Calculation: A Practical Guide

In the realm of cataract surgery, achieving optimal visual outcomes is paramount. While surgical skill, advanced technology, and high-end branded intraocular lenses (IOLs) play crucial roles, the cornerstone of success exists in a precisely accurate IOL power calculation. If you are content with achieving a mere 90% of your refractive targets, this book may not be for you. However, for those seeking to elevate their quality of surgery and achieve remarkable results, this guide is an invaluable resource.

This practical book delves into the intricacies of IOL power calculation, offering insights that can transform your approach to cataract surgery. Discover the small yet significant details that can make all the difference in achieving accurate IOL power determinations. From foundational techniques to cutting-edge methodologies in this age of artificial intelligence (AI), this book encompasses a wide spectrum of tools, technologies, and approaches suitable for various settings—be it private practices, small clinics, large hospitals, or even remote health facilities engaged in charitable work.

Equip yourself with the knowledge to enhance your surgical outcomes and provide the best possible care for your patients. Whether you're a very experienced eye surgeon or just starting your journey, this guide is designed to help you reach new heights in IOL power calculation.

Contents

Editor and Contributors

About the Editor

Gede Pardianto is a consultant ophthalmologist at the Sabang Merauke Eye Center (SMEC), Prima Vision Eye Hospital, and Star Premiere Eye Center (SPEC). He serves as associate professor and chairman of residency program at Department of Ophthalmology and Vision Sciences, Universitas Prima Indonesia. He graduated as an MD and ophthalmologist from Universitas Airlangga and earned his PhD by (Summa) Cum Laude from Universitas Sumatera Utara. He has published in more than 100 national and international publications, serves as an editor for 2 journals with more than 80 editorial works, reviewer for 20 international journals with more than 200 reviews, has contributed to more than 400 international papers, and has edited and authored several books and chapters, including editor of 2 books published by Springer Nature. He is the course director of 40 episodes of Maestro Lecture World Series. He was also a panelist and chair in many international conferences and has received many honors, trophies, awards, and medals.

Contributors

Steve A. Arshinoff Department of Ophthalmology and Vision Sciences, University of Toronto, Toronto, ON, Canada

Febrina Art Universitas Sriwijaya, Palembang, Indonesia

Tommy T. Atmaja Sabang-Merauke Eye Center (SMEC), Tanjung Pinang, Indonesia

Anil Boyaju Tilganga Institute of Ophthalmology, Kathmandu, Nepal

Budiman Universitas Padjadjaran, Bandung, Indonesia
Cicendo National Eye Hospital, Bandung, Indonesia

Bandung Eye Center, Bandung, Indonesia

Dago Vision Care, Bandung, Indonesia

Eric R. Chen Department of Ophthalmology, Baylor College of Medicine, Cullen Eye Institute, Houston, TX, USA

Muhammad Edrial IEC Eye Care, Jakarta, Indonesia

Muhammad Zidny Fahmi JEC Java @ Surabaya, JEC Eye Hospitals & Clinics, Surabaya, Indonesia

Sanchay Gupta Department of Ophthalmology, Baylor College of Medicine, Cullen Eye Institute, Houston, TX, USA

Syahira Halisa Sabang-Merauke Eye Center (SMEC), Malang, Indonesia

Sultan Hasanuddin JEC ORBITA, Makassar, Indonesia

Universitas Hasanuddin, Makassar, Indonesia

Johan A. Hutauruk JEC Eye Hospitals & Clinics, Jakarta, Indonesia

Nashrul Ihsan JEC Eye Hospitals & Clinics, Jakarta, Indonesia

John Steven Jarstad Morsani School of Medicine, University of South Florida, Tampa, FL, USA

Andrew Maximillian Herman Knoch Universitas Padjadjaran, Bandung, Indonesia

Cicendo National Eye Hospital, Bandung, Indonesia

Bandung Eye Center, Bandung, Indonesia

Douglas D. Koch Department of Ophthalmology, Baylor College of Medicine, Cullen Eye Institute, Houston, TX, USA

Evelyn Komaratih Department of Ophthalmology, Universitas Airlangga, Surabaya, Indonesia

Vidyapati Widiarto Mangunkusumo JEC Eye Hospitals & Clinics, Jakarta, Indonesia

Florence Meilani Manurung JEC Eye Hospitals & Clinics, Jakarta, Indonesia

Faraby Martha Cipto Mangunkusumo Hospital, Jakarta, Indonesia

Universitas Indonesia, Jakarta, Indonesia

Gede Pardianto Department of Ophthalmology and Vision Sciences, Universitas Prima Indonesia, Medan, Indonesia

Sabang Merauke Eye Center (SMEC), Medan, Indonesia

Prima Vision Eye Hospital, Medan, Indonesia

Star Premiere Eye Center (SPEC), Medan, Indonesia

Rinanto Prabowo Dr. Yap Eye Hospital, Yogyakarta, Indonesia

Ferdian Ramadhan Klinik Utama Sumenep, Sumenep, Indonesia

Rio Rhendy Cipto Mangunkusumo Hospital, Jakarta, Indonesia
Universitas Indonesia, Jakarta, Indonesia

Setiyo Budi Riyanto JEC Eye Hospitals & Clinics, Jakarta, Indonesia

Ricky E. Rooroh KMN Eye Care, Jakarta, Indonesia

Sagar Ruit Tilganga Institute of Ophthalmology, Kathmandu, Nepal

Sanduk Ruit Tilganga Institute of Ophthalmology, Kathmandu, Nepal

Satenla Ruit Tilganga Institute of Ophthalmology, Kathmandu, Nepal

Emma Rusmayani JEC Eye Hospitals & Clinics, Jakarta, Indonesia

Muhammad Bayu Sasongko Department of Ophthalmology, Faculty of Medicine, Public Health, and Nursing, Universitas Gadjah Mada, Yogyakarta, Indonesia

Sindy B. Sembiring Department of Ophthalmology and Vision Sciences, Universitas Prima Indonesia, Medan, Indonesia
Sabang Merauke Eye Center (SMEC), Medan, Indonesia

Swechha Sharma Tilganga Institute of Ophthalmology, Kathmandu, Nepal

Sharita Rosalyne Siregar JEC Eye Hospitals & Clinics, Jakarta, Indonesia

Novita Sitompul Priangan Medical and Eye Center, Bandung, Indonesia

Darmawan M. Sophian Saruni Eye Clinic, Pandeglang, Banten, Indonesia

Triana Budi Sulistya Universitas Brawijaya, Malang, Indonesia

Chinmayi H. Vyas Department of Surgery, Vitreoretinal Surgery Service, McMaster University, Hamilton, ON, Canada

Li Wang Department of Ophthalmology, Baylor College of Medicine, Cullen Eye Institute, Houston, TX, USA

Hadi Prakoso Wreksoatmodjo IEC Eye Care, Jakarta, Indonesia

Jessica Zarwan Cipto Mangunkusumo Hospital, Jakarta, Indonesia
Universitas Indonesia, Jakarta, Indonesia

Abbreviations

a0	Power Prediction Curve or Corneal Power
a1	Anterior Chamber Depth
a2	Axial Length
AAO	American Academy of Ophthalmology
AC IOL	Anterior Chamber IOL
AC	Anterior Chamber
ACA	Anterior Corneal Astigmatism
ACCP	Average Central Corneal Power
ACD	Anterior Chamber Depth
A-Constant	ACD-Constant
ACP	Average Corneal Power
ACW	Anterior Chamber Width
AI	Artificial Intelligence
AL	Axial Length
ALK	Automated Lamellar Keratoplasty
ALP	Actual Lens Position
AnnCP	Annular Ring of Corneal Power
ANSI	American National Standards Institute
APACRS	Asia Pacific Association of Cataract and Refractive Surgery
AQD	Aqueous Depth
A-Scan	Amplitude Mode Scan/Display
ASE	Aphakic Spherical Equivalent
ASCRS	American Society of Cataract and Refractive Surgery
AS-OCT	Anterior Segment Optical Coherence Tomography
ASSORT	Alpins Statistical System for Ophthalmic Refractive Surgery Techniques
ATA	Angle to Angle
ATR	Against-the-Rule Astigmatism
AXL	Axial Length
A/B Scan	Amplitude/Brightness Mode Scan/Display
BCE	Before the Common Era

BID	bis in die, or twice a day
B-scan	Brightness Mode Scan/Display
BSS	Balanced Salt Solution
BUII	Barrett Universal II
CA	California
CACD	Cornea/Calculated Anterior Chamber Depth
CCC	Continuous Curvilinear Capsulorhexis
CCP	Central Corneal Power
CCT	Central Corneal Thickness
CD	Corneal Diameter
CDC	Cataract Diagnostic Center
CEDOF	Continuous Extended Depth of Focus
CH	Corneal Hysteresis
CLR	Crystalline Lens Rises
CMAL	Cooke Modified Axial Length
CME	Cystoid Macular Edema
CPCS	Conventional Phacoemulsification Cataract Surgery
CRS	Corneal Refractive Surgery
CSR	Cataract Surgical Rate
cSt	Centistoke
CT	Corneal Thickness
CTR	Capsular Tension Ring
CXL	Corneal Collagen Crosslinking
D	Diopter
DALK	Deep Anterior Lamellar Keratoplasty
dB	Decibels
DCNN	Deep Convolutional Neural Network
DISCOVER	Determination of Feasibility of Intraoperative Spectral-Domain Microscope Combined/Integrated OCT Visualization during En Face Retinal and Ophthalmic Surgery
DMEK	Descemet Membrane Endothelial Keratoplasty
DSAEK	Descemet Stripping Automated Endothelial Keratoplasty
ECCE	Extracapsular Cataract Extraction
ECL	Endothelial Cell Loss
ECP	Effective Corneal Power
EDOF	Extended-Depth-of-Focus
EffRP	Effective Refractive Power
EKR	Equivalent Keratometry Readings
ELP	Effective Lens Position
EMR	Electronic Medical Records
ENLIGHTEN	Enhanced Light Energy Technology
ESCRS	European Society of Cataract and Refractive Surgeons
EUA	Examination Under Anaesthesia
EuReCCa	European Registry on Childhood Cataract

EUREQUO	European Registry of Quality Outcomes for Cataract and Refractive Surgery
EVO	Emmetropia Verifying Optical
FDA	Food and Drug Administration
FD-OCT	Fourier-Domain Optical Coherence Tomography or Frequency-Domain Optical Coherence Tomography
FLACS	Femtosecond Laser Assisted Cataract Surgery
fs	Femtosecond
HM	Hand Movement
HOA	High Order Aberration
Hoffer QST	Kenneth J. Hoffer Q/Giacomo Savini/Leonardo Taroni
HSM	Heparin Surface Modification
HWTW	Horizontal White to White
IC	Intracameral
ICL	Implantable Collamer Lens
IFIS	Intraoperative Floppy Iris Syndrome
ILM	Inner Limiting Membrane
ILO	Interlenticular Opacification
ILP	Internal Lens Position
iOCT	intraoperative Optical Coherence Tomography
IOL	Intraocular Lens
IPCL	Implantable Phakic Intraocular Lenses
IRB	Intraoperative Refractive Biometry
ISO	International Organization for Standardization
IWA	Intraoperative Wavefront Aberrometry
JRA	Juvenile Rheumatoid Arthritis
K	Keratometric or Keratometry Reading
kHz	Kilohertz
KLEx	Keratorefractive Lenticule Extraction
Kpost	Post-LASIK/PRK Keratometry Readings
KS	Kamiya-Shimizu
LAL	Light Adjustable Lens
LASIK	Laser In-Situ Keratomileusis
LDD	Light Delivery Device
LEC	Lens Epithelial Cell
LF	Lens Factor
LISA-PPV	Ensemble Artificial Intelligence-Based Thick Intraocular Lens Calculation Formula for Vitrectomized Eyes
LOCS	Lens Opacities Classification System
LP	Light Perception
LRI	Limbal Relaxing Incisions
LSF	Ladas Super Formula
LT	Lens Thickness
LVC	Laser Vision Correction
MAE	Mean Absolute Error

MBE	Mean Bias Error
ME	Mean (Prediction or Bias) Error
MedAE	Median Absolute Error
MHz	Megahertz
MICS	Micro Incision Cataract Surgery
MIGS	Microinvasive Glaucoma Surgeries
ML	Machine Learning
mm	Millimeter
MMD	Micro Medical Device
MR	Manifest Refraction
m/s	Meter/Second
NC	No Cataract
NCP	Net Corneal Power
NK	Nakamura-Kamiya
NET	Feedforward Neural Networks
NRR	No Rotation Recommended
NSAID	Nonsteroidal Anti-Inflammatory Drug
NULEX	Non-ultrasonic Lens Extraction
NVG	Neovascular Glaucoma
NY	New York
OBBCGS	Optical Biometry Based Cataract Grading System
OBEC	Optical Biometry Examined Cataract
OBUC	Optical Biometry Unexamined Cataract
OCOS	Online Calculation & Ordering System
OCT	Optical Coherence Tomography
OLCR	Optical Low Coherence Reflectometry
OMEC	Outreach Microsurgical Clinic
ONH	Optic Nerve Head
ORA	Optiwave Refractive Analysis
OT	Operating Theatre
OVD	Ophthalmic Viscosurgical Devices
pACD	Individualized Anterior Chamber Depth
PAS	Peripheral Anterior Synechiae
PCA	Posterior Corneal Astigmatism
PCI	Partial Coherence Interferometry
PCO	Posterior Capsule Opacification
PE	Prediction Errors
PEARL	PrEsbyopic Allogenic Refractive Lenticule
PEARL-DGS	Postoperative spherical Equivalent prediction using ARtificial intelligence and Linear Algorithms by Guillaume Debellemanière, Damien Gatinel, and Alain Saad
PEX	Pseudoexfoliation
pIOL	Phakic Intraocular Lens
PIONEER	Prospective Intraoperative and Perioperative Ophthalmic Imaging with Optical Coherence Tomography

PK	Penetrating Keratoplasty
PKA	Posterior Corneal Astigmatism
PMMA	Polymethyl-Methacrylate
PRK	Photorefractive Keratectomy
PROMs	Patient-Reported Outcome Measures
ps	Picosecond
PXF	Pseudoexfoliation
RA	Residual Astigmatism
RBF	Radial Basis Function
recCP	Reconstructed Corneal Power
REG	Linear Regression
RK	Radial Keratotomy
RLE	Refractive Lens Extraction
RMS	Root Mean Square
RNFL	Retinal Nerve Fiber Layer
RPE	Retinal Pigment Epithelium
RRG2	Reanalysis of Refractive Growth 2
SA	Spherical Aberration
SAA	Steve A. Arshinoff
SaMD	Software as a Medical Device
SD	Standard Deviation
SD-OCT	Spectral-Domain Optical Coherence Tomography
SE	Spherical Equivalent
SF	Surgeon Factor
SIA	Surgery-Induced Astigmatism or Surgically Induced Astigmatism
Sim-K	Simulated Keratometry
SMILE	Small Incision Lenticule Extraction
SNR	Signal-to-Noise Ratio
SRK	Sanders-Ritzlaff-Kraff (Drs. Donald R. Sanders, John A. Retzlaff, and Manus C. Kraff)
SRK/T	Sanders-Retzlaff-Kraff/Theoretical
SS-OCT	Swept-Source Optical Coherence Tomography
STS	Sulcus to Sulcus
TCA	Total Corneal Astigmatism
TCP	Total Corneal Power
TCRP	Total Corneal Refractive Power
TD-OCT	Time-Domain Optical Coherence Tomography
TILP	Theoretical Internal Lens Position
TIO	Tilganga Institute of Ophthalmology
tIOL	Toric Intraocular Lenses
TK	Total Keratometry
TNP	True Net Power
TPIOL	Toric Phakic Intraocular Lens
True K	True Keratometry
TX	Texas

UBM	Ultrasound Biomicroscopy
UDVA	Uncorrected Distance Visual Acuity
UGH	Uveitis-Glaucoma-Hyphema
ULIB	User Group for Laser Interference Biometry
US	United States
USD	United States Dollar
USG	Ultrasonography
UV	Ultraviolet
UV-A	Ultraviolet-A
VRF	Voytsekhivskyy Regression Function
VRF-G	Voytsekhivskyy Regression Function-Gender
WHO	World Health Organization
WK	Wang-Koch Axial Length Adjustments
WK1	First Linear Wang-Koch Axial Length Adjustment
WKA	Wang-Koch Adjustment
WTR	With-the-Rule Astigmatism
WTW	White to White
XGBoost	eXtreme Gradient Boosting
YAG	Yttrium Aluminum Garnet
ΔMR	Surgical Induced Change in Manifest Refraction
μJ	Microjoule

Chapter 1
History of Intraocular Lens and IOL Power Calculation

Johan A. Hutauruk and Gede Pardianto

1.1 Introduction

The development of intraocular lenses (IOLs) represents one of the most remarkable advancements in ophthalmology. From their early beginnings to today's highly sophisticated designs, IOLs have revolutionized the treatment of cataracts and refractive errors. Alongside these advancements, the evolution of IOL power calculation has transformed cataract surgery from a simple vision-restoring procedure into a precise refractive surgery, allowing surgeons to deliver exceptional visual outcomes and reduce patients' dependence on spectacles [1, 2].

In this chapter, we review the historical development of intraocular lenses and the progression of IOL power calculation formulas, underscoring their transformative impact on the field of cataract and refractive surgery.

All authors declare no financial interest.

J. A. Hutauruk (✉)
JEC Eye Hospitals & Clinics, Jakarta, Indonesia
e-mail: johan.hutauruk@jec.co.id

G. Pardianto
Department of Ophthalmology and Vision Sciences, Universitas Prima Indonesia, Medan, Indonesia

Sabang Merauke Eye Center (SMEC), Medan, Indonesia

Prima Vision Eye Hospital, Medan, Indonesia

Star Premiere Eye Center (SPEC), Medan, Indonesia

G. Pardianto (ed.), *Intraocular Lens (IOL) Power Calculation*,
https://doi.org/10.1007/978-981-92-1223-1_1

1.2 The Birth of IOL

1.2.1 Sir Nicholas Harold Lloyd Ridley and the First IOL

The origins of the IOL can be traced to the 1940s, when Sir Nicholas Harold Lloyd Ridley, an English ophthalmologist, made a pivotal observation that paved the way for a revolution in cataract surgery. During World War II, Ridley noticed that Royal Air Force pilots who suffered eye injuries from shattered cockpit canopies—made of polymethyl methacrylate (PMMA)—often retained fragments in their eyes without triggering severe inflammation. This remarkable biocompatibility sparked Ridley's visionary idea: If PMMA could remain inert inside the eye, perhaps it could serve as the material for an artificial lens to restore sight after cataract removal. That insight marked the beginning of modern IOL development [1–3].

On November 29, 1949, at St. Thomas' Hospital in London, Ridley performed an extracapsular cataract extraction on a 45-year-old woman and implanted a Perspex IOL. However, according to his resident, Peter Choyce, Ridley promptly removed the lens due to concerns about its stability. The lens was designed without haptics, compromising its stability and leading to a significant myopic refractive error of −21 diopters (D). Additionally, its sterilization using cetrimide was suspected to have contributed to the development of postoperative uveitis [1, 3–5].

Despite early complications such as lens dislocation and chronic inflammation due to lack of proper fixation and biocompatibility understanding, Ridley's invention marked a pivotal moment in ophthalmology [4, 5].

1.2.2 Evolution of IOL Design

- 1950s–1960s: Early lenses, like Ridley's, were anterior chamber (AC) lenses, which often caused significant complications such as uveitis, glaucoma, and hyphema (termed the "uveitis-glaucoma-hyphema (UGH) syndrome") [2, 4, 5].
- 1970s: Introduction of posterior chamber (PC) lenses provided better anatomical positioning and stability, reducing complications.
- 1980s–1990s: Advances in materials like foldable acrylic and silicone allowed for smaller incisions and safer surgery. Development of single-piece and three-piece designs improved lens fixation and visual outcomes [2].
- 2000s–present: Modern IOLs offer enhanced refractive solutions, including toric, multifocal, extended depth-of-focus (EDOF), and accommodating lenses. Improved biocompatibility, edge designs to reduce posterior capsule opacification (PCO), and aspheric optics further refined outcomes [2, 6].

1.3 The Evolution of IOL Power Calculation

The success of IOL implantation is not solely dependent on surgical technique or lens design, but critically on accurately determining the appropriate lens power. Over time, IOL power calculation has evolved from basic estimations to sophisticated mathematical models integrated with cutting-edge technology (Table 1.1) [7, 8].

Table 1.1 IOL formulas, their generations, and their ELP prediction [7, 8, 11, 12, 15, 16, 18]

Generation	Formulas	Year	ELP prediction
First	Svyatoslav Nikolayevich Fyodorov M.C. Colenbrander James (Jim) P. Gills and Tom Lloyd Henry M. Clayman Richard D. Binkhorst Donald R. Sanders, John A. Retzlaff, and Manus C. Kraff (SRK)	1967–1980s	4 mm (constant)
Second	Modified Binkhorst SRK II	1980s	Using AL (single predictor)
	Kenneth J. Hoffer (1)		
Third	SRK/T	1988	Using AL and K-reading
	Jack T. Holladay 1		
	Hoffer Q		
Fourth	Holladay 2	1990s–2010	Using AL, K-reading, ACD, and Lens Thickness (LT)
	Thomas Olsen		
	Graham D. Barrett Universal II (BUII)		
	Wolfgang Haigis		
Newer	Jack X. Kane Ladas Super Formula PEARL-DGS Warren E. Hill-RBF OKULIX Emmetropia Verifying Optical (EVO) Oleksiy V. Voytsekhivskyy Regression Function-Gender (VRF-G)	~2010s–2020s	Using AL, K, ACD, LT, plus Central Corneal Thickness (CCT), AI, Gender, etc.

1.3.1 *First-Generation Formulas*

The accuracy of IOL power calculation is largely determined by the effective lens position (ELP). The method for determining ELP has evolved over time. Before the 1980s, the ELP was a constant value of 4 mm in every patient and every IOL, including anterior chamber IOL (AC IOL). This was the birth of the first regression and theoretical formulas: [8, 9]

1.3.1.1 Empirical or Regression Formulas

In the 1950s and 1960s, IOL power selection was largely empirical. Surgeons relied on average axial-lengths (AL) and keratometry (K)-readings, often resulting in high degrees of postoperative refractive error: [4, 8, 9]

- Gills formula (1978) is a simplified, and empirically fitted regression-based formula, not a purely theoretical one.
- The SRK (Sanders-Retzlaff-Kraff) formula, introduced in the late 1970s (launched in 1980), was one of the first attempts at a systematic approach to lens power calculation. The SRK I formula was a linear regression formula that included AL and K-reading but was relatively crude by modern standards.

1.3.1.2 Theoretical Formulas

As understanding of ocular anatomy and optics improved, theoretical formulas emerged:

- Binkhorst formula (1970s): One of the first theoretical formulas, incorporating anterior chamber depth (ACD) to estimate the ELP.
- Fyodorov (from the 1970s and published in 1975), Colenbrander (1973), Hoffer-Colonbrander (1974), and Clayman (1979) were among these theoretical formulas [8, 9].

1.3.2 *Second-Generation Formulas*

In the 1980s, the second-generation formulas used AL, a single variable predictor, as a scaling factor to determine the ELP. These formulas include: SRK II (regression formula, 1988), and previous theoretical formulas include: modified Binkhorst or Binkhorst II (1981) and Hoffer (1982) [8–10].

1.3.3 *Third-Generation Formulas*

From 1988, third-generation formulas, including: Holladay 1 (1988), SRK/T (1990), and Hoffer Q (1990), incorporated two variable predictors, AL and K-reading, to improve the accuracy of the scaling factors of ELP. Third-generation formulas optimized outcomes for normal eyes but struggled with extremes in AL or corneal curvature [9, 10].

1.3.4 *Fourth-Generation Formulas*

From 1990 onward, fourth-generation ELP formulas, such as: Haigis (developed from the 1990s and published in 2000) and Holladay 2 (1996), were improved by adding two more variables, pre-op ACD and LT. In addition, fourth-generation formulas incorporated additional biometric parameters such as white-to-white (WTW) or corneal diameter (CD) to enhance ELP prediction [5]. Other fourth-generation formulas in the service are Barrett Universal II (BUII, 2010–2013), and Olsen (2010–2011) [10, 11].

1.4 The Era of Optical Biometry

The introduction of optical biometry, first by the launching of partial coherence interferometry (PCI) in the late 1990s with devices like the IOLMaster (Carl Zeiss Meditec, Dublin, CA), marked a major leap forward in measurement precision. Noncontact, highly accurate AL, K-reading, and ACD measurements significantly improve refractive outcomes [11–14].

Optical low coherence reflectometry (OLCR) launched in 2008. Lenstar LS900 (Haag-Streit, Köniz, Switzerland) and Aladdin (Topcon, Tokyo, Japan) are among the known OLCR in service [13].

Since the 2010s, swept-source optical coherence tomography (SS-OCT), including: IOLMaster 700 (Carl Zeiss Meditec, Dublin, CA), Eyestar 900 (Haag-Streit, Köniz, Switzerland), ARGOS (Movu, Aichi, Japan), ANTERION (Heidelberg Engineering, Heidelberg, Germany), and CASIA2 (Tomey Corporation, Nagoya, Japan) significantly improve IOL power calculation [13, 14].

In 2015, a Scheimpflug-based optical biometer was launched. Pentacam AXL (Oculus Optikgeräte, Wetzlar, Germany) uses Scheimpflug camera combined with PCI. It integrates AL measurement into the previous Pentacam platform (2000s). On the other hand, the Galilei G6 (Ziemer, Biel, Switzerland) combines a dual rotating Scheimpflug camera to perform axial biometry [7, 13].

First, optical biometry machines provide many standard IOL calculation formulas in their system. Modern formulas that emerge in the age of optical biometry include:

- BUII: A sophisticated formula considering posterior corneal curvature, lens position, and other biometric factors, delivering highly accurate results across a wide range of eyes [11, 12].
- Olsen: Utilizes ray tracing and a C-constant to predict ELP more reliably [11, 12, 16, 17].
- Hill-RBF (radial basis function, version 1.0 (2016), version 2.0 (2018), and version 3.0 (2020)): An artificial intelligence (AI)-driven algorithm that uses pattern recognition and a large database to predict IOL power without relying on traditional theoretical optics [11, 12, 15, 16].
- Kane formula (2017): Combines theoretical optics, AI, and regression analysis to deliver excellent accuracy, particularly in post-refractive surgery eyes [11, 12, 16].
- Ladas super formula (2015–2019), and the postoperative spherical quivalent prediction using ARtificial intelligence and linear algorithms by Guillaume Debellemanière, Damien Gatinel, and Alain Saad or PEARL-DGS (2021)—other examples of hybrid and AI-enhanced formulas pushing the boundaries of prediction accuracy [11, 12].

1.5 Intraoperative Aberrometry

Intraoperative aberrometry supports phaco surgeons to calculate the IOL power intraoperatively, furthermore to determine the axis of toric IOL, and give accurate guidance to place it correctly [7].

1.6 IOL Power Calculation in Special Situations

Throughout the history of IOL power calculation, some calculation methods need armaments, adjustments, additional predictive factors, etc., to improve their accuracy:

- Post-refractive surgery eyes: Accurate IOL calculation in these eyes remains challenging. Methods like the Barrett True-K (2008–2015), Haigis-L (2008), and American Society of Cataract and Refractive Surgery (ASCRS) online calculators are commonly used [19, 20].
- In case of long eyes or high myopic eyes, the Wang-Koch Adjustment (2011) can enhance the accuracy of Holladay 1, SRK/T, Hoffer Q, and Haigis formulas in IOL power calculation for high myopia. The similar concept is still used, though newer formulas (e.g., Barrett True-K, Haigis-L, and Olsen) [21].

- Pediatric IOL calculation: Requires consideration of ocular growth and refractive changes over time [22].
- Toric and multifocal IOLs: Require meticulous measurement of corneal astigmatism, posterior corneal curvature, and careful patient selection to ensure optimal outcomes. Beyond the toric calculators, some armaments like the Toric Results Analyzer Calculator or AstigmatismFix from Drs. John Berdahl and David Hardten (2012), the Alpins Statistical System for Ophthalmic Refractive Surgery Techniques (ASSORT) Toric Calculator from Dr. Noel Alpins (2014–2015), and the Baylor Normogram (2010–2012) play an important role for helping some formulas in toric IOL power calculation [23–25].
- Some challenging cases, and the need of new engineered IOLs such us multifocal and toric IOLs, nondiffractive isofocal optic technology, EDOF, light adjustable lens (LAL), light delivery device (LDD), enhanced light energy technology (ENLIGHTEN), and "lens-in-a-lens" designs need to be resolved by using newer biometry machines and latest IOL power calculation formulas, such as: Double K Modification, Hoffer Q Savini/Taroni (Hoffer QST), Hoffer Double AL, SRK/$T_{corrected}$ K, Shammas PL, Shammas No-History, Barrett Toric, Barrett True K Toric, Barrett Rx, Bayesian Additive Regression Trees (BART), FullMonte, Abulafia-Koch, Ladas AI, Clarke Neural Network, Panacea, T2 (updated version of SRK/T), Telomere Restriction Fragments (TRF), User Group for Laser Interference Biometry (ULIB), Kristian Naeser 2, Sramka, Voytsekhivskyy Regression Function (VRF), Maloney, and Wang-Koch-Maloney, Masket, and by add "TK" to some formulas [11–13, 16–18, 23–26].
- Nowadays, some AI-driven formulas emerge to play an important role in IOL power calculation. Hill-RBF 3.0, EVO 2.0, Kane Formula, PEARL-DGS, Hoffer QST, Ladas Super 2.0/Ladas AI, ZEISS AI IOL Calculator, Zhu-Lu Formula, etc., are among them [27, 28].
- Online IOL calculators are appearing in increasing numbers every day, adding to the variety of available formula options. IOL manufacturers are also keeping up by providing their own online IOL formula services to support doctors who use their products [28, 29].
- Beyond current sophisticated biometers, the latest conventional formulas, and the most advanced AI-assisted online formulas, that nowadays the surgeons are able to calculate the IOL power through AI-chat engine (ChatGPT, etc), as a comparative back-up, especially for some challenging or special cases, to assure and reconfirm that the conventional calculations were right.

The history of intraocular lenses (IOLs) and IOL power calculation is a testament to human ingenuity and the relentless drive for excellence in ophthalmology. From Sir Harold Ridley's pioneering implantation to today's advanced premium IOL designs, AI-driven formulas, and IOL power calculation through AI-chat engine, this field has transformed cataract surgery into a highly predictable refractive procedure. As technology continues to evolve, the vision of fully customized, patient-specific visual rehabilitation is rapidly becoming a reality.

References

1. Apple DJ, Sims J. Harold Ridley and the invention of the intraocular lens. Surv Ophthalmol. 1996;40(4):279–92. https://doi.org/10.1016/s0039-6257(96)82003-0. PMID: 8658339.
2. Packard R. The history of innovation in cataract surgery. In: Pardianto G, Tassignon MJ, editors. Innovation in cataract surgery. Singapore: Springer; 2024. p. 1–34. https://doi.org/10.1007/978-981-97-5192-1_1.
3. Margo CE. Harold Ridley: the development of a plastic implantable lens. In: Marmor M, Albert D, editors. Foundations of ophthalmology. Cham: Springer; 2017. p. 169–81. https://doi.org/10.1007/978-3-319-59641-9_14.
4. Leffle CT, Spalton D. Harold Ridley's first intraocular lens implant. In: Leffler CT, editor. A new history of cataract surgery part 2: from 1751 through the modern era. Wayenborgh; 2024.
5. Leffler CT, Spalton D, Grzybowski A, Schwartz SG. The ophthalmologist's time machine: Chapter 23 Harold Ridley and the first intraocular lens. Nov 2024. https://theophthalmologist.com/subspecialties/the-ophthalmologists-time-machine-chapter-23.
6. Arbisser LB. Intraocular lens selection in cataract surgery. In: Pardianto G, Tassignon MJ, editors. Innovation in cataract surgery. Singapore: Springer; 2024. p. 103–21. https://doi.org/10.1007/978-981-97-5192-1_7.
7. Dhawlikar NS, Dai YL, Hughes KV, Rao NK. IOL power calculation in special situations. In: Pardianto G, editor. The intraocular lens power calculation. Medan: Anak Sudarti Foundation; 2022. p. 43–73. https://bit.ly/TheIOLPowerCalculation
8. Sanders DR, Retzlaff J, Kraff MC. Comparison of the SRK II formula and other second generation formulas. J Cataract Refract Surg. 1988;14(2):136–41. https://doi.org/10.1016/s0886-3350(88)80087-7.
9. Hoffer KJ. The Hoffer Q formula: a comparison of theoretic and regression formulas. J Cataract Refract Surg. 1993;19(6):700–12. https://doi.org/10.1016/s0886-3350(13)80338-0.
10. Retzlaff J, Sanders DR. SRK formula history. In: Aramberri J, Hoffer KJ, Olsen T, Savini G, Shammas HJ, editors. Intraocular lens calculations. Essentials in ophthalmology. Cham: Springer; 2024. p. 767–74. https://doi.org/10.1007/978-3-031-50666-6_53.
11. Moshirfar M, Sulit CA, Brown AH, Irwin C, Ronquillo YC, Hoopes PC. Comparing the accuracy of the Kane, Barrett Universal II, hill-radial basis function, emmetropia verifying optical, and Ladas super formula intraocular lens power calculation formulas. Clin Ophthalmol. 2023;17:2643–52. https://doi.org/10.2147/OPTH.S417865. PMID: 37701462; PMCID: PMC10494915.
12. Yasar II, Yasar S, Al Barri L, Darabus DM, Tîrziu AT, Munteanu M, Stanca HT. Comparative analysis of intraocular lens power calculation formulas (Kane, Barrett Universal II, Hill-Radial Basis Function, and Ladas Super Formula): Which one is more accurate? J Clin Med. 2025;14(7):2443. https://doi.org/10.3390/jcm14072443. PMID: 40217893; PMCID: PMC11989757.
13. Pathak M, Sahu V, Kumar A, Kaur K, Gurnani B. Current concepts and recent updates of optical biometry – a comprehensive review. Clin Ophthalmol. 2024;18:1191–206. https://doi.org/10.2147/OPTH.S464538. PMID: 38711575; PMCID: PMC11073143.
14. Szalai E, Csutak A. Comparative analysis of two optical biometry devices: high wavelength swept source OCT versus partial coherence interferometry. Int Ophthalmol. 2022;42(2):627–34. https://doi.org/10.1007/s10792-021-02036-0. Epub 2021 Oct 11. PMID: 34633606; PMCID: PMC8882571.
15. Darcy K, Gunn D, Tavassoli S, Sparrow J, Kane JX. Assessment of the accuracy of new and updated intraocular lens Power Calculation formulas in 10930 eyes from the UK national health service. J Cataract Refract Surg. 2020;46(1):2–7. https://doi.org/10.1016/j.jcrs.2019.08.014. PMID: 32050225.
16. Stopyra W, Langenbucher A, Grzybowski A. Intraocular lens power calculation formulas-a systematic review. Ophthalmol Ther. 2023;12(6):2881–902. https://doi.org/10.1007/s40123-023-00799-6. Epub 2023 Sep 12. PMID: 37698825; PMCID: PMC10640516.

17. Wei LQ, Fu YH, Pan WH, Nie L, Chen Y, Liu GF, Qian ZB. Accuracy of optimized Sirius ray-tracing method in intraocular lens power calculation. Int J Ophthalmol. 2022;15(2):228–32. https://doi.org/10.18240/ijo.2022.02.06. PMID: 35186681; PMCID: PMC8818452.
18. Hipólito-Fernandes D, Elisa Luís M, Gil P, Maduro V, Feijão J, Yeo TK, Voytsekhivskyy O, Alves N. VRF-G, a new intraocular lens power calculation formula: a 13-formulas comparison study. Clin Ophthalmol. 2020;14:4395–402. https://doi.org/10.2147/OPTH.S290125. PMID: 33364744; PMCID: PMC7751728.
19. Vilaltella M, Cid-Bertomeu P, Serés-Noriega T, Huerva V. Accuracy of 12 IOL power calculation formulas in highly myopic eyes. Int Ophthalmol. 2025;45(1):264. https://doi.org/10.1007/s10792-025-03608-0. PMID: 40560233; PMCID: PMC12198256.
20. Yeo TK, Heng WJ, Pek D, Wong J, Fam HB. Accuracy of intraocular lens formulas using total keratometry in eyes with previous myopic laser refractive surgery. Eye (Lond). 2021;35(6):1705–11. https://doi.org/10.1038/s41433-020-01159-5. Epub 2020 Aug 31. PMID: 32868880; PMCID: PMC8169843.
21. Bernardes J, Raimundo M, Lobo C, Murta JN. A comparison of intraocular lens power calculation formulas in high myopia. J Refract Surg. 2021;37(3):207–11. https://doi.org/10.3928/1081597X-20201123-01. Epub 2021 Mar 18. PMID: 34038295.
22. Khokhar S, Rani D. Innovations in paediatric cataract surgery. In: Pardianto G, Tassignon MJ, editors. Innovation in cataract surgery. Singapore: Springer; 2024. p. 219–46. https://doi.org/10.1007/978-981-97-5192-1_16.
23. Park DY, Lim DH, Hwang S, Hyun J, Chung TY. Comparison of astigmatism prediction error taken with the Pentacam measurements, Baylor nomogram, and Barrett formula for toric intraocular lens implantation. BMC Ophthalmol. 2017;17(1):156. https://doi.org/10.1186/s12886-017-0550-z. PMID: 28836956; PMCID: PMC5571625.
24. Shukhaev SV, Boiko EV, Kudlakhmedov SS. Sravnitel'naya otsenka tochnosti rascheta toricheskikh intraokulyarnykh linz [Comparative assessment of the accuracy of toric intraocular lens calculations]. Vestn Oftalmol. 2022;138(1):5–12. Russian. https://doi.org/10.17116/oftalma20221380115. PMID: 35234415.
25. Sharma AC, Khetan A. Comparing IOLM700 TK, Berdahl and Hardten astigmatism fix calculator and Barrett Rx formula in managing residual astigmatism due to toric intraocular lens misalignment. Indian J Ophthalmol. 2022;70(2):413–9. https://doi.org/10.4103/ijo.IJO_1760_21. PMID: 35086207; PMCID: PMC9024007.
26. Lwowski C, Pawlowicz K, Hinzelmann L, Adas M, Kohnen T. Prediction accuracy of IOL calculation formulas using the ASCRS online calculator for a diffractive extended depth-of-focus IOL after myopic laser in situ keratomileusis. J Cataract Refract Surg. 2020;46(9):1240–6. https://doi.org/10.1097/j.jcrs.0000000000000238. PMID: 32379087.
27. Stopyra W, Voytsekhivskyy O, Grzybowski A. Accuracy of 7 artificial intelligence-based intraocular lens power calculation formulas in extremely long caucasian eyes. Am J Ophthalmol. 2025;271:337–46. https://doi.org/10.1016/j.ajo.2024.10.033. Epub 2024 Nov 12. PMID: 39536848.
28. Savini G, Hoffer KJ. Online intraocular lens power calculators. In: Pardianto G, Tassignon MJ, editors. Innovation in cataract surgery. Singapore: Springer; 2024. p. 123–38. https://doi.org/10.1007/978-981-97-5192-1_8.
29. Buonsanti D, Raimundo M, Findl O. Online intraocular lens calculation. Curr Opin Ophthalmol. 2024;35(1):11–6. https://doi.org/10.1097/ICU.0000000000001014. Epub 2023 Nov 3. PMID: 37922421.

Chapter 2
Fundamental Knowledge and Definitions in Intraocular Lens Power Calculation

Gede Pardianto, Syahira Halisa, Sindy B. Sembiring, and Tommy T. Atmaja

2.1 Introduction

In understanding the calculation of the intraocular (IOL) power, there are many terms that must be well understood by cataract surgeons, especially for phacoemulsification (phaco) surgeons. A profound understanding of the terminologies used is crucial because in many aspects, a good understanding can help a surgeon obtain accurate IOL power calculations, the results of which will raise the chances of patients obtaining maximum visual function and benefiting from successful surgery [1, 2].

Understanding different fundamental knowledge and definitions in IOL power calculations should be a part of comprehensive learning for every prospective phaco

---

All authors declare no financial interest.

G. Pardianto (✉)
Department of Ophthalmology and Vision Sciences, Universitas Prima Indonesia, Medan, Indonesia

Sabang Merauke Eye Center (SMEC), Medan, Indonesia

Prima Vision Eye Hospital, Medan, Indonesia

Star Premiere Eye Center (SPEC), Medan, Indonesia

S. Halisa
Sabang-Merauke Eye Center (SMEC), Malang, Indonesia

S. B. Sembiring
Department of Ophthalmology and Vision Sciences, Universitas Prima Indonesia, Medan, Indonesia

Sabang Merauke Eye Center (SMEC), Medan, Indonesia

T. T. Atmaja
Sabang-Merauke Eye Center (SMEC), Tanjung Pinang, Indonesia

G. Pardianto (ed.), *Intraocular Lens (IOL) Power Calculation*,
https://doi.org/10.1007/978-981-92-1223-1_2

surgeon. This is also important for any professions responsible for assisting the measurement and calculations of IOL power, such as technicians and nurses [1, 3, 4].

In the digital era of advanced technology and digital intelligence, coupled with increasingly high patient expectations regarding the surgical outcomes, calculating the IOL power is crucial for the phaco surgeon, who has no choice but to master it as excellently as possible [2, 5, 6].

2.2 Biometry in General

Biometry is a part of anthropometry, which is a mathematical measurement carried out on living creatures. This measurement covers various aspects of certain living creatures, which can include height, weight, head circumference, arm length, leg length, chest circumference, abdominal circumference, etc. Biometry is used for measurement in various important aspects, such as research, science, statistics, population, logistic supply, health, medicine and aviation safety, sports, immigration and border security, etc. [7, 8]

2.3 Eye Biometry

In the field of ophthalmology, biometry plays a crucial role in helping ophthalmologists reach diagnosis, enabling treatment and surgical decisions, as well as patient follow-up. In ophthalmology, biometry is carried out using various tools, such as optical coherence tomography (OCT), confocal biomicroscopy, Scheimpflug cameras, interferometry, ultrasound biomicroscopy (UBM), ultrasonography (USG), specular microscope, corneal topography, aberrometer, interferometer, etc., to obtain calculation values and important data from the eyelids, cornea, anterior chamber, pupil, crystalline lens, vitreous, retina, macula, retinal nerve fiber layer (RNFL), optic nerve head (ONH), refractive status, and general eyeball condition [8–10].

2.4 Biometry in Cataract Surgery

Cataract surgery has reached many advances. Initially, the primary objective of cataract surgery was to overcome total blindness due to the cataractous lens. Over time, with the advancement of knowledge and technology, cataract surgery has reached the goal of higher level of vision. Nowadays, cataract surgery has become a refractive surgery expected to not only enable patients to reach maximum visual function but also for fast surgical recovery. Today, cataract surgery has a target of zero diopter (D) in distance, intermediate, and near visions. With heightened surgical outcome expectations, proper knowledge and skills in calculating IOL power become even more crucial [4, 8, 9, 11].

2.5 IOL Power Calculation in Today's Cataract Surgery

In the early days of IOL power calculation, to help surgeons determine the power of the IOL that would be implanted, axial length (AL or AXL) was the most important calculation to measure. *AL* is the distance (in mm) from the corneal tear film surface to the posterior part of the eye ball. For many years, the UBM was the gold standard for AL measurement, with two different methods available [8, 12, 13].

In more recent years, optical biometry is used for most cataract cases due to its accuracy. In UBM, the measurement aligns with the internal limiting membrane (ILM) known as the AL-ILM, while in optical biometry, the measurement aligns with the retinal pigment epithelium (RPE) or Bruch's membrane, known as the AL-RPE [12, 14, 15]. Since traditional IOL power calculators or formulas were developed during the era of UBM, which means any AL-RPE measurement should be adjusted to AL-ILM by subtracting the retinal thickness by approximately 300 μm for each eye [12, 15].

AL plays a significant role in the precision and accuracy of IOL power calculation. A cohort study reported that the average AL in the normal eye increases from 16.8 mm in infants to 23.6 mm in adults [16]. By measuring the valid value of AL, commonly in normal adult eyes, phaco surgeons may choose any formulas to calculate the right IOL power to gain the best result. Based on AL, the vintage formulas that may be accurate are:

(a) For AL <20 mm: Hoffer Q, and Holladay 2.
(b) For AL 20–22 mm: Hoffer Q.
(c) For AL 22–24.5 mm: Holladay 1, Hoffer Q, and SRK/T (Sanders-Retzlaff-Kraff/Theoretical).
(d) For AL 24.5–26 mm: Holladay 1.
(e) For AL >26 mm: SRK/T [12, 17–19].

What if the AL measurement goes wrong? The role of AL is so important because every 1 mm error in AL measurement could impact postoperative refraction:

(a) Above 30 mm AL could miss 1.75 D per 1 mm.
(b) About 20–30 mm AL could miss 2.35 D per 1 mm.
(c) Below 20 mm AL could miss about 3.75 D per 1 mm [17].

2.6 Biometry of the Cornea for IOL Power Calculation

K1 and K2 are the two basic terms in corneal biometry or keratometry. Keratometry measures the radius of the anterior corneal curvature, presented in millimeters (mm). This assessment is usually converted into the power maps of Dioptric or Diopter (D). *K1* represents the flattest meridian of the anterior corneal curvature, while *K2* determines the steepest meridian of the anterior corneal curvature. K1 and K2 are generally orthogonal, or close to orthogonal. The mathematical formula for *average corneal power* (ACP) is (K1 + K2)/2 D [20].

The next definition in keratometry is *white-to-white* (WTW) or horizontal white-to-white (HWTW). It ultimately represents the *horizontal corneal diameter* (HCD). WTW is determined by the horizontal distance between two limbi (nasal and temporal border of the cornea) [21, 22].

Central corneal power (CCP) refers to the power of the cornea, determined by measuring the radius of the corneal anterior surface curvature from a central area with a predetermined diameter, generally approximated to be 3 mm, to represent an average pupil diameter [22, 23].

Combined surface refers to the single hypothetical representation of the corneal surface as a combination of the anterior and posterior corneal surfaces. It requires some given assumptions about the ratio of the corneal anterior and posterior curvature radii. For a certain ratio, the approximated representative corneal refractive index, which is smaller than the refractive indices of the corneal material and aqueous humor, is calculated. This approximated representative corneal refractive index differs for each IOL power calculation formula [23]. Previously, the standardized refractive index was usually determined as 1.3375, while the geometric ratio of posterior/anterior corneal curvature was accepted as 0.822 and the *corneal thickness* (CT) as 500 μm [24].

Some have calculated the corneal refractive index as approximately 1.3315 [25]. *Simulated keratometry* (Sim-K) measurements characterize the corneal curvatures in the 3-mm central area. It is obtained from the corneal anterior curvature using the 1.3375 index [26]. The steep Sim-K reading is the steepest meridian of the cornea. *The total corneal refractive power* (TCRP) or *total corneal power* (TCP) value is calculated by using the air refractive index (1.000), corneal refractive index (1.376), and aqueous humor refractive index (1.336) using Snell's law without depending on any precedented assumptions. More recently, to calculate the TCRP or TCP, the ray-tracing method is performed on both anterior and posterior corneal surfaces [27]. Scheimpflug imaging helps to provide *true net power* (TNP), which is calculated as the refractive power of the cornea based on both the anterior and posterior surfaces [12].

Astigmatisms are categorized into corneal keratometric and internal astigmatisms. The result of the unequal curvature along both of the two principal meridians of the anterior cornea generates corneal keratometric astigmatism. Internal astigmatism (IA happens due to the components of refractive astigmatism behind the cornea. The *total corneal astigmatism* (TCA) is described by the sum of the anterior and posterior corneal surfaces [27]. Compared to the anterior surface, the toricity of the posterior corneal surface has a greater impact. The corneal posterior surface is generally steeper than the anterior surface with a smaller radius of curvature, commonly yielding a negative dioptric power. Posterior cornea contributes an average of about 0.3 D of against-the-rule astigmatism (ATR). Failure in computing the number of posterior corneal astigmatism can result in overcorrection of with-the-rule astigmatism (WTR) or undercorrection of ATR. In refractive surgery aimed to correct astigmatism, only calculating the anterior surface of the cornea without taking the posterior surface into account can compromise the outcome [27, 28].

The *equivalent keratometry reading* (EKR) is obtained from the corneal diameters, which range from 1.0 to 7.0 mm. The EKR value at 4.5 mm was determined to be the most closely matched to conventional K values [24–27]. Central topography is a tool that takes the anterior refractive powers to evaluate the corneal topography, and to detect any visually relevant central corneal asymmetries by averaging the topographic data of 3.4–5.4 mm diameter of the central cornea with 3-zone keratometry on corneal radii of 6–11 mm. Meanwhile, the *average central corneal power* (ACCP) is defined as the average of the mean powers of the central cornea [22, 26, 29]. *Total keratometry* (TK) is a tool that combines the unique telecentric keratometry measurement of the anterior corneal surface with the measurement of the posterior corneal surface by using Swept-Source Optical Coherence Tomography (SS-OCT) [22].

The *No-History* method is a viable alternative tool for performing IOL power calculation without relying on any prior history of refractive surgery when the data is not available [30].

2.7 Anterior Chamber Measurement

The *anterior chamber depth* (ACD) refers to the distance between the anterior surface of the cornea and the anterior surface of the lens [31, 32]. Some studies have described ACD as the distance between the corneal endothelium and the anterior capsule of the crystalline lens [31–33]. However, this definition has since been corrected as the definition of *aqueous depth* (AQD). In the case of ACD, the central thickness of the cornea is taken into account [34, 35].

2.8 Lens Measurement

The *lens thickness* (LT) is measured as the distance from the anterior capsule apex to the posterior capsule apex of the crystalline lens [36].

Actual lens position (ALP) refers to the physical distance that is measured from the anterior corneal surface to the anterior IOL surface. Meanwhile, the *internal lens position* (ILP) is defined as the physical distance between the posterior corneal surface and the anterior IOL surface [37]. Both ALP and ILP are *physical lens position* (PLP).

Effective lens position (ELP) is defined as the distance from the cornea to the anterior surface of the IOL 3 months after the surgery, plus the distance to the principal point or central point of the principal plane of the IOL. In other words, ELP refers to the distance from the anterior corneal vertex to the principal point of the IOL, which is correctly implanted, 3 months after surgery. ELP is very important to predict the postoperative IOL position within the eye. If the final IOL position is closer to the cornea, it results in myopia, while if the posterior is closer to the principal point, it results in hyperopia [35, 37].

Over time, ELP has an even greater role as a variable in IOL power calculation. Modern IOL power calculation explores AL, K reading, WTW or HWTW, CCT, preop ACD, and LT to determine more accurate ELP to achieve accurate calculations [38–40].

Posterior shift of the IOL could increase hyperopia, while the anterior shift of IOL position could increase myopia. In the case of short AL in short eye, IOL position tends to be slightly more posterior, which is why some surgeons opt to add +0.5 to +1.00 to the IOL power calculation [12].

In the capsular bag, ELP is typically 5.20 mm, while in the sulcus, it would be estimated to be 4.70 mm. If the surgeon decides to place the IOL in the sulcus during surgery, IOL power reduction may be needed due to the anterior displacement of the IOL relative to the plan. For example:

(a) Below 9 D, it may be reduced by 0 D.
(b) Between 9.5–17 D, it may be reduced by 0.5 D.
(c) Between 17.5–27 D, it may be reduced by 1 D.
(d) Between 27–35 D, the power may be reduced by 1.5 D [13, 29].

2.9 IOL Factors in Biometry

IOL factor is mostly known as the *lens constant*. It is a feature used to achieve ELP, IOL power, and a particular refractive aim by considering the IOL type, material, design, shape, and in vivo seating in the capsular bag or other designated location (e.g., the AC IOL), usually around 4–6 weeks postoperatively [41, 42]. Surgical factors such as preoperative and postoperative medication, incision (size, shape, position), capsulorhexis size and centration, inadequate OVD removal, AC (too deep, too shallow, collapse, etc.), IOL dislocation, postop capsular bag contraction and fibrosis, etc. may also affect final ELP [12, 13].

The *A-constant* is a specific value for each IOL and is unitless; it depends on multiple variables, including the IOL material, the refractive index, style, shape, and the predicted position of the lens within the eye. It was initially designated as the lens constant for the Sanders-Ritzlaff-Kraff or Donald R. Sanders, John A. Retzlaff, and Manus C. Kraff (SRK) formula, specified by the manufacturer, and used in order to achieve higher rates of accuracy [41].

ACD-constant refers to a specific value of lens factor. *Individualized ADC* (pACD) is designated as the lens constant for the Hoffer Q formula. It represents the average distance between the anterior surface of the cornea and the anterior surface of the IOL after surgery. Variations in ACD significantly affect the IOL's position and refractive outcome [12]. Surgeons should maintain postoperative ACD as it is not too shallow, especially in short eye cases, and it is not too deep, especially in long eye cases [8].

The *C-constant* refers to the ratio of the distance between the center of IOL and the preoperative anterior lens capsule relative to the preoperative crystalline lens thickness. It is useful to predict the IOL position or ELP from the preoperative dimension and position of the natural crystalline lens, where the empty capsular bag will encapsulate and fixate an in-the-bag implanted IOL. In other words, the C-constant is related to where exactly the IOL will rest in an empty capsular bag [3, 13].

Corneal ACD *(CACD) constant* is a derived value, designed as a component within the vergence-based regression function (VRF) formula. This crucial factor is specifically used to optimize the calculation of IOL power [4, 13].

The *surgeon factor* (SF) is the specific distance from the pseudophakic anterior iris plane to the principal plane of the thin IOL. This value at some points differs from one surgeon to another. It was first designed in 1988 as a lens constant for Holladay 1 formula and can now be used to achieve better ELP results [12, 42]. As surgeon techniques become more and more consistent over time, surgeon factors should have less value.

The *lens factor* (LF) describes the distance between the iris plane and the second principal plane of the IOL (in the thick lens model). Initially, it was designed as a lens constant for the Barrett Universal formula and used together with AL and K to predict the ELP [43].

The *prediction error* (PE) is the difference between the predicted postoperative refraction and the actual postoperative refraction. The *mean bias error* (MBE) or *mean (prediction) error* (ME) represents the average of the difference between the predicted and actual postoperative refraction. *Mean absolute error* (MAE) is a metric used to assess the accuracy of a formula in predicting the required IOL power [13]. The *standard deviation* (SD) is a statistical measure needed to assess the dispersion or spread of PE [10, 13]. *Median absolute error* (MedAE) refers to a statistical measure used to evaluate the accuracy of different IOL calculation formulas. Meanwhile, the *root mean square* (RMS) is a statistical measure used to evaluate the accuracy of different IOL power calculation formulas [13]. More accurately, the measurement and the formula, PE, ME, and MAE for every case of cataract surgery would be zero or very close to zero [8, 13].

The International Organization for Standardization (ISO) Standard or *ISO permitted tolerance* had determined some standards to ensure accuracy for IOL manufacturing tolerances:

(a) Power 0 to <15 D, permitted tolerance is ±0.3 D.
(b) Power >15 to <25 D, permitted tolerance is ±0.4 D.
(c) Power >25 to <30 D, permitted tolerance is ±0.5 D.
(d) Power >30 D, permitted tolerance is ±1.00 D [44].

The current standard for toric IOL from the American National Standards Institute (ANSI) is approved as ANSI Z80.30-2010. It regulates optical and mechanical properties, labeling, biocompatibility, sterility, shelf life, and clinical investigation standards for toric IOLs. The guideline for toric IOLs:

(a) Total dioptric *spherical power and cylindrical power error* should be less than or equal to 0.30–0.50 D for most power ranges.
(b) The combined angular error of the toric marks and the orthogonality between meridians of toricity should be 5° or less.
(c) The rotational stability of a toric IOL is a change of 5° or less in rotation for at least 90% of eyes on spaced consecutive visits of at least 3 months apart [45].

2.10 Innovation and Engineering in Biometry

Regression refers to a set of calculation or statistical methods used to examine the relationship between variables, in early age of IOL power calculation like the SRK formula, were traditionally based on simplified mathematical models of the eye and relied on constants derived from a limited number of cases. Over time, the regression principle using statistical analysis of large datasets of pre- and postoperative refractive data, identifying precise relationships between AL, K, WTW, ACD, etc. Basically, this analysis helps to minimize PE, ME, and MAE and improve the predictability of refractive outcomes after cataract surgery [4, 8, 12, 13].

Theoretical in IOL power calculation refers to mathematical equations and concepts that are based on optical principles and a simplified model of the eye, rather than solely relying on regression analysis of clinical data [1, 2, 13].

Vergence is a calculation method that refers to the measurement of the convergence or divergence of light rays as they pass through optical elements. Vergence describes how light rays are converging (coming together) or diverging (spreading out). When light passes through the eye, it would be desirably refracted (bent) by the cornea and the IOL precisely to the macula. The vergence formula calculates the total vergence of the light and determines the IOL power [8, 13].

Ray tracing is a method for calculating the path of a single ray of light through a given optical system. As a ray passes through an optical system, starting at a given point and at a specified angle relative to the system's optical axis, it is refracted at each optical surface, causing the ray to change direction [3, 26, 46, 47]. In terms of ray tracing, *exact ray tracing* is based on Snell's law of refraction, while *paraxial ray tracing* is based on Gaussian optics. Paraxial ray tracing simplifies IOL calculations by assuming that all light rays travel close to the optical axis at small angles [48, 49].

Thin-lens formulas are based on the understanding that the cornea and the IOL act as single refracting planes within the optical system of the eye. These formulas evolve from Fyorodov, Colenbrander, Binkhorst, SRK/T, Holladay, Hoffer, Haigis, VRF, etc. [8, 12].

Artificial intelligence (AI) leverages computers and machines to mimic the problem-solving and decision-making capabilities of the human mind [50]. Artificial "know-how" refers to science and engineering that allows the manufacturing of intelligent machines to understand and mimic human intelligence [51]. AI is the cutting-edge technology and engineering-based algorithm and statistical model to solve problems that will progressively become more important now and in the future. Some parts of ophthalmology in which AI has the potential to grow are in the field of IOL power calculation (through advanced machine learning algorithms), automated image analysis, and predictive modeling for surgical planning and outcome. Through the integration of technological advancements and clinical expertise, IOL selection can provide more customization for each patient, particularly through the incorporation of visual behavior analysis, biometric data integration, and defocus curve comparisons. There is plenty of room for growth in refining capabilities through technological advancements, which require contributions and collaborations between clinicians and researchers. The presence of AI is inevitable here in IOL power calculation, and it could be the mainstream technology in the future of IOL power calculation [3, 5].

2.11 Types of Biometry Machines

The *ultrasonographic (USG) biometry* or ultrasound biometry plays an important role in IOL power calculations. It uses an ultrasonic scanning mode display (*A-scan* or amplitude mode scan/display), which gives a one-dimensional measurement, such as AL [52], and *B-scan* or brightness mode scan/display, which gives a two-dimensional image [52, 53]. B-scan plays an important role in the IOL power calculation in eyes with AL that is longer than 26 mm.

To increase its accuracy, USG biometry is enhanced by using the immersion technique, where an ultrasound probe is firmly fixated in a shell filled with balanced salt solution (BSS). Instead of touching the cornea directly, it provides an A-scan measurement to be taken through the shell water bath, thereby eliminating approximately 0.14–0.28 mm corneal compression, which occurs with the contact or applanation technique and can lead to erroneous measurements, because the compression applied by different technicians to different patients is variable, and therefore cannot be mathematically accounted for. For optimal ultrasonic biometry, surgeons should use the immersion vector A/B-scan technique to measure the refractive AL [54].

The *optical biometry* refers to a rapid and highly accurate measurement method using automated noncontact and noninvasive technology [4, 55].

(a) *Partial coherence interferometry* (PCI) is a kind of instrument that measures AL as the distance from the anterior corneal apex to the retinal pigment epithelium. PCI uses a 780–820 nm wavelength infrared laser to measure AL [37, 38]. PCI in the market includes IOL Master 500 (Carl Zeiss Meditec, Dublin, CA) and AL Scan (Nidek Co, Aichi, Japan).
(b) *Optical low coherence reflectometry* (OLCR) is a kind of technology based on interferometry, which is engineered to detect and localize reflectors with an 820 nm wavelength super-luminescent diode to measure AL [40]. OLCR in the market includes Lenstar LS900 (Haag-Streit, Köniz, Switzerland) and Aladdin (Topcon, Tokyo, Japan).
(c) *SS-OCT* provides corneal tomography by using a tunable swept laser, which eliminates the deployment of a spectrometer, providing faster scan speeds and potentially greater and better sensitivity at deeper scanning depths compared to spectral domain OCT (SD-OCT). *Corneal topography* is the engineering in mapping and evaluating the curvature and shape of the corneal surface, while corneal tomography maps and evaluates a three-dimensional section of the corneal structures. *Corneal tomography* is engineered for the evaluation and examination of the anterior and posterior structures and curvatures of the cornea, beyond endothelial pachymetric imaging [56]. SS-OCT uses a 1050–1070 nm wavelength swept-source to collect cross-sectional images of the entire eye. The system uses three OCT images to measure AL and ACD for every single calculation [57, 58]. SS-OCT in the market includes IOLMaster 700 (Carl Zeiss Meditec, Dublin, CA), ANTERION (Heidelberg Engineering, Heidelberg, Germany), ARGOS (Movu, Aichi, Japan), Eyestar 900 (Haag-Streit, Köniz, Switzerland), and CASIA2 (Tomey Corporation, Nagoya, Japan) . Newer SD-OCT for biometry includes MS-39 and MS-39 AL (CSO, Florence, Italy). It is combined with placido disc topography.
(d) *Scheimpflug-based optical biometer* is basically a Scheimpflug-based anterior segment topographer that may be used to perform any measurements of biometry data, including anterior and posterior corneal curvature, corneal topography, corneal pachymetry, corneal diameter and pupillary diameter, ACD, lens density, LT, and AL. It also provides formulas for IOL power calculation. Pentacam AXL (Oculus Optikgeräte, Wetzlar, Germany) uses a Scheimpflug camera combined with PCI. Meanwhile, the Galilei G6 (Ziemer, Biel, Switzerland) combines a dual rotating Scheimpflug camera, a placido disc topographer, and an OCT-based A-scan. It performs axial biometer by using 880 nm wavelength light based on OLCR [12].

2.12 Result of Surgery

Target refraction represents the desired refractive result of surgery in order to achieve the best uncorrected visual acuity for distance vision, intermediate vision, and reading vision [59, 60]. Some surgeons call it desired refraction [61].

Emmetropia or 0 (zero) D correction will be the goal for most patients and surgeons; however, some may benefit from being postoperatively left intentionally mild myopic (or, rarely, hypermetropic), depending on the patient's preference and the refraction of the fellow eye. Anisometropia should be below 3 D. The monovision or intentional postoperative anisometropia can eliminate the need for glasses after surgery, but should generally be less than 3 D and should be well explained to the patient before the surgery, including presenting all options to the patient.

Target refraction in terms of *spherical aberration* (SA) is still a topic of debate. By considering patient preferences, anisometropia, and the SA, surgeons can not only optimize visual outcome but, most importantly, patient satisfaction [62].

SA happens when incoming light rays end up focusing at different points after passing through a spherical lens. *Positive SA* has more optical power away from the optical axis to the periphery. *Negative SA* has less optical power away from the optical axis toward the periphery [63].

SA causes a dysphotopic halo or a blurry image. Based on SA, the IOL power calculation should be well-tuned and the expected residual SA should be carefully calculated:

(a) If SA is 0 (zero), target refraction is plano or zero D.
(b) If SA is positive, target refraction is −0.25 D for every 0.10 μm of SA.
(c) If SA is negative, target refraction is +0.25 D for every 0.10 μm of SA [64].

Surgery-induced astigmatism or *surgically induced astigmatism* (SIA) refers to astigmatism that is a direct result of surgery. SIA relates to the incision width as the main factor, and also depends upon the length, type, location, and structure of the incision, etc. It influences the refractive outcome [65].

Residual astigmatism (RA) refers to astigmatism that remains after an astigmatism-correcting surgery. RA can be caused by incorrect axis or rotation of a toric IOL, incorrect marking of the cornea, inaccurate preoperative biometry and IOL measurements, unanticipated SIA, uncalculated posterior corneal curvature, etc. [66]

Spherical equivalent (SE) refers to a spherical power that is calculated by adding the spherical (myopic or hypermetropic) error and ½ the cylindrical (astigmatism) components of the patient's refractive error [67]. *Aphakic SE* (ASE) is a measurement factor to be assessed during surgery. It is very crucial in intraoperative IOL power calculation (see intraoperative biometry below in this chapter) [13].

Defocus curve refers to the curve that plots visual acuity against different levels of defocus (measured in D). Binocular photopic defocus curves are graphs that determine how well the visual acuity is at various distances. A good defocus curve for a particular IOL should be obtained as good 6 m or 20 feet distance vision (near emmetropia, around 0.00 D), a secondary peak in the 60–66 cm intermediate range (e.g., around −1.50 D to −2.50 D), and potentially a third peak or acceptable vision at near (25–40 cm) distance. The curve should be relatively smooth; in this term, some minimal dips or fluctuations indicate visual disturbances. The defocus curve helps surgeons assess the optical performance of different IOLs. In this modern era, this information is definitely crucial for counseling patients and selecting the most appropriate lens for their visual needs and lifestyle [8].

In some challenging situations, we may need to perform *intraoperative optical refractive biometry*, intraoperative OCT (iOCT), and intraoperative aberrometry for IOL power estimation, without K and AL using optical retinoscopy [68, 69]. A *wavefront* is defined as the physical propagation of a ray of light. The term *aberrations* refers to the distortions of any visual waves caused by any irregularities of the optical mechanism. Intraoperative (wavefront) aberrometry helps surgeons in refractive measurements, IOL axis adjustment, and precisely accurate IOL placement [70, 71].

2.13 How Things Can Go Wrong

So many factors may lead to unfavored results, including instrument error, index of refraction error, and formula error. The other factors are usually correlated with a combination of human factors (technician or patient) and technical factors, such as: time pressure (rushing in performing the surgery), lack of training, lack of accessible guidelines, fatigue, patient predisposition such as dry eye or many other eye abnormalities, lack of fixation, mechanical failure of instrumentation, wrong A-constant selection, wrong formula used, wrong K-readings entered by hand (90 degrees out), biometry printout stuck in the wrong patient's notes, incorrectly labeled IOL, wrong patient in theater, reversed IOL optic, wrong IOL implanted (e.g.: 25.5 D implanted instead of 22.5 D or +30 D instead of +3.00 D), the required IOL power not available on the surgery day, etc. [62]

2.14 Special Attention in Special Conditions

IOL power calculation is a long journey. We need to do it preoperatively, and sometimes still require refinement intraoperatively or postoperatively. In order to do "successful one-step surgery," we need to do IOL power calculation thoroughly [72, 73].

The calculation should be verified *by two separate instruments, or repeat the keratometry measurement* if:

(a) The corneal power is less than 41.00 D, or greater than 47.00 D.
(b) There is a history of previous keratorefractive surgery. Errors in keratometry due to flat cornea after keratorefractive surgery can affect IOL power calculation.
(c) ACP between the two eyes is more than 0.09 D.
(d) The patient is not able to fixate adequately.
(e) Corneal astigmatism is greater than 2.50 D.
(f) Corneal diameter is less than 10.75 mm or more than 13.00 mm.
(g) The patient has a problem in cooperation or understanding [13, 73].

General rule suggests acquiring at least 5 consistent AL readings. For A-scan biometry, it is necessary to acquire 8–10 consecutive reading with SD <0.05. It is compulsory to consider a *second person or a different person to remeasure both eyes' AL* if:

(a) The AL is less than 21.30 mm, or greater than 26.60 mm in the fellow eye.
(b) The AL is greater than 26.00 mm, and there is a poor retinal spike or wide variability in the readings. In this case, a B-scan should be performed to seek a peripapillary posterior staphyloma. Simultaneously, the AL to the center of the macula should be measured by vector A-scan.
(c) The AL difference between the two eyes is greater than 0.33 mm, which is not correlated with the patient's oldest refraction.
(d) The AL measurement of one eye does not correlate with the patient's refractive error. This may be caused by very steep or flat corneas.
(e) There's a wide variability in individual AL readings obtained [72, 73].

A *second person should repeat the AL measurements, the keratometry readings, and reperform the IOL power calculations for both eyes*, if:

(a) The difference of the IOL power for target emmetropia is greater than 3.00 D compared to the anticipated value.
(b) The IOL power difference between the two eyes is greater than 1.00 D.
(c) The patient had prior keratorefractive surgery, and the calculated IOL power is less than +17.00 D or greater than +23.00 D [72].

2.15 Surgeons' Clinical Suggestions in IOL Power Calculation

Different cases might need a different approach. Here are some clinical approaches that have been *previously* used:

(a) In managing patients with high myopia or long eyes undergoing cataract surgery, the Wang-Koch adjustment has become a valuable tool in IOL power calculations. This adjustment can improve the accuracy of IOL power, leading to excellent refractive outcomes and lower refractive surprises. The Wang-Koch adjustment can be employed in conjunction with the Holladay 1, SRK/T, Hoffer Q, and Haigis formulas [4, 8, 12].
(b) In eyes with extreme corneal diameters, corneal curvatures, and AL, there is no perfect formula to accurately determine IOL power [8, 12, 69].
(c) It is advisable to use several formulas to calculate the suitable IOL power. To streamline calculations, it could be beneficial to utilize one IOL power calculation formula selected by the surgeon for the majority of surgeries and employ a wider range of formulae only in specific cases [1, 2, 69].

(d) Interferometers accurately measure AL in eyes containing silicone oil, but the silicone mode must be employed. Assessments of the surgically modified corneal contour through traditional keratometry result in considerable overvaluation of the power following myopic keratorefractive surgery, thus necessitating an inquiry into any previous keratorefractive surgery history. The American Society of Cataract and Refractive Surgery (ASCRS) tool for postrefractive eyes is the formula of choice [38, 40, 69].
(e) In cases of sulcus-fixated IOL or anterior chamber IOL, some IOL power calculation adjustments are needed (see ELP above in this chapter) [1, 2, 8].
(f) For in-the-sulcus IOL implantation, BUII, SRK/T, Holladay 2, and Hoffer Q are among the recommended formulas [12].
(g) In the implantation of anterior chamber IOL (AC IOL), the appropriate A-constant is used along with SRK, or SRK II formulas. Other formulas to consider are Binkhorst II and Colenbrander-Hoffer) [74]. If the AC IOL is a phakic IOL (pIOL), the common formula used is the formula of van der Heijde. For implantable collamer lens (ICL), surgeons can choose the EVO ICL formula via the internet [12].
(h) Changing IOL with a different lens constant to a different place in the eye requires a change of IOL power. For example, from a one-piece in-the-bag IOL with 118.80 lens constant to an anterior chamber IOL with 115.50 lens constant requires a change of IOL power of −3.30 D [75] (See lens constant above in this chapter).
(i) Achieving ultimate accuracy in outcomes is almost not possible, unless IOLs are available in 0.1 D or 0.2 D steps [8, 69].
(j) If a refractive surprise arises after IOL implantation, a second IOL may be placed in the sulcus, utilizing 1.2 times the myopic SE refractive error and 1.5 times the hyperopic spherical SE error, should IOL exchange be deemed challenging or unsuitable. The Barrett suite of formulas for IOL power calculation can likewise determine the power of the secondary IOL [1, 4].
(k) With current monofocal IOLs, it is hard to achieve excellent near, intermediate, and distance visions at the same time without correction in the majority of cases. Monovision vision is useful in reducing glasses dependence after bilateral cataract surgery, followed by IOL implantation [69].
(l) A little bit of myopia may be more desirable for patients after cataract surgery than a little bit of hypermetropia [8, 12].
(m) Pseudophakic monovision or mini-monovision is an option that may correct a dominant eye with target refraction 0 D distance vision, and the other eye is focused at near with −0.75 to −1.75 D of myopia. -1.50 D is the mode. This technique is a low-cost option for patients who would like to reduce dependence on spectacles postoperatively [13, 76].
(n) Many surgeons tend to use the SRK/T formula for AL >21.5 mm and the Hoffer Q formula for AL <21.5 mm previously, and recently many surgeons tend to use the Haigis formula [8, 77].
(o) In everyday practice, many surgeons tend to use the SRK/T formula, as well as in cases of long AL in myopic eyes [78].

(p) With the newer multifocal IOL lens designs, alignment of the optical modifications of the lens with the eye's visual axis is necessary to achieve better visual outcomes, as lens decentration can degrade optical performance and induce visual distortions. These newer devices can also measure the distance between the visual axis of the eye and both the corneal apex and the pupillary center. Assessing the angles alpha and kappa may be important when determining whether a particular lens design will provide optimal visual outcomes in that eye. This may be especially important in hyperopic eyes, which have been shown to have greater variation in these values [12, 62]. Olsen, Holladay 2, BUII, Hoffer Q, SRK/T, and Haigis can be used as preferred formulas for multifocal IOLs [12].

(q) In accordance with the IOL power calculation process, while performing biometric measurements using an optical biometer, at the same time we can differentiate the grade of cataracts using that optical biometer. This particular effort is useful in surgical planning for those who are learning phacoemulsification or are in transition to certain techniques in the field of cataract surgery. Gede Pardianto (2009) introduced Optical Biometry Based Cataract Grading System (OBBCGS) [79, 80]:

    1. No Cataract (NC).
    2. Optical Biometry Examined Cataract (OBEC).
    3. Optical Biometry Unexamined Cataract (OBUC).

    This particular grading system, combined with IOL power calculation using optical biometry, was presented at the 2010 European Society of Cataract and Refractive Surgeons (ESCRS) Congress in Paris [79]. This grading system is very useful for posterior segment studies or researches combined with IOL power calculation in patients undergoing phacoemulsification [79, 80].

    In daily practice, NC is almost similar to Lens Opacities Classification System (LOCS) III's NC0, C0, and P0. This classification is suitable for refractive lens extraction (RLE) phacoemulsification plan. On the other hand, OBEC is almost similar to LOCS III's NC1-3, C1-3, P1-3 It is suitable for low-energy phacoemulsification plan and is safe for learning a phacoemulsification procedure, and in transition to microincision cataract surgery (MICS) and femtosecond laser cataract surgery (FLACS). Nowadays, it might be suitable for learning a noncavitating cataract removal procedure or nonultrasonic lens extraction (ZEISS NULEX/ZEISS MICOR 700, Carl Zeiss Meditec, Dublin, CA). Meanwhile, OBUC is almost similar to LOCS III's NC4-5, C4-5, P4-5, which need examination by applanation ultrasound biometry. This grading is suitable for high-energy and more maneuverable phacoemulsification plan [79, 81].

(r) Mixing and matching contralateral implantation of different multifocal IOLs (e.g., EDOF, diffractive, and refractive IOLs) could enhance vision and patient's satisfaction [81, 82]. Nowadays, BUII is a favorable formula among Haigis, Holladay 2, SRK/T, and Kane for this strategical plan [82, 83].

(s) Simplifying the process of minimizing PE, ME or MBE, SD, and RMS in single-optimized IOL power predictions, offering more precision and accuracy in IOL power calculation [84, 85].
(t) Dysphotopsia, particularly negative dysphotopsia, is a common complaint after cataract surgery and can be associated with various IOL designs. LAL is a good choice for cases that have a higher risk of postoperative refractive surprise and/or accurate postoperative refraction is needed. If dysphotopsia is caused by SA, it needs advanced IOL power calculation (see SA above) [12, 62, 63, 69].
(u) In case of keratoconus, some surgeons suggest BUII, Kane, Haigis, Olsen, Holladay 1 with Wang Koch Adjustment, and SRK/T with K adjustment [12, 86, 87].
(v) In pediatric cataract cases, SRK/T, Holladay 1, Holladay 2, BUII, and Hoffer Q are still formulas of choice, while some surgeons use a simple rule of thumb as: Target refraction = 7—age (in years). On other hand, undercorrection has been recommended for years. The younger the age, the greater the undercorrection. Therefore, undercorrection has to be done carefully, especially in unilateral cases, as greater undercorrection tends to lead to anisometropia, as well as amblyopia. The alternative percentages of undercorrection of IOL implantation in children are as follows [12, 19, 88]:

- <6 months: 20%
- 6 months–1 year: 15%
- 1 year: 10%
- 2 years 5%
- 3 years: 4%
- 4 years: 3%
- 5 years: 2%
- >5 years: no under correction.

See Chap. 5 for more advanced IOL calculation in pediatric cataract cases.
(w) In cases of retinal disorders, especially in postvitrectomy cataract surgery, BUII, Olsen, EVO, Kane, Ladas Super Formula, Haigis, Hill-RBF, Hoffer Q, Holladay 1, and SRK/T can be considered [12, 87, 89]. See Chap. 9 for more advanced IOL calculation in vitrectomized eyes.
(x) Regarding that the posterior shift of the IOL could increase hyperopia, while the anterior shift of the IOL position could increase myopia (see ELP above), it is better if surgeons pay attention not to fill the AC too shallow or too deep at the conclusion of surgery, compared to the preoperative condition of the AC, especially in cases of high myopia [8, 12, 87].
(y) In rare cases, such as combined high AL and K reading, or other challenging cases, the use of AI chat is recommended to confirm conventional calculations (see Chap. 21).

(z) In general, IOL power calculation needs multiple specific parameters or measurement variables to determine the ELP. Each IOL formula with its principle (vergence, ray tracing, AI, etc.) can only work if all measurement variables needed are available properly. And with the help of a particular lens constant, IOL formulas are able to provide correct IOL power [8, 12, 13, 87].

2.16 Additional Information

(a) AI-assisted IOL calculators [3, 5, 12, 59]:

- Hill-RBF 3.0.
- EVO 2.0.
- Kane Formula.
- PEARL-DGS.
- Hoffer QST.
- LSF: Ladas Super 2.0/Ladas AI.
- ZEISS AI IOL Calculator.
- Zhu-Lu Formula.
- Alternatively, surgeons can use some AI chat applications, even by only submitting any measurement value from a biometry machine's screen or printout. It is truly worth trying to confirm that conventional formulas were right, especially in some special cases.

(b) List of online calculators [12, 59]:

- Asia Pacific Association of Cataract and Refractive Surgery (APCRS) Barrett's formulas: https://apacrs.org/
- ASCRS: https://ascrs.org/tools/post-refractive-iol-calculator
- ASSORT Web: www.assort.com
- Barrett Toric Calculator: www.ascrs.org/tools/barrett-toric-calculator
- BUII: https://calc.apacrs.org/barrett_universal2105/
- Cooke Formula K6: https://cookeformula.com
- ESCRS All Formulas: https://iolcalculator.escrs.org
- EVO Formula: https://www.evoiolcalculator.com/start.aspx
- Hill-RBF: https://rbfcalculator.com/online/index.html
- Hoffer QST: https://HofferQST.com
- Holladay 2: https://www.hic-soap.com/calc/
- IOL Con: https://iolcon.org
- Kane Formula: https://www.iolformula.com
- Karmona Formula: https://karmona-iol.com
- LSF (Ladas 2.0/Ladas AI): https://www.iolcalc.com
- Nallasamy Formula: https://lenscalc.com
- Panacea: http://www.panaceaiolandtoriccalculator.com/downloads.html
- PEARL-DGS: https://iolsolver.com/main, including for complex eyes:

– Postmyopic laser vision correction.
– Posthyperopic laser vision correction.
– Post radial keratotomy (RK).
– Post implantable collamer lens (ICL).
– Nonphysiological cornea.

- ULIB: http://ocusoft.de/ulib/c1.htm

(c) Manufacturer's online toric calculators [12, 59]:

- Alcon: https://www.acrysoftoriccalculator.com
- Bausch + Lomb: https://envista.toriccalculator.com
- Biotech: http://biotechcalculators.com
- Hanita: https://calc.hanitalenses.com/toric-iol-calculator-v5-01/
- Hoya: www.hoyatoric.com
- Johnson & Johnson Vision: https://tecnistoriccalc.com
- Kowa: https://avanseetoriccalculator.com
- Omni: http://www.omnilens.in/portfolio/toric-calculator/
- Ophtec: https://calculator.ophtec.com/calculator-choice
- Physiol: https://www.physioltoric.eu
- Rayner: https://www.raytrace.rayner.com
- STAAR Surgical/Online Calculation & Ordering System (OCOS) for EVO ICL: https://evo-ocos.staarag.ch/live/
- VSY: https://easytoriccalculator.com
- ZEISS: https://zcalc.meditec.zeiss.com

In the future and in the age of AI, IOL power calculation is expected to be performed more easily, faster, cheaper, and even more accurately to support cataract surgery for patients, surely with very satisfying results [12, 87].

References

1. Stopyra W, Langenbucher A, Grzybowski A. Intraocular lens power calculation formulas-a systematic review. Ophthalmol Ther. 2023;12(6):2881–902. https://doi.org/10.1007/s40123-023-00799-6. Epub 2023 Sep 12. PMID: 37698825; PMCID: PMC10640516.
2. Stopyra W, Cooke DL, Grzybowski A. A review of intraocular lens power calculation formulas based on artificial intelligence. J Clin Med. 2024;13(2):498. https://doi.org/10.3390/jcm13020498. PMID: 38256632; PMCID: PMC10816994.
3. Olsen T. Calculation of intraocular lens power: a review. Acta Ophthalmol Scand. 2007;85(5):472–85. https://doi.org/10.1111/j.1600-0420.2007.00879.x. Epub 2007 Apr 2. PMID: 17403024.
4. Pardianto G. What was known about biometry and IOL Power Calculation? In: Pardianto G, editor. The intraocular lens power calculation. Medan: Anak Sudarti Foundation; 2022. p. 11–23. ISBN 978-623-6763-50-6, e-ISBN 978-623-6763-51-3.
5. Nuliqiman M, Xu M, Sun Y, Cao J, Chen P, Gao Q, Xu P, Ye J. Artificial intelligence in ophthalmic surgery: current applications and expectations. Clin Ophthalmol. 2023;20(17):3499–511. https://doi.org/10.2147/OPTH.S438127. PMID: 38026589; PMCID: PMC10674717.

6. Lindegger DJ, Wawrzynski J, Saleh GM. Evolution and applications of artificial intelligence to cataract surgery. Ophthalmol Sci. 2022;2(3):100164. https://doi.org/10.1016/j.xops.2022.100164. PMID: 36245750; PMCID: PMC9559105.
7. Casadei K, Kiel J. Anthropometric measurement. [Updated 2022 Sep 26]. In: StatPearls [Internet]. Treasure Island (FL): StatPearls Publishing; 2024 Jan-. Available from: https://www.ncbi.nlm.nih.gov/books/NBK537315/.
8. Pardianto G, editor. The intraocular lens power calculation. Anak Sudarti Foundation: Medan; 2022. ISBN 978-623-6763-50-6, e-ISBN 978-623-6763-51-3
9. Scholtz SK, Langenbucher A. Die Berechnung des menschlichen Auges – zur Evolution der Biometrie in der Kataraktchirurgie [Calculating the human eye – the evolution of biometry for cataract surgery]. Klin Monbl Augenheilkd. 2020;237(8):933–7. German. https://doi.org/10.1055/a-1002-0136. Epub 2019 Oct 10. PMID: 31600819.
10. Ganesh D, Lin SR. Global metrics on ocular biometry: representative averages and standard deviations across ten countries from four continents. Eye (Lond). 2023;37(3):511–5. https://doi.org/10.1038/s41433-022-01961-3. Epub 2022 Feb 21. PMID: 35190667; PMCID: PMC9905050.
11. Kuriakose RK, Gulati R, Bains H, Ramaprasad A, Chan NK, Basti S. Change in major ocular biometry parameters axial length and keratometry in adults over time. J Cataract Refract Surg. 2023;49(5):474–8. https://doi.org/10.1097/j.jcrs.0000000000001144. PMID: 36700942.
12. Pardianto G. Pocket e-book series: a supplement to the intraocular lens power calculation. Medan: Anak Sudarti Foundation; 2024.
13. Pardianto G, Anastasia R, Purworini D. Patient selection and maintenance of standards to improve the safety of immediate sequential bilateral cataract surgery in tropical regions. Cureus. 2025;17(8):e91356. Published 2025 Aug 31. https://doi.org/10.7759/cureus.91356.
14. Hitzenberger CK. Optical measurement of axial length by laser Doppler interferometry. Invest Ophthalmol Vis Sci. 1991;32:616–24. PMID: 2001935.
15. Goto S, Maeda N, Noda T, Ohnuma K, Koh S, Iehisa I, Nishida K. Comparison of composite and segmental methods for acquiring optical axial length with swept-source optical coherence tomography. Sci Rep. 2020;10:4474. https://doi.org/10.1038/s41598-020-61391-7. PMID: 32161358; PMCID: PMC7066125.
16. Gordon RA, Donzis PB. Refractive development of the human eye. Arch Ophthalmol. 1985;103:785–9. https://doi.org/10.1001/archopht.1985.01050060045020. PMID: 4004614.
17. Norrby S. Sources of error in intraocular lens Power Calculation. J Cataract Refract Surg. 2008;34:368–76. https://doi.org/10.1016/j.jcrs.2007.10.031. PMID: 18299059.
18. Vanderveen DK, Trivedi RH, Nizam A, Lynn MJ, Lamber SR. Infant Aphakia Treatment Study Group. Predictability of intraocular lens power calculation formulae in infantile eyes with unilateral congenital cataract: results from the Infant Aphakia Treatment Study. Am J Ophthalmol. 2013;156:1252–60.e2. https://doi.org/10.1016/j.ajo.2013.07.014. Epub 2013 Sep 4. PMID: 24011524; PMCID: PMC4140419.
19. Vasavada V, Shah SK, Vasavada VA, Vasavada AR, Trivedi RH, Srivastava S, et al. Comparison of IOL power calculation formulae for pediatric eyes. Eye. 2016;30:1242–50. https://doi.org/10.1038/eye.2016.171. Epub 2016 Aug 5. PMID: 27494083; PMCID: PMC5023817.
20. Yu JG, Zhong J, Mei ZM, Zhao F, Tao N, Xiang Y. Evaluation of biometry and corneal astigmatism in cataract surgery patients from Central China. BMC Ophthalmol. 2017;17(1):56. https://doi.org/10.1186/s12886-017-0450-2. PMID: 28446167; PMCID: PMC5405481.
21. Hoffer KJ. Clinical results using the Holladay 2 intraocular lens power formula. J Cataract Refract Surg. 2000;26(8):1233–7. https://doi.org/10.1016/s0886-3350(00)00376-x. PMID: 11008054.
22. Lawless M, Jiang JY, Hodge C, Sutton G, Roberts TV, Barrett G. Total keratometry in intraocular lens Power Calculations in eyes with previous laser refractive surgery. Clin Experiment Ophthalmol. 2020;48(6):749–56. https://doi.org/10.1111/ceo.13760. PMID:32279436.

23. Preussner PR, Olsen T, Hoffmann P, Findl O. Intraocular lens calculation accuracy limits in normal eyes. J Cataract Refract Surg. 2008;34(5):802–8. https://doi.org/10.1016/j.jcrs.2008.01.015. PMID: 18471636.
24. Borasio E, Stevens J, Smith GT. Estimation of true corneal power after keratorefractive surgery in eyes requiring cataract surgery: BESSt formula. J Cataract Refract Surg. 2006;32(12):2004–14. PIMD: 17137976.
25. Olsen T. On the calculation of power from curvature of the cornea. Br J Ophthalmol. 1986;70(2):152–4. https://doi.org/10.1136/bjo.70.2.152.
26. Savini G, Hoffer KJ, Lomoriello DS, Ducoli P. Simulated keratometry versus total corneal power by ray tracing: a comparison in prediction accuracy of intraocular lens power. Cornea. 2017;36(11):1368–72. https://doi.org/10.1097/ICO.0000000000001343. PMID: 28991853.
27. Peyman A, Dastborhan Z, Peyman M. Astigmatic treatment with photorefractive keratectomy: Investigations of non-keratometric ocular astigmatism. J Curr Ophthalmol. 2017;29(2):98–102. https://doi.org/10.1016/j.joco.2016.12.001. PMID: 28626818; PMCID: PMC5463002.
28. Koch DD, Ali SF, Weikert MP, Shirayama M, Jenkins R, Wang L. Contribution of posterior corneal astigmatism to total corneal astigmatism. J Cataract Refract Surg. 2012;38(12):2080–7. https://doi.org/10.1016/j.jcrs.2012.08.036. PMID:23069271.
29. Mehta R, Aref AA. Intraocular lens implantation in the ciliary sulcus: challenges and risks. Clin Ophthalmol. 2019;13:2317–23. https://doi.org/10.2147/OPTH.S205148. PMID: 31819356; PMCID: PMC6885568.
30. Shammas HJ, Shammas MC. No-history method of intraocular lens power calculation for cataract surgery after myopic laser in situ keratomileusis. J Cataract Refract Surg. 2007;33(1):31–6. https://doi.org/10.1016/j.jcrs.2006.08.045. PMID: 17189790
31. Yan PS, Lin HT, Wang QL, Zhang ZP. Anterior segment variations with age and accommodation demonstrated by slit-lamp-adapted optical coherence tomography. Ophthalmology. 2010;117:2301–7. https://doi.org/10.1016/j.ophtha.2010.03.027. Epub 2010 Jun 29. PMID: 20591484.
32. Ning X, Yang Y, Yan H, Zhang J. Anterior chamber depth - a predictor of refractive outcomes after age-related cataract surgery. BMC Ophthalmol. 2019;19(1):134. https://doi.org/10.1186/s12886-019-1144-8. PMID: 31238910; PMCID: PMC6591866.
33. Khorrami-Nejad M, Moradi R, Akbarzadeh Baghban A, Khosravi B. Effect of axial length and anterior chamber depth on the peripheral refraction profile. Int J Ophthalmol. 2021;14(2):292–8. https://doi.org/10.18240/ijo.2021.02.17. PMID:33614460. PMCID: PMC7840374.
34. Hoffer KJ. Definition of ACD. Letter to the Editor General correspondence. Ophthalmology. 2011;118(7):1484. https://doi.org/10.1016/j.ophtha.2011.03.009. PMID: 21724050.
35. Tamaoki A, Kojima T, Tanaka Y, Hasegawa A, Kaga T, Ichikawa K, Tanaka K. Prediction of effective lens position using multiobjective evolutionary algorithm. Transl Vis Sci Technol. 2019;8(3):64. https://doi.org/10.1167/tvst.8.3.64. PMID: 31293818; PMCID: PMC6602360.
36. Shammas J, Shammas MC. Measuring the cataractous lens. J Cataract Refract Surg. 2015;41(9):1875–9. https://doi.org/10.1016/j.jcrs.2015.10.036. PMID: 26603396.
37. Gatinel D, Debellemanière G, Saad A, Dubois M, Rampat R. Determining the theoretical effective lens position of thick intraocular lenses for machine learning-based IOL power calculation and simulation. Transl Vis Sci Technol. 2021;10(4):27. https://doi.org/10.1167/tvst.10.4.27. PMID: 34004006; PMCID: PMC8088222.
38. Martinez-Enriquez E, Pérez-Merino P, Durán-Poveda S, Jiménez-Alfaro I, Marcos S. Estimation of intraocular lens position from full crystalline lens geometry: towards a new generation of intraocular lens power calculation formulas. Sci Rep. 2020;8:9829. https://doi.org/10.1038/s41598-018-28272-6.
39. Xia T, Martinez CE, Tsai LM. Update on Intraocular Lens Formulas and Calculations. Asia Pac J Ophthalmol (Phila). 2020;9(3):186–93. https://doi.org/10.1097/APO.0000000000000293. PMID: 32501896; PMCID: PMC7299214.

40. Olsen T, Corydon L, Gimbel H. Intraocular lens power calculation with an improved anterior chamber depth prediction algorithm. J Cataract Refract Surg. 1995;21:313–9. https://doi.org/10.1016/s0886-3350(13)80140-x. PMID: 7674170.
41. Eldaly MA, Mansour KA. Personal A-constant in relation to axial length with various intraocular lenses. Indian J Ophthalmol. 2014;62(7):788–91. https://doi.org/10.4103/0301-4738.138300. PMID: 25116771; PMCID: PMC4152648.
42. Holladay JT, Prager TC, Ruiz RS. A three-part system for refining intraocular lens Power Calculations. J Cataract Refract Surg. 1988;14:17–24. https://doi.org/10.1016/s0886-3350(88)80059-2. PMID: 3339543.
43. Barrett GD. An improved universal theoretical formula for intraocular lens power prediction. J Cataract Refract Surg. 1993;19:713–20. https://doi.org/10.1016/s0886-3350(13)80339-2. PMID: 8271166.
44. Stewart P. Meeting higher patient expectations with the Softec HD: the major advantages of this lens are its 0.25 D increments and stated manufacturing tolerances. Cataract Refract Surg Today. 2007;10:68–70.
45. Chang DH. ANSI Standard for toric IOLs. Cataract Refract Surg Today. 2013;6:32.
46. Preussner PR, Wahl J, Lahdo H, Dick B, Findl O. Ray tracing for intraocular lens calculation. J Cataract Refract Surg. 2002;28:1412–9. https://doi.org/10.1016/s0886-3350(01)01346-3. PMID: 12160812.
47. Gjerdrum B, Gundersen KG, Lundmark PO, Aakre BM. Refractive precision of ray tracing IOL calculations based on OCT data versus traditional IOL calculation formulas based on reflectometry in patients with a history of laser vision correction for myopia. Clin Ophthalmol. 2021;15:845–57. https://doi.org/10.2147/OPTH.S298007. PMID: 33664562; PMCID: PMC7924114.
48. Satou T, Shimizu K, Tsunehiro S, Igarashi A, Kato S, Koshimizu M, Niida T. Development of a new intraocular lens Power Calculation method based on lens position estimated with optical coherence tomography. Sci Rep. 2020;10(1):6501. https://doi.org/10.1038/s41598-020-63546-y. PMID: 32300162; PMCID: PMC7162886.
49. Olsen T, Hoffmann P. C constant: new concept for ray tracing-assisted intraocular lens Power Calculation. J Cataract Refract Surg. 2014;40(5):764–73. https://doi.org/10.1016/j.jcrs.2013.10.037. PMID: 24767910.
50. IBM Cloud Education. 2020. Available at: https://www.ibm.com/cloud/learn/what-is-artificial-intelligence.
51. McCarthy J. 2004. Available at: https://homes.di.unimi.it/borghese/Teaching/AdvancedIntelligentSystems/Old/IntelligentSystems_2008_2009/Old/IntelligentSystems_2005_2006/Documents/Symbolic/04_McCarthy_whatisai.pdf.
52. Cass K, Thompson CM, Tromans C, Wood IC. Evaluation of the validity and reliability of A-scan ultrasound biometry with a single use disposable cover. Br J Ophthalmol. 2002;86(3):344–9. https://doi.org/10.1136/bjo.86.3.344. PMID: 11864896; PMCID: PMC1771057.
53. Yang QH, Chen B, Peng GH, Li ZH, Huang YF. Accuracy of axial length measurements from immersion B-scan ultrasonography in highly myopic eyes. Int J Ophthalmol. 2014;7(3):441–5. https://doi.org/10.3980/j.issn.2222-3959.2014.03.10.
54. Trivedi RH, Wilson ME. Axial length measurements by contact and immersion techniques in pediatric eyes with cataract. Ophthalmology, 2021;118(3):498–502. https://doi.org/10.1016/j.ophtha.2010.06.042. Epub 2010 Oct 29. PMID: 21035871; PMCID: PMC3052929.
55. Silitonga AR, Pardianto G. Fundamentals of phaco innovations: definitions and basic understanding. In: Pardianto G, Tassignon MJ, editors. Innovation in cataract surgery. Singapore: Springer; 2024. p. 35–54. https://doi.org/10.1007/978-981-97-5192-1_2.
56. Ambrósio R Jr, Belin MW. Imaging of the cornea: topography vs tomography. J Refract Surg. 2010;26(11):847–9. https://doi.org/10.3928/1081597X-20101006-01. PMID: 21053870.
57. Whang WJ, Yoo YS, Kang MJ, et al. Predictive accuracy of partial coherence interferometry and swept-source optical coherence tomography for intraocular lens Power Calculation. Sci

Rep. 2018;8:13732. https://doi.org/10.1038/s41598-018-32246-z. PMID: 30214016; PMCID: PMC6137182.
58. Cummings AB, Naughton S, Coen AM, Brennan E, Kelly GE. Comparative analysis of swept-source optical coherence tomography and partial coherence interferometry biometers in the prediction of cataract surgery refractive outcomes. Clin Ophthalmol. 2020;14:4209–20. https://doi.org/10.2147/OPTH.S278589. PMID: 33293790; PMCID: PMC7719307.
59. Savini G, Hoffer KJ. Online intraocular lens power calculators. In: Pardianto G, Tassignon MJ, editors. Innovation in cataract surgery. Singapore: Springer; 2024. p. 123–38. https://doi.org/10.1007/978-981-97-5192-1_8.
60. Schuster AK, Schlichtenbrede FC, Harder BC, Beutelspacher SC, Jonas JB. Target refraction for best uncorrected distance and near vision in cataract surgery. Eur J Ophthalmol. 2014;24(4):509–15. https://doi.org/10.5301/ejo.5000414. Epub 2013 Dec 16. PMID: 24366766.
61. Tappin MJ, Ferguson VMG. Per-operative retinoscopy as a predictor of final post-operative refraction. Eye. 1999;13:559–61. https://doi.org/10.1038/eye.1999.138. PMID: 10692931.
62. Astbury N, Ramamurthy B. How to avoid mistakes in biometry. Community Eye Health. 2006;19(60):70–1. PMID: 17515971; PMCID: PMC1871684.
63. Holladay JT. Spherical Aberration: The Next Frontier: Only understanding the math can ophthalmologists target the ideal correction for their patients. Cataract Refract Surg Today. 2006;11:95–102.
64. Beiko G. Customizing the Correction of Spherical Aberration: Undercorrection with aspheric IOLs may help patients achieve optimal outcomes. Cataract Refract Surg Today. 2006;11:92–4.
65. Yang J, Wang X, Zhang H, Pang Y, Wei RH. Clinical evaluation of surgery-induced astigmatism in cataract surgery using 2.2 mm or 1.8 mm clear corneal micro-incisions. Int J Ophthalmol. 2017;10(1):68–71. https://doi.org/10.18240/ijo.2017.01.11. PMID: 28149779; PMCID: PMC5225351.
66. Berdahl J. Correcting residual astigmatism after the implantation of a Toric IOL: tips for determining whether to rotate the IOL or perform laser vision correction. Refract Surg Today. 2012;6:42–6.
67. Calvo-Sanz JA, Bonnin-Arias C, Arias-Puente A. Clinical application of bicylindric intraocular lens power calculation method. Indian J Ophthalmol. 2020;68(6):1073–8. https://doi.org/10.4103/ijo.IJO_1237_19. PMID: 32461432; PMCID: PMC7508133.
68. Ianchulev T, Salz J, Hoffer K, Albini T, Hsu H, Labree L. Intraoperative optical refractive biometry for intraocular lens power estimation without axial length and keratometry measurements. J Cataract Refract Surg. 2005;31(8):1530–6. https://doi.org/10.1016/j.jcrs.2005.01.035. PMID: 16129287.
69. Srinivas SP, Young AL, Behndig A, Chang DF, Dhubhghaill SN, Eom Y, Fan AH, Findl O, Gundersen KG, Khanna RC, Kohnen T, Mah FS, Miller KM, Nanavaty MA, Nuijts R, Oshika T, Pardianto G, Reus NJ, Ruit S, Sharma N, Venkatesh R, Zhang M, Zheng K, Rao SK, Alió JL. Controversies, consensuses and guidelines on modern cataract surgery by the Academy of Asia-Pacific Professors of Ophthalmology (AAPPO). Asia Pac J Ophthalmol (Phila). 2025;6:100224. https://doi.org/10.1016/j.apjo.2025.100224. PMID: 40628343.
70. Marcos S. Aberrometry: basic science and clinical applications. Bull Soc Belge Ophtalmol. 2006;302:197–213. PMID: 17265799.
71. Kaufman AR, Pineda R 2nd. Intraoperative aberrometry: an update on applications and outcomes. Curr Opin Ophthalmol. 2023;34(1):48–57. https://doi.org/10.1097/ICU.0000000000000915. Epub 2022 Oct 20. PMID: 36484210.
72. Knox Cartwright NE, Johnston RL, Jaycock PD, Tole DM, Sparrow JM. The Cataract National Dataset electronic multicentre audit of 55,567 operations: when should IOLMaster biometric measurements be rechecked? Eye. 2010;24(5):894–900. https://doi.org/10.1038/eye.2009.196. Epub 2009 Aug 14. PMID: 19680278.

73. Zaldivar R, Schultz M, Davidori J. Intraocular lens calculation in patients with extreme myopia. J Cataract Refract Surg. 2000;26:668–74. https://doi.org/10.1016/s0886-3350(00)00367-9. PMID: 10831895.
74. Villada JR, Raj PS, Akingbehin T. Calculation of the power of anterior chamber implants. Br J Ophthalmol. 1992;76(5):303–6. https://doi.org/10.1136/bjo.76.5.303. PMID: 1390516; PMCID: PMC504263.
75. Lahood B. The lens constant. Cataract Refract Surg Today. 2021;6:64–6.
76. Goldberg DG, Goldberg MH, Shah R, Meagher JN, Ailani H. Pseudophakic mini-monovision: high patient satisfaction, reduced spectacle dependence, and low cost. BMC Ophthalmol. 2018;18(1):293. https://doi.org/10.1186/s12886-018-0963-3. PMID: 30413145; PMCID: PMC6230294.
77. Hill WE. Something borrowed, something new: improved accuracy for IOL power calculations. The Charles D. Kelman Innovator's Lecture presented at: ASCRS/ASOA Symposium and Congress; April 28, 2014; Boston, MA
78. Fang X, Ben S, Dong Y, Chen X, Xue W, Wang Y. Outcomes of the Haigis-L formula for calculating intraocular lens power in extreme long axis eyes after myopic laser in situ keratomileusis. Eye. 2021;6(11) https://doi.org/10.1097/j.jcrs.0000000000000238. PMID: 32379087.
79. Pardianto G. MataPedia for ophthalmologist. Medan: Perdana; 2014. ISBN 978-602-8935-62-3.
80. Khurana AK. Disorder of the lens and cataract. In: Modern system of ophthalmology series. New Delhi: CBD Publishers & Distributors Pvt. Ltd; 2024. p. 44. eISBN 978-93-546-6463-2.
81. Pardianto G, Suyar MSS, Purworini D. Preventing post phacoemulsification infection with intracameral levofloxacin administrative. J Neonatal Surg. 2025;14(9S):143–7. https://doi.org/10.52783/jns.v14.2639.
82. Gunenc U, Celik L. Long-term experience with mixing and matching refractive array and diffractive CeeOn multifocal intraocular lenses. J Refract Surg. 2008;24(3):233–342. https://doi.org/10.3928/1081597X-20080301-04. PMID: 18416257.
83. Xiong T, Chen H, Fan W. Comparison of bilateral implantation of an extended depth of focus lenses and a blend approach of extended depth of focus lenses and bifocal lenses in cataract patients. BMC Ophthalmol. 2023;23(1):476. https://doi.org/10.1186/s12886-023-03228-1. PMID: 37990306; PMCID: PMC10664382.
84. Gatinel D, Debellemanière G, Saad A, Rampat R, Wallerstein A, Gauvin M, Malet J. A new method to minimize the standard deviation and root mean square of the prediction error of single-optimized IOL Power Formulas. Transl Vis Sci Technol. 2024;13(6):2. https://doi.org/10.1167/tvst.13.6.2. PMID: 38837172; PMCID: PMC11160955.
85. Gatinel D, Debellemanière G, Saad A, Brenner LF, Gauvin M, Wallerstein A, Malet J. Impact of the minimization of standard deviation before zeroization of the mean bias on the performance of IOL Power Formulas. Transl Vis Sci Technol. 2024;13(10):22. https://doi.org/10.1167/tvst.13.10.22. PMID: 39392436; PMCID: PMC11472891.
86. Felipe A, Artigas JM, Díez-Ajenjo A, García-Domene C, Alcocer P. Residual astigmatism produced by toric intraocular lens rotation. J Cataract Refract Surg. 2011;37(10):1895–901. https://doi.org/10.1016/j.jcrs.2011.04.036. Epub 2011 Aug 23. PMID: 21865007.
87. Dhawlikar NS, Dai YL, Hughes KV, Rao NK. IOL power calculation in special situations. In: Pardianto G, editor. The intraocular lens power calculation. Medan: Anak Sudarti Foundation. 2022; 43–73. ISBN 978-623-6763-50-6, e-ISBN 978-623-6763-51-3.
88. Khokhar S, Rani D. Innovations in paediatric cataract surgery. In: Pardianto G, Tassignon MJ, editors. Innovation in cataract surgery. Singapore: Springer; 2024. p. 20169–246. https://doi.org/10.1007/978-981-97-5192-1_16.
89. Hipólito-Fernandes D, Elisa Luís M, Gil P, Maduro V, Feijão J, Yeo TK, Voytsekhivskyy O, Alves N. VRF-G, a new intraocular lens Power Calculation Formula: a 13-formulas comparison study. Clin Ophthalmol. 2020;14:4395–402. https://doi.org/10.2147/OPTH.S290125. PMID: 33364744; PMCID: PMC7751728.

Chapter 3
The Formulas: From Basics to Online Settings and the Era of Artificial Intelligence

Novita Sitompul and Triana Budi Sulistya

3.1 The Basics of IOL Formulas

3.1.1 Historical Foundations

The journey to accurately calculate intraocular lens (IOL) power began in the 1960s, as surgeons sought to replace bulky aphakic glasses with precise lens implants. Early formulas relied on basic optical principles but often failed in real-world settings due to oversimplified assumptions about eye anatomy [1]. A major breakthrough came in 1980 with the SRK formula, developed by Sanders, Retzlaff, and Kraff. This formula used a simple equation—linking axial length (AL) and corneal curvature (keratometry, or K)—to estimate IOL power [2]. Though imperfect, it laid the foundation for modern IOL calculations.

By the late 1980s, surgeons realized that one formula could not suit all eyes. Pioneers such as Jack T. Holladay and Kenneth J. Hoffer introduced refinements to address extremes in eye anatomy. Holladay's insistence on incorporating anterior chamber depth (ACD) and effective lens position (ELP) into calculations led to the Holladay 1 formula (1988). The Holladay 1 formula (1988) introduced "surgeon factor" to personalize calculations [3], while Hoffer's Q-formula improved outcomes for eyes with shorter AL [4]. These advances shifted IOL calculations from generic equations to tools adaptable to individual patient features.

All author declare no financial interest.

N. Sitompul (✉)
Priangan Medical and Eye Center, Bandung, Indonesia

T. B. Sulistya
Universitas Brawijaya, Malang, Indonesia

G. Pardianto (ed.), *Intraocular Lens (IOL) Power Calculation*,
https://doi.org/10.1007/978-981-92-1223-1_3

3.1.2 Mathematical Principles

All IOL formulas solve a core problem, calculating the lens power needed to focus light onto the retina. The equation depends on three critical variables:

1. AL: Measured via ultrasound or Amplitude Mode Scan/Display (A-scan) or optical biometry (e.g., IOL-Master (Carl Zeiss Meditec, Dublin, CA)).
2. K reading: Corneal curvature, a proxy for refractive power.
3. ELP: The postoperative position of the IOL relative to the cornea.

Early formulas treated ELP as A-constant, leading to errors in eyes with shallow or deep anterior chambers [5]. For example, the SRK II formula adjusted the A-constant based on AL but ignored ACD, resulting in refractive surprises particularly in long eyes [6]. The Haigis formula (1990s) addressed this by using three independent constants (a0, a1, a2) to model ELP as a function of ACD and AL, significantly improving accuracy in long eyes [7].

3.1.3 Generational Classifications

IOL formulas are often categorized into generations based on their complexity and input parameters:

1. Third-generation formulas (e.g., Holladay 1, Sanders-Retzlaff-Kraff/Theoretical (SRK/T), Hoffer Q): Incorporate AL, K, and ACD, with ELP derived from regression analysis.
2. Fourth-generation formulas (e.g., Haigis, Barrett Universal II): Integrate additional variables such as lens thickness (LT), white-to-white (WTW) distance, and corneal asphericity.

The Barrett Universal II (BUII) formulaBarrett Universal II (BUII) formulaIntraocular lens (IOL) formulasclassifications (2010) stands out as a modern benchmark. It combines ray-tracing optics with a flexible eye model, improving accuracy in complex cases, such as eyes with prior laser vision correction [8]. Studies show it outperforms older formulas, reducing postoperative vision errors [9].

3.2 Transition to Online Settings

3.2.1 The Personalization Revolution

The shift toward personalized constants marked another leap forward. Surgeons could now optimize formula constants (e.g., A-constant, surgeon factor (SF)) based on their outcomes, a practice validated by studies showing reduced mean absolute error (MAE) in refractive outcomes [10]. This principle of "formula customization" bridged the gap between theoretical precision and real-world surgical variability.

3.2.2 The Digital Revolution in IOL Calculations

The turn of the twenty-first century marked a seismic shift in IOL power calculation, driven by the convergence of optical biometry and internet connectivity. The introduction of devices like the IOLMaster (Carl Zeiss Meditec, Dublin, CA) in the 1990s replaced manual A-scan ultrasound with optical coherence-based AL measurements, reducing human error and improving reproducibility [11]. This technological leap set the stage for online calculators, which transformed static formulas into dynamic, data-driven tools.

Platforms such as the American Society of Cataract and Refractive Surgery (ASCRS) IOL Calculator (2008) allowed surgeons to compare multiple formulas (e.g., Holladay 2, BUII) in real time, accounting for variables such as prior refractive surgery or irregular corneas [8]. For the first time, surgeons could leverage computational power to refine preoperative planning at the click of a button.

3.2.3 Advantages of Cloud-Based Platforms

Online calculators democratized access to the latest formula updates. For example, the BUII, hosted on a cloud platform since 2013, automatically integrates surgeon-specific constants and global outcome data to optimize predictions [12]. This dynamic approach proved transformative for complex cases:

- A 2016 study showed that combining the Barrett formula with online toric IOL calculators reduced postoperative astigmatism outliers by 38% compared to manual methods [13].

Integration with electronic medical records (EMR) further streamlined workflows. Systems such as Zeiss Callisto Eye (Carl Zeiss AG, Dublin, CA) and the Alcon Verion Image Guided System (Alcon Laboratories, Inc., Fort Worth, TX) are now directly synchronized with surgical planning and biometric software, reducing transcription errors and enabling "one-stop" preoperative assessments [15].

3.2.4 Challenges and Adaptations

Despite their benefits, online tools introduced new challenges:

1. Data security: Storing patient biometric data on cloud servers raised concerns about Health Insurance Portability and Accountability Act (HIPAA) compliance and cybersecurity [16].
2. Internet dependency: Surgeons in areas with poor connectivity faced difficulties accessing real-time tools.
3. Surgeon reliance: Overdependence on automated outputs risked eroding manual calculation skills. A 2019 survey found that 62% of trainees could not explain the mathematical principles behind common formulas [17].

Hybrid models emerged to address these issues. For instance, the OCULUS Keratograph allows offline biometry storage with cloud synchronization once connectivity is restored [18]. Organizations such as the ASCRS also launched training programs to help surgeons master both digital tools and manual calculations [19].

Integrating artificial intelligence (AI) into online platforms represents the next frontier. Tools such as Clarity (Alcon Laboratories, Inc., Fort Worth, TX) now combine traditional formulas with machine learning (ML) algorithms trained on millions of global surgeries, offering real-time adjustments based on surgeon-specific outcomes [20]. As these systems evolve, they promise further to narrow the gap between theoretical precision and real-world variability.

3.3 Artificial Intelligence and the Future

3.3.1 The Rise of AI in IOL Calculations

The integration of artificial intelligence (AI) into ophthalmology marks a paradigm shift in intraocular lens (IOL) calculations. While traditional formulas rely on linear regression and theoretical optics, AI leverages ML to analyse vast, heterogeneous datasets—identifying patterns imperceptible to human researchers [21]. This capability is particularly transformative for complex cases, such as eyes with prior refractive surgery, irregular corneas, or rare anatomical features. For instance, the PEARL-DGS formula (Postoperative spherical Equivalent prediction using ARtificial intelligence and Linear algorithms) is an open-source, machine-learning–based sum-of-segments thick-lens formula. Developed and validated on several thousand eyes, it predicts the theoretical internal lens position (TILP) and achieves refractive-prediction accuracy comparable to other state-of-the-art formulas such as Barrett Universal II, EVO 2.0, and Olsen [14, 22].

3.3.2 ML Techniques and Applications

AI-driven IOL tools employ diverse ML architectures:

- Random forest models excel at handling nonlinear relationships between variables (e.g., AL, corneal asphericity) [24].
- Neural networks mimic human cognition, iteratively refining predictions through layers of interconnected nodes. These models power platforms such as LENSAR, which adjust IOL power in real time during femtosecond laser-assisted cataract surgery [24].
- Ensemble learning combines multiple algorithms to reduce error margins. The Hoffer AI Formula, for example, merges outputs from 10+ models to optimize outcomes for paediatric cataracts [25].

In one machine-learning study, the absolute errors of the ML method were lower than those of Barrett Universal II; although the difference was not statistically significant, the authors concluded that their method was non-inferior to Barrett Universal II [27].

3.3.3 AI-Driven Clinical Platforms

Commercial AI tools are now integral to preoperative planning:

- *Alcon Clarity* (Alcon Laboratories, Inc., Fort Worth, TX): Integrates optical biometry with ML algorithms to recommend IOL power, astigmatism management, and intraoperative adjustments [27].
- *Zeiss Veracity Surgical Planner* (Carl Zeiss Meditec, Dublin, CA): Uses AI to analyze historical surgeon-specific outcomes, tailoring formula constants to individual practice patterns. ZEISS VERACITY Surgery Planner minimizes the risk of transcription errors or inaccurate diagnostic data affecting surgery or outcomes. It cross-references data from multiple platforms to ensure every detail is accounted for overlooking [28]. The ZEISS VERACITY Surgery Planner reduces the risk of transcription errors and inaccurate diagnostic data affecting surgical outcomes. By cross-referencing data from multiple platforms, it helps ensure that no detail is overlooked [29].
- *EyeTelligence* (Bausch + Lomb, Bridgewater, NJ): EyeTelligence can help analyze the data and provide the details we need to counsel them. For example, the software can alert us to a high-angle alpha or kappa via an app on our smartphone so we can consider this information when evaluating a multifocal or extended depth of focus (EDOF) IOL. Similarly, the software can notify us of a high root mean square, indicating a significant magnitude of higher-order aberrations. EyeTelligence also analyzes anterior corneal topography and can alert us

if asymmetric or irregular astigmatism is present found [29]. EyeTelligence (Bausch + Lomb, Bridgewater, NJ): This platform analyses biometric and topographic data to support preoperative counselling. It can flag a large angle alpha or kappa—accessible via a smartphone app—which is relevant when evaluating a multifocal or extended depth of focus (EDOF) IOL, and can highlight an elevated root-mean-square value indicating a clinically significant magnitude of higher-order aberrations. By analysing anterior corneal topography, it also identifies asymmetric or irregular astigmatism that may affect IOL selection [30]

These platforms also address global disparities in surgical access. In rural India, Aravind Eye Care System deployed an AI model that reduced refractive errors by 35% in settings with limited access to optical biometers [30].

3.3.4 Ethical and Practical Challenges

Despite its promise, AI adoption faces hurdles:

1. The "Black Box" dilemma: Many ML models lack transparency, making it difficult to audit decision-making processes [31].
2. Data bias: Models trained on Western populations may underperform in diverse ethnic groups. A 2023 audit found that 78% of AI IOL studies used datasets from Europe or North America [32].
3. Surgeon reliance: Overdependence on AI risks deskilling; 45% of surgeons in a 2023 survey admitted deferring to AI even when clinical intuition suggested alternative approaches [33].

Regulatory frameworks are evolving to address these concerns. The World Health Organization (WHO)'s 2021 guidelines advocate for "clinician-in-the-loop" AI, ensuring human oversight, while the Food and Drug Administration (FDA)'s SaMD (Software as a Medical Device) standards mandate rigorous validation across diverse populations [34].

3.3.5 Future Directions and Innovations

The next generation of AI tools aims to transcend static predictions:

- Adaptive AI: Systems such as Netra.AI update in real time using global surgical outcomes, refining predictions as new data emerges. Netra.AI analyzes images from portable, technician-operated fundus camera devices to assess referable DR grading through a cloud-based web portal. The solution utilizes advanced AI algorithms, developed in collaboration with leading retina experts, employing a four-step deep convolutional neural network (DCNN). This neural network aids in detecting DR stages and annotating lesions based on pixel density in the fundus images. The solution can be expanded to other retinal conditions, including glaucoma and biometry [35].

- Multimodal integration: Combining biometry with optical coherence tomography (OCT), aberrometry, and genetic data to personalize IOL power for conditions such as age-related macular degeneration [36].
- Surgical robotics: Robotic surgery, also referred to as robot-assisted surgery, has seen major growth over the past 20 years. The development of systems such as the da Vinci Surgical System (Intuitive Surgical Inc., Sunnyvale, CA, USA) has given surgeons greater precision and control, allowing them to perform minimally invasive surgeries with improved results and dexterity. These technologies are transforming how surgeons plan, execute, and monitor surgical procedures, resulting in improved patient outcomes and fewer complications. As these technologies evolve, they will not only transform the practice of surgery but also redefine the way healthcare is delivered, ultimately leading to a new era of robotic cataract surgery [37].

3.4 Conclusions

The journey of IOL calculations has transformed cataract surgery from a skill guided by basic math to a precise science powered by technology. Early formulas, such as the SRK and Holladay 1, used simple measurements to estimate lens power. Over time, tools like the Barrett Universal II introduced advanced math and computers to handle complex eye shapes. Today, AI analyzes millions of surgeries to predict outcomes more accurately, even for challenging cases. While AI offers exciting possibilities, its success depends on collaboration—combining smart machines with the experience and judgment of surgeons.

Looking forward, AI will keep improving as it learns from global data, helping surgeons achieve better patient results. At the same time, simpler tools will ensure that even surgeons in remote areas can access these advances. By blending tradition with innovation, the future promises cataract surgeries that are precise and personalized, making a clear vision achievable for everyone.

References

1. Fyodorov SN, Galin MA, Linksz A. Calculation of the optical power of intraocular lenses. Investig Ophthalmol. 1975;14(8):625–8.
2. Sanders DR, Retzlaff J, Kraff MC. Comparison of the SRK II formula and other second generation formulas. J Cataract Refract Surg. 1988;14(2):136–41. https://doi.org/10.1016/s0886-3350(88)80087-7. PMID: 3351749.
3. Holladay JT, Prager TC, Chandler TY, Musgrove KH, Lewis JW, Ruiz RS. A three-part system for refining intraocular lens power calculations. J Cataract Refract Surg. 1988;14(1):17–24. https://doi.org/10.1016/s0886-3350(88)80059-2. PMID: 3339543.

4. Hoffer KJ. The Hoffer Q formula: a comparison of theoretic and regression formulas. J Cataract Refract Surg. 1993;19(6):700–12. https://doi.org/10.1016/s0886-3350(13)80338-0. PMID: 8271165.
5. Olsen T. Prediction of the effective postoperative (intraocular lens) anterior chamber depth. J Cataract Refract Surg. 2006;32(3):419–24. https://doi.org/10.1016/j.jcrs.2005.12.139. PMID: 16631049
6. Wang L, Koch DD. Modified axial length adjustment formulas in long eyes. J Cataract Refract Surg. 2018;44(11):1396–7. https://doi.org/10.1016/j.jcrs.2018.07.049. Epub 2018 Sep 28. PMID: 30274847.
7. Tassignon MJ. IOL power calculation for the Bag-in-the-Lens (BIL) implantation technique. In: Pardianto G, editor. The intraocular lens power calculation. Medan: Anak Sudarti Foundation; 2022. p. 85–93.
8. Barrett GD. Intraocular lens calculation formulas for new intraocular lens implants. J Cataract Refract Surg. 1987;13(4):389–96. https://doi.org/10.1016/s0886-3350(87)80037-8.
9. Kane JX, Van Heerden A, Atik A, Petsoglou C. Accuracy of 3 new methods for intraocular lens power selection. J Cataract Refract Surg. 2017;43(3):333–9. https://doi.org/10.1016/j.jcrs.2016.12.021. PMID: 28410714.
10. Aristodemou P, Knox Cartwright NE, Sparrow JM, Johnston RL. Formula choice: Hoffer Q, Holladay 1, or SRK/T and refractive outcomes in 8108 eyes after cataract surgery with biometry by partial coherence interferometry. J Cataract Refract Surg. 2011;37(1):63–71. https://doi.org/10.1016/j.jcrs.2010.07.032. PMID: 21183100.
11. Haigis W, Lege B, Miller N, Schneider B. Comparison of immersion ultrasound biometry and partial coherence interferometry for intraocular lens calculation according to Haigis. Graefes Arch Clin Exp Ophthalmol. 2000;238(9):765–73. https://doi.org/10.1007/s004170000188. PMID: 11045345.
12. Abulafia A, Koch DD, Holladay JT, Wang L, Hill W. Pursuing perfection in intraocular lens calculations: IV. Rethinking astigmatism analysis for intraocular lens-based surgery: Suggested terminology, analysis, and standards for outcome reports. J Cataract Refract Surg. 2018;44(10):1169–74. https://doi.org/10.1016/j.jcrs.2018.07.027. PMID: 30243391.
13. Abulafia A, Hill WE, Koch DD, Wang L, Barrett GD. Accuracy of the Barrett True-K formula for intraocular lens power prediction after laser in situ keratomileusis or photorefractive keratectomy for myopia. J Cataract Refract Surg. 2016;42(3):363–9. https://doi.org/10.1016/j.jcrs.2015.11.039. Epub 2016 Mar 19. PMID: 27006324.
14. Lundström M, Manning S, Barry P, Stenevi U, Henry Y, Rosen P. The European registry of quality outcomes for cataract and refractive surgery (EUREQUO): a database study of trends in volumes, surgical techniques and outcomes of refractive surgery. Eye Vis (Lond). 2015;2:8. https://doi.org/10.1186/s40662-015-0019-1. PMID: 26613089; PMCID: PMC4660846.
15. Melles RB, Holladay JT, Chang WJ. Accuracy of intraocular lens calculation formulas. Ophthalmology. 2018;125(2):169–78. https://doi.org/10.1016/j.ophtha.2017.08.027. Epub 2017 Sep 23. PMID: 28951074.
16. Kruse CS, Frederick B, Jacobson T, Monticone DK. Cybersecurity in healthcare: a systematic review of modern threats and trends. Technol Health Care. 2017;25(1):1–10. https://doi.org/10.3233/THC-161263. PMID: 27689562.
17. Arshinoff SA, Gupta R. IOL power calculation in standard eyes. In: Pardianto G, editor. The intraocular lens power calculation. Medan: Anak Sudarti Foundation; 2022. p. 33–41.
18. Savini G. Intraocular lens power calculations formulas. In: Pardianto G, editor. The intraocular lens power calculation. Medan: Anak Sudarti Foundation; 2022. p. 25–31.
19. Shetty N, Sathe P, Aishwarya FM, Shetty R. Comparison of intraocular lens power prediction accuracy of formulas in American Society of Cataract and Refractive Surgery post-refractive surgery calculator in eyes with prior radial keratotomy. Indian J Ophthalmol. 2023;71(9):3224–8. https://doi.org/10.4103/IJO.IJO_3417_22.
20. Tran E, Shah N, Caballero Ortiz S, Kyveris A, Berg G, Chan T. Visual performance and refractive stability of Clareon® monofocal intraocular lens implanted with an automated delivery

system. Clin Ophthalmol. 2025;19:3933–9. Published 2025 Oct 24. https://doi.org/10.2147/OPTH.S545977.
21. Ting DSW, Pasquale LR, Peng L, Campbell JP, Lee AY, Raman R, Tan GSW, Schmetterer L, Keane PA, Wong TY. Artificial intelligence and deep learning in ophthalmology. Br J Ophthalmol. 2019;103(2):167–75. https://doi.org/10.1136/bjophthalmol-2018-313173. Epub 2018 Oct 25. PMID: 30361278; PMCID: PMC6362807.
22. Debellemanière G, Dubois M, Gauvin M, Wallerstein A, Brenner LF, Rampat R, Saad A, Gatinel D. The PEARL-DGS formula: the development of an open-source machine learning–based thick IOL calculation formula. Am J Ophthalmol. 2021;232:58–69. https://doi.org/10.1016/j.ajo.2021.05.004. PMID: 33992611.
23. Redden LD, Grubauer B, Hoffmann P, et al. Response to comment on: intraocular lens power calculation-comparing big data approaches to established formulas. Am J Ophthalmol. 2025;276:397–9. https://doi.org/10.1016/j.ajo.2025.03.045.
24. Wortz G, Gupta PK, Weinstock JR. Comparative outcomes of robotic laser arcuate keratotomy and toric intraocular lenses for the management of lower magnitude astigmatism at the time of cataract surgery. Clin Ophthalmol. 2025;19:3401–8. Published 2025 Sep 15. https://doi.org/10.2147/OPTH.S543462.
25. Al Shamrani M, Al TS. Update of intraocular lens implantation in children. Saudi J Ophthalmol. 2012;26(3):271–5. https://doi.org/10.1016/j.sjopt.2012.05.005. Epub 2012 Jun 7. PMID: 23961005; PMCID: PMC3729693.
26. Yamauchi T, Tabuchi H, Takase K, Masumoto H. Use of a machine learning method in predicting refraction after cataract surgery. J Clin Med. 2021;10(5):1103. https://doi.org/10.3390/jcm10051103. PMID: 33800825; PMCID: PMC7961666.
27. Breyer DRH, Saad A. Refractive cataract surgery with advanced technology intraocular lens (AT-IOL). In: Pardianto G, Tassignon MJ, editors. Innovation in cataract surgery. Singapore: Springer; 2024. p. 311–35. https://doi.org/10.1007/978-981-97-5192-1_21.
28. Solomon K.D., Scott, M.C. Commanding your cataract workflow. A schematic of the ZEISS cataract workflow with ZEISS VERACITY surgery planner 2023. https://crstoday.com/veracity-cataract-workflow. Accessed 26 Nov 2025.
29. Lobanoff M, Hovanesian J.A, Fram N.R. EyeTelligence. 2023. https://crstoday.com/articles/june-2023/ai-models-for-iol-calculation. Accessed 26 Nov 2025.
30. AI in Healthcare Series Workshop: 11 – Applications of AI: Experiences from Aravind Eye Care System. Dr R. Kim, Chief Medical Officer of the Aravind Eye Hospital (Madurai, India), discusses his experience of using AI in ophthalmology, including the real-time deployment of AI in the screening of diabetic retinopathy. Available from: https://youtu.be/wrf3bg5hwEg?si=_kQSCtCnl1_nhXJm.
31. Topol EJ. High-performance medicine: the convergence of human and artificial intelligence. Nat Med. 2019;25(1):44–56. https://doi.org/10.1038/s41591-018-0300-7. Epub 2019 Jan 7. PMID: 30617339.
32. Ravindranath R, Stein JD, Hernandez-Boussard T, Fisher AC, Wang SY; SOURCE Consortium. The impact of race, ethnicity, and sex on fairness in artificial intelligence for glaucoma prediction models. Ophthalmol Sci. 2024;5(1):100596. https://doi.org/10.1016/j.xops.2024.100596. PMID: 39386055; PMCID: PMC11462200.
33. Müller S, Jain M, Sachdeva B, Shah PN, Holz FG, Finger RP, Murali K, Wintergerst MWM, Schultz T. Artificial intelligence in cataract surgery: a systematic review. Transl Vis Sci Technol. 2024;13(4):20. https://doi.org/10.1167/tvst.13.4.20. PMID: 38618893; PMCID: PMC11033603.
34. World Health Organization. Ethics and Governance of AI in Health. 2021. Available from: https://www.who.int/publications/i/item/9789240029200. Accessed 26 Nov 2025.
35. Netra.AI. This Intel-powered Netra.AI solution can detect diabetic retinopathy in just 2 minutes. 2021. Available from: https://indianexpress.com/article/technology/tech-news-technology/intel-powered-netra-ai-solution-diabetic-retinopahty-7223916/. Accessed 26 Nov 2025.

36. Venkatapathappa P, Sultana A, K S V, Mansour R, Chikkanarayanappa V, Rangareddy H. Ocular pathology and genetics: transformative role of artificial intelligence (AI) in anterior segment diseases. Cureus. 2024;16(2):e55216. https://doi.org/10.7759/cureus.55216. PMID: 38435218; PMCID: PMC10908431.
37. George T, Ekn J, Christopher G. Revolutionizing surgery: the impact of AI and robotics on modern medicine. 2024. https://www.researchgate.net/publication/387410487_Revolutionizing_Surgery_The_Impact_of_AI_and_Robotics_on_Modern_Medicine/citations. Accessed 26 Nov 2025.

Chapter 4
Calculation in Normal Eyes

Setiyo Budi Riyanto and Sultan Hasanuddin

4.1 Anatomy of the Eyes

An anatomical window into the vascular and neurological systems, the eye is an intriguing and intricate organ that can show systemic disease. Our sense of sight accounts for almost 80% of our sensory input [1]. The internal architecture of the globe is partitioned into three distinct anatomical compartments: the anterior and posterior chambers, as well as the vitreous cavity. The peripheral boundaries of the anterior chamber (AC) are defined by the drainage angle, while its internal dimensions are demarcated anteriorly by the corneal endothelium and posteriorly by the iris surface and the crystalline lens. The iris's posterior surface, the zonular fibers' anterior surface, the central surface of crystalline lens, and the ciliary processes' peripheral surfaces all serve to define the posterior chamber. The ciliary body, zonular fibers, and the posterior side of the crystalline lens define the vitreous chamber anteriorly, whereas the retina and optic nerve define it posteriorly [2].

Structurally, the ocular globe is organized into three concentric tunics: an external fibrous envelope (comprising the cornea, sclera, and lamina cribrosa), a medial uveal tract (encompassing the iris, the ciliary body's dual components—pars plicata and pars plana—and the choroid), and an internal neurosensory layer

All authors declare no financial interest.

S. B. Riyanto (✉)
JEC Eye Hospitals & Clinics, Jakarta, Indonesia

S. Hasanuddin
JEC ORBITA, Makassar, Indonesia

Universitas Hasanuddin, Makassar, Indonesia

G. Pardianto (ed.), *Intraocular Lens (IOL) Power Calculation*,
https://doi.org/10.1007/978-981-92-1223-1_4

(consisting of the retinal pigment epithelium alongside the photoreceptor and neuronal networks). Complementing this structural framework are three distinct intraocular fluid media [3]:

1. Aqueous humor: This transparent, low-viscosity medium functions as a specialized physiological solution, primarily composed of water and a precise balance of electrolytes that mirrors the osmolarity of interstitial fluids.
2. Vitreous humor: This transparent, viscoelastic hydrogel is characterized by a sophisticated three-dimensional scaffolding of collagen fibrils. Within this fibrillar matrix, the interstitial voids are occupied by highly polymerized glycosaminoglycans—specifically hyaluronic acid—which facilitate significant water retention and structural integrity.
3. Ocular hematology and hemodynamics: Beyond its systemic roles, the vascular compartment—predominantly localized within the choroid—is a critical determinant of intraocular pressure homeostasis. The choroidal circulation is distinguished by having the highest blood flow rate per unit of tissue mass in the human body. Notably, the minimal oxygen desaturation observed in efferent choroidal blood suggests that its physiological utility extends beyond mere metabolic support for the outer retina.

Cranial Nerve III the oculomotor nerves, which course This nerve divides into superior and inferior divisions immediately prior to entering the orbit after passing through its interdural cistern and entering the cavernous sinus ceiling slightly below the anterior clinoid process. Both divisions enter the superior orbital fissure's central compartment by traveling medially just lateral to the optic strut. Sensory innervation the orbit is connected to the first two branches of the trigeminal nerve. The ophthalmic nerve, the smallest branch of the trigeminal nerve, splits into the lacrimal, frontal, and nasociliary nerves before entering the superior orbital fissure. It is lodged in the dura mater of the lateral wall of the cavernous sinus. In addition, other sensory innervations to the eye are the lacrimal nerve, frontal nerve, nasociliary nerve, ciliary ganglion, maxillary nerve, and abducens nerve [4].

Situated in the immediate retro-pupillary space, posterior to the aqueous chamber, the lens is a specialized biconvex optical element. In the emmetropic adult eye, it provides approximately 20.00 D of refractive power, representing one-third of the globe's total 60.00 D convergent capacity. The equatorial span of the human lens, initially measuring 6.5 mm at birth, demonstrates progressive enlargement throughout early adulthood. Following this developmental phase, the lens maintains a relatively constant equatorial diameter of 9–10 mm throughout the remainder of the adult lifespan. In the neonatal phase, the lens exhibits an anteroposterior diameter of roughly 3.0 mm. This axial dimension remains dynamic throughout adulthood, doubling its initial width to approximately 6.0 mm by age 80 as a result of continuous secondary fiber accretion. While the aging lens exhibits a more pronounced anterior convexity—which typically increases optical convergence—the overall refractive stability of the eye is preserved. This is achieved through a structural remodeling of the lens's internal refractive gradient, effectively counteracting the dioptric shift induced by the altered surface curvature [1].

The lens capsule, epithelial cells, lens fibers, and zonules are the four components that make up the lens. The lens zonules, which are connected between the pars plana and the equatorial lens capsule, normally hold the lens hanging on the ciliary body. Light with wavelengths as long as 1200 nm can pass through the lens due to its transparency. The tight and ordered structure of the lens fiber and the high solubility of lens proteins are necessary for maintaining lens transparency [5]. The lens may adapt in order to capture sharp retinal images of objects at various distances. The ciliary body and lens work together to achieve accommodation. The Helmholtz accommodation theory states that the ciliary muscles relax as one looks at far-off things, causing the lens zonules to become tense and flattened. Conversely, the ciliary muscle contracts and the lens zonules relax for crisp close vision, increasing the lens's convexity [6].

4.2 Physiology of the Eyes

The retina is the sensitive screen that forms the image in the human eye, which functions similarly to a camera. Cone-shaped and cylindrical cells make up this screen, which is the area of the eye that is sensitive to light. Cylindrical cells are color-sensitive except for red, while cone-shaped cells are color-sensitive. These cells are activated by exposure to light. Color and light are perceived by the brain as a result of these nerve sensations traveling through the visual nerve fibers [2, 7]. In the eye, light travels through several layers. These layers include the outer lattice-like layer, the inner granular layer, the inner lattice-like layer, the pigment layer, and the inner nucleated layer. A light-sensitive material found in cone-shaped, cylindrical cells breaks down in the smallest amount of light. The material created by this breakdown activates the cells' membranes, which are then sent to the nervous system. A total of 900,000 nerve fibers connect the retina's 125 million cylindrical and 5.5 million cone-shaped cells to the brain [7]. Melanin, a black pigment produced by the retinal pigment layer, has a similar function to black inside a camera in that it stops light from being reflected inside the eyeball, which is crucial for clear vision. Without pigment, the production of distinct dark and bright spots—which are essential for precise vision—is inhibited and light is reflected in all directions inside the eyeball. In addition to lacking eye pigment, those with albinism have visual acuity of just 15–20% [7].

Afferent signals from the optic nerves converge at the optic chiasm, a central landmark where contralateral and ipsilateral fibers integrate. This anatomical reconfiguration transforms the bilateral neural input into the postchiasmatic optic tracts, facilitating the transmission of binocular information to the lateral geniculate nucleus. Neural transmission of visual data is characterized by a dual-projection system: The nasal afferents cross the midline to the contralateral cortex, whereas the temporal fibers bypass decussation, maintaining an ipsilateral course. This precise axonal sorting facilitates the integration of binocular information within the primary visual cortex of each hemisphere. Downstream from the chiasm, the optic tracts maintain a precise topographical arrangement of binocular data from the opposite hemifield. Upon synapsing within the laminated architecture of the thalamic lateral geniculate body, this refined neural information is propagated via optic radiations to the occipital cortex for complex visual interpretation. In addition to the thalamic route, visual signals are channeled into the brainstem's pretectal and collicular architecture to govern reflexive tracking and focusing. Concurrently, a subset of retinal projections targets the hypothalamic suprachiasmatic nuclei, establishing the neurological foundation for circadian regulation and systemic homeostasis [8].

The lateral geniculate nucleus is characterized by a six-layered neuronal network designed for the rigorous spatial and functional organization of visual data. By employing this laminar architecture, the thalamus achieves a systematic integration of neural impulses, ensuring that color, contrast, and motion cues are appropriately categorized before their subsequent interpretation by the striate cortex. The ipsilateral temporal visual field provides information to layers II, III, and V, whereas the contralateral nasal visual fields provide information to layers I, IV, and VI. Magnocellular neurons make up layers I and II, whereas parvocellular neurons make up layers III, IV, V, and VI to provide interest. Within the retinal architecture, visual information is bifurcated into distinct parvocellular and magnocellular channels. The parvocellular system is dedicated to the transduction of color and fine structural detail. In contrast, the magnocellular system prioritizes the transmission of motion-related data and luminance-based contrast, facilitating the rapid detection of environmental shifts prior to higher-order cortical analysis. The lateral geniculate nucleus maintains a strict functional segregation, with a four-to-two ratio of parvocellular to magnocellular layers. This arrangement ensures the simultaneous transmission of color and motion-sensitive information to the visual cortex. In the final stage of the primary visual pathway, the cortex synthesizes these parallel cues, enabling the brain to interpret the multifaceted properties of the visual field [8].

4.3 Calculation of Intraocular Lens in Normal Eyes

When the natural crystalline lens of the eye becomes opaque due to cataracts or other degenerative processes, an artificial lens known as an intraocular lens (IOL) is used to replace it. The structural makeup of the eye lens is made up of 35% proteins and 65% water, which denature with age and reduce transparency. Advanced IOL materials and design are being developed in response to the growing need for specialized and customized solutions. A variety of high-quality intraocular lenses are now available that can effectively prevent side effects following IOL implantation and surgery, filter particular wavelengths, and offer accommodation capabilities, all made possible by advancements in ocular technology. Among the cutting-edge IOLs currently available on the market are injectable, shape-memory, and adjustable models [9, 10].

The two primary components of IOLs are haptics and optics. Haptics are the extensions of the center optics that are held in position, whereas optics is the central region that is in charge of refraction. Single-piece and three-piece haptic IOL designs are typically utilized in cataract surgery. Because all components are made of the same material (acrylic, silicone, or polymethyl-methacrylate (PMMA)), single-piece IOLs—also known as one-piece IOLs—get their name. In contrast, PMMA held a 12% market share and silicone only 3% by 2017, with hydrophilic and hydrophobic PMMA accounting for 85% of the IOL distribution worldwide. Both stiff (PMMA) and foldable acrylic materials are available, as are hydrophobic and hydrophilic acrylics [10, 11].

The accuracy of intraocular lens (IOL) power estimation is fundamentally predicated on the precision of preoperative biometric parameters. Key variables, including axial length (AL), keratometry (K), and anterior chamber depth (ACD), serve as the critical inputs for IOL calculation formulas; the synergistic reliability of these measurements and the chosen mathematical model dictates the predictability of the postoperative refractive state [12].

4.3.1 Keratometry or K as Corneal Refractive State

Keratometry is a technique that uses the cornea's curvature to quantify its power. A manual or automated keratometer can be used to make this measurement, which is given in diopters. Keratometry relies on the assumption of corneal spherocylindricity, utilizing a fixed ratio to correlate anterior and posterior curvatures. While this facilitates rapid IOL power estimation, it overlooks individual variations in posterior corneal astigmatism, potentially impacting the precision of refractive outcomes in specialized clinical cases [12]. The determination of corneal refractive power is traditionally predicated on the anterior surface's curvature, an approach that inherently lacks absolute precision. This methodology operates under the paraxial approximation, treating the cornea as a perfectly spherical optical mirror and assuming a static, invariant ratio between the anterior and posterior corneal radii. A virtual image of the object is then produced by the cornea working as a perfect convex mirror. This predicts the corneal curvature, which is subsequently utilized to measure the power of the cornea. The fundamental flaw with the majority of keratometers is that they don't give enough details to reliably determine corneal curvature [13].

4.3.2 The AL

The distance between the corneal anterior surface and the retinal pigment epithelium (RPE) is known as the AL, and it is expressed in millimeters. Either optical biometry or ultrasound biometry (achieved by direct contact or immersion) can be used to quantify the AL [14]. In the majority of current formulas, it is arguably the most crucial parameter. The impact of biometric inaccuracies on refractive outcomes is nonlinear and highly dependent on globe dimensions. In short eyes, the sensitivity of IOL power estimation is significantly amplified; a marginal error in measurement can alter the required IOL power by a factor of 2.5–3.0 times more than in longer, myopic eyes. Ocular ultrasonography utilizes the reflection of mechanical waves to determine axial dimensions based on the transit time of a pulse from the cornea to the retina. The velocity of sound propagation is critically dependent on the tissue's acoustic density; it is significantly higher in the crystalline lens and cornea (approximately 1641 m/s) compared to the aqueous and vitreous humors, where it travels at a reduced rate of 1532 m/s [13].

4.3.3 A-Constant

The lens power (LP) , AL, and K are related theoretically by the A-constant. The lens's power and the A-constant fluctuate roughly in a 1:1 ratio. A-constant is actually very varied and reliant on a number of elements, including the type of IOL, IOL material, IOL position, surgeon, incision method, incision placement, AL and K measurement modification, and even the way biometry is performed. It is added as a constant to the proper formula after being set for a certain surgeon, IOL, and scan machine [13, 14].

4.3.4 Effective Lens Position (ELP)

ELP represents the effective optical distance of the lens implant behind the cornea, a parameter that superseded the traditional ACD due to the latter's failure to accurately predict the final position of "in-the-bag" IOLs. This evolution in positional predictability has allowed for the systematic division of IOL formulas into distinct generations, each characterized by an increasing number of biometric variables used to estimate the ELP [13].

4.4 SRK (Sanders, Retzlaff, and Kraff) Formula

The SRK formula for IOL power calculation was introduced by Drs. Donald R. Sanders, John A. Retzlaff, and Manus C. Kraff, where $P = A - 2.5L - 0.9K$, where P is the intraocular lens power required to achieve emmetropia, A is A-constant, L is the eye's axial length, and K is the term that refers to average anterior curvature of the cornea, and it is called keratometry. For common normal eyes, the SRK formula was an advancement over the first-generation theoretical formulations that came before it. The original SRK equation was modified to create SRK II as a secondary generation formula, which offered improved accuracy in eyes with ALs of >26 mm and <22 mm. Since some hyperopic eyes had deep AC and some extremely myopic eyes had small AC, it was later shown that ACD did not always correspond well with AL [15].

In 1990, the Sanders-Retzlaff-Kraff/Theoretical (SRK/T) formula, as one of the third-generation formulas, was introduced. By fusing the benefits of the theoretical model and the linear regression model, the SRK/T formula improves accuracy. The formula employs a combination of the corneal refractive index and mean retinal thickness to compute the functional ACD through the A-constant. This approach ensures that the calculation accounts for the refractive power of the anterior segment while compensating for the posterior axial dimensions, thereby refining the accuracy of the IOL power prediction. Effective lens location is not considered by SRK/T. The SRK/T formula is more accurate than the other third-generation formulas in longer eyes, typically AL >26.0 mm, according to several studies [15, 16].

4.5 Hoffer Q and Hoffer Q/Giacomo Savini/Leonardo Taroni (Hoffer QST) Formulas

Kenneth J. Hoffer published this formula in 1993. The fundamental Hoffer formula, which is a significant modification of Colenbrander's formula, serves as the core vergence formula. The Hoffer Q formula operates on a specialized ELP prediction equation that leverages the axial length and the tangent of the corneal power. This computational framework is designed to establish a personalized anterior chamber depth (pACD) for each patient. By utilizing these core biometric inputs, the formula mitigates the inaccuracies of earlier models, providing a more robust estimation of the IOL's final refractive plane. [15, 17] The Hoffer QST is a new formula that was further refined by Hoffer, Savini, and Taroni. This is an advancement of the Hoffer Q formula from 1993 that uses algorithms to improve accuracy in long eyes and artificial intelligence (AI) to improve ELP prediction. Numerous recent studies currently that depending on the parameters selected (mean absolute error (MAE), median absolute error (MedAE), standard deviation (SD), %±0.50 D, etc.), the Hoffer QST formula stands at the forefront of IOL power prediction, offering results that equal or exceed the precision of contemporary AI-driven and paraxial models [17].

4.6 Holladay Formula

Three components make up Holladay's initial formula (Holladay 1) by Dr. Jack Holladay. A collection of data screening criteria makes up the first section. Identifying the unlikely AL and K measurements and warning users to confirm the data and potential negative consequences are the goals. The formula's core architecture utilizes a modified second-generation framework to improve refractive outcomes. Specifically, it leverages Fyodorov's equation to calculate corneal height as a function of AL and K, thereby refining the ELP prediction. This methodological advancement serves to minimize the discrepancy between predicted and actual post-operative lens positions, particularly in eyes with variant corneal topographies. A customized "surgeon factor" (SF) is utilized to compensate for systematic biases that may arise from an individual's operative profile. This personalized lens constant serves to calibrate the IOL power formula against real-world postoperative data, effectively bridging the gap between theoretical models and the specific surgical environment to minimize refractive surprises. Although it is not public, the Holladay 2 formula can be purchased as a component of the Holladay IOL Consultant software. Besides AL and K, it needs the patient's age, phakic preop ACD, lens thickness (LT), and corneal diameter (CD). With additional characteristics, the Holladay 2 was able to accurately calculate and understand the subtleties of disproportionate eyes [17].

4.7 T2 Formula

The T2 formula, an update to the SRK/T formula, was also derived using regression analysis based on actual postoperative outcomes in order to reduce systematic error from corneal height estimation. For AL 24.5–26 mm, the T2 formula showed the lowest absolute error. While another study showed comparable outcomes between the T2 and Haigis, T2 also had a lower absolute error when compared to SRK/T, Hoffer Q, and Holladay 2. The method still has the drawback of being reliant on only two variables, even though the T2 was an improvement over the SRK/T [18].

4.8 Haigis Formula

This method from Wolfgang Haigis can be applied to a variety of eyes because it uses three variables. The three factors are associated with ACD (a1), AL (a2), and power prediction curve (a0), which shifts the curve up or down. This formula is more applicable to a broad range of AL eyes since it requires the following parameters: AL, corneal power, and ACD. The term "double analysis" refers to this formula approach [15, 17].

4.9 Olsen C Formula

Ray tracing refers to a novel physical method in the Olsen formula by Thomas Olsen. In order to enhance implant position prediction, this model now incorporates LT measurements. The formula's C-constant, which is utilized to precisely predict the IOL location, is a feature exclusive to this method. An estimate of the empty capsular bag that will contain the replacement IOL is produced by this constant. The corneal power, ACD, and LT are the only prerequisites needed to complete this computation [15].

4.10 Barrett Universal II (BUII) Formula

This formula is a thick lens formula by Dr. Graham D. Barrett. It uses a "lens factor" or LF to calculate the depth of the AC. Both AL and K affect this LF. One important aspect of this formula is that it uses the location of the IOL's major plane of refraction as a pertinent variable. The two fundamental parameters needed for this calculation are corneal power and AL. Other alternative parameters are the white-to-white (WTW) corneal diameter, LT, and ACD [15].

4.11 Hill-Radial Basis Function (RBF) Formula

Based on RBF principle, which is comparable to a neural network, Dr. Warren E. Hill introduced Hill-RBF in 2016. The limitations and advantages of a lens-position evaluation are not present in the Hill-RBF formula since it is a data-driven approach to calculate IOL power. It makes use of a sophisticated type of data interpolation and MATLAB-developed pattern recognition. The RBF calculator identifies coherent patterns in complex biometric datasets by processing a multitude of known clinical examples. This methodology effectively maps the relationship between ocular dimensions and refractive outcomes, transforming a seemingly random distribution of data into a robust predictive model. Consequently, the RBF-based approach offers enhanced precision, particularly in outlier cases that fall outside the predictive range of conventional formulas. The predictive accuracy of this formula has been rigorously calibrated for an IOL power spectrum of +6.00 D to +30.00 D. This optimization was achieved utilizing biometric datasets derived from the Lenstar LS 900 optical biometer (Haag-Streit, Köniz, Switzerland), specifically in conjunction with the Alcon SN60WF biconvex intraocular lens (Alcon Laboratories, Inc., Fort Worth, TX). Such hardware-specific tuning ensures maximum refractive predictability within standard clinical ranges [19].

Beyond standard dioptric powers, the formula has undergone independent calibration for high-convexity implants up to +35.00 D. Furthermore, for low-power and meniscus-style applications, the algorithm demonstrates high fidelity when paired with biometric data from the aforementioned optical biometer, specifically for the Alcon MA60MA extended-range IOL (Alcon Laboratories, Inc., Fort Worth, TX) within a refractive span of +5.00 D to −5.00 D. When combined with data from other devices, the Hill-RBF online calculator (https://rbfcalculator.com/online/index.html) can produce biometry data that are clinically comparable to that of the

LENSTAR LS 900. The utility of this predictive model extends beyond specific brand-name implants to encompass a wide array of IOL platforms with comparable optical architectures. For dioptric powers between +5.00 D and − 5.00 D, the formula remains highly effective for alternative meniscus-design IOLs. Similarly, for the more common range of +6.00 D to +35.00 D, its algorithmic strengths can be leveraged for various biconvex IOL models, ensuring consistent refractive accuracy across different manufacturing platforms. The variables AL, K, ACD, LT, WTW, central corneal thickness (CCT), and gender are used in the Hill-RBF 3.0 model [19, 20].

4.12 Karmona Formula

David Carmona González of Spain created and coded Karmona, the most recent of these IOL power calculation formulas, which was engineered within the Shiny-RStudio ecosystem (Version 1.1.423; R Foundation, Boston, MA) during a sustained development cycle from 2018 to 2021. This model represents a paradigm shift in IOL power calculation, relying exclusively on pure artificial intelligence. Unlike traditional frameworks, it operates independently of Gaussian optics and paraxial theory, instead utilizing complex neural networks to discern refractive patterns directly from empirical datasets. Its foundation is a combination of two machine learning models known as cubist decision trees and regularized Bayesian neural networks. Out of 11 nonlinear regression models, these were chosen as the most effective. They were then adjusted, which improved their metrics. Ultimately, a machine learning (ML) technique that integrated predictions from various methodologies produced an ensembled model [21].

AL, K, WTW, ACD, and central radius of the anterior corneal surface are among the data inputs used by Karmona. Optional factors include posterior corneal central radius, rear to front central radius of corneal surface ratio, anterior segment depth (the sum of ACD and LT), LT, and gender. Using a database of just 386 eyeballs with standard AL (22.0–25.0 mm), Karmona has been introduced as a novel technique. Since the formula uses nonconventional data inputs, such as the ratio of the anterior segment depth and the central radius of the rear to front surface of the cornea, as a separate unique parameter, it may have been created to improve accuracy and precision in extremely short or long and atypical eyes [19].

4.13 Nallasamy Formula

Tingyang Li, Joshua Stein, and Nambi Nallasamy released a new formula in 2022. Two layers made up the ensemble ML model used by Nallasamy et al. The predictive model utilizes a layered ensemble architecture to optimize refractive outcomes. In the primary stratum, a suite of level-1 base learners is trained using preoperative biometric inputs and IOL power to target the postoperative refraction. The subsequent second layer consists of a meta-model that processes the outputs of these initial learners as its input features. Consequently, the level-2 meta-model refines the predictions of the primary layer to produce the final anticipated refraction, leveraging five core mandatory variables—AL, K, ACD, WTW, and LT—alongside the optional parameter of CCT [22].

References

1. Ludwig PE, Jessu R, Czyz CN. Physiology, eye. [Updated 2023 Jul 17]. In: StatPearls [Internet]. Treasure Island (FL): StatPearls Publishing; 2025 Jan-. Available from: https://www.ncbi.nlm.nih.gov/books/NBK470322/.
2. Rehman I, Hazhirkarzar B, Patel BC. Anatomy, head and neck, eye. [Updated 2023 Jul 24]. In: StatPearls [Internet]. Treasure Island (FL): StatPearls Publishing; 2025 Jan-. Available from: https://www.ncbi.nlm.nih.gov/books/NBK482428/.
3. Galloway NR, Amoaku WMK, Galloway PH, Browning AC. Basic anatomy and physiology of the eye. In: Common eye diseases and their management; 2016. p. 1–7. https://doi.org/10.1007/978-3-031-08450-8_2.
4. Lieber S, Fernandez-Miranda JC. Anatomy of the orbit. J Neurol Surg B Skull Base. 2020;81(4):319–32. https://doi.org/10.1055/s-0040-1715096.
5. Hejtmancik JF, Shiels A. Overview of the lens. Prog Mol Biol Transl Sci. 2015;134:119–27. https://doi.org/10.1016/bs.pmbts.2015.04.006.
6. Ruan X, Liu Z, Luo L, Liu Y. The structure of the lens and its associations with the visual quality. BMJ Open Ophthalmol. 2020;5(1):e000459. Published 2020 Sep 18. https://doi.org/10.1136/bmjophth-2020-000459.
7. Brous A. A study of the physiology of the human eye, a careful and meticulous study. Eurasian J Sci Technol. 2021;1(2):100–5. https://doi.org/10.48309/EJST.2021.285020.1017.
8. Sánchez López de Nava A, Somani AN, Salini B. Physiology, vision. [Updated 2023 May 1]. In: StatPearls [Internet]. Treasure Island (FL): StatPearls Publishing; 2025 Jan-. Available from: https://www.ncbi.nlm.nih.gov/books/NBK538493/.
9. Luo C, Wang H, Chen X, Xu J, Yin H, Yao K. Recent advances of intraocular lens materials and surface modification in cataract surgery. Front Bioeng Biotechnol. 2022;10:913383. Published 2022 Jun 8. https://doi.org/10.3389/fbioe.2022.913383.
10. Vacalebre M, Frison R, Corsaro C, et al. Current state of the art and next generation of materials for a customized intraocular lens according to a patient-specific eye power. Polymers (Basel). 2023;15(6):1590. https://doi.org/10.3390/polym15061590.
11. Zhong X, Long E, Chen W, et al. Comparisons of the in-the-bag stabilities of single-piece and three-piece intraocular lenses for age-related cataract patients: a randomized controlled trial. BMC Ophthalmol. 2016;16:100. https://doi.org/10.1186/s12886-016-0283-4.
12. Sridhar MS. Anatomy of cornea and ocular surface. Indian J Ophthalmol. 2018;66(2):190–4. https://doi.org/10.4103/ijo.IJO_646_17.
13. Nenning M, Findl O. History of optical biometry. In: Pardianto G, editor. The intraocular lens power calculation. Medan: Anak Sudarti Foundation; 2022. p. 1–9.
14. Song AL, Rizzuti A. Optical biometry. [Updated 2023 Apr 17]. In: StatPearls [Internet]. Treasure Island (FL): StatPearls Publishing; 2025 Jan-. Available from: https://www.ncbi.nlm.nih.gov/books/NBK580549/.
15. Kramer B, Toric IOL. Power calculation and managing residual astigmatism. In: Pardianto G, editor. The intraocular lens power calculation. Medan: Anak Sudarti Foundation; 2022. p. 75–84.

16. Cooke DL, Cooke TL. Comparison of 9 intraocular lens power calculation formulas. J Cataract Refract Surg. 2016;42(8):1157–64. https://doi.org/10.1016/j.jcrs.2016.06.029.
17. Savini G, Hoffer KJ. Online intraocular lens power calculators. In: Pardianto G, Tassignon MJ, editors. Innovation in cataract surgery. Singapore: Springer; 2024. p. 123–38. https://doi.org/10.1007/978-981-97-5192-1_8.
18. Xia T, Martinez CE, Tsai LM. Update on intraocular lens formulas and calculations. Asia Pac J Ophthalmol (Phila). 2020;9(3):186–93. https://doi.org/10.1097/APO.0000000000000293.
19. Stopyra W, Cooke DL, Grzybowski A. A review of intraocular lens power calculation formulas based on artificial intelligence. J Clin Med. 2024;13(2):498. https://doi.org/10.3390/jcm13020498.
20. Kane JX, Van Heerden A, Atik A, Petsoglou C. Intraocular lens power formula accuracy: comparison of 7 formulas. J Cataract Refract Surg. 2016;42(10):1490–500. https://doi.org/10.1016/j.jcrs.2016.07.021.
21. Carmona González D, Palomino BC. Accuracy of a new intraocular lens power calculation method based on artificial intelligence. Eye (Lond). 2021;35(2):517–22. https://doi.org/10.1038/s41433-020-0883-3.
22. Li T, Stein J, Nallasamy N. Evaluation of the Nallasamy formula: a stacking ensemble machine learning method for refraction prediction in cataract surgery. Br J Ophthalmol. 2023;107(8):1066–71. https://doi.org/10.1136/bjophthalmol-2021-320599.

Chapter 5
IOL Calculation in Pediatric Cataract

Florence Meilani Manurung and Hadi Prakoso Wreksoatmodjo

5.1 Introduction

Intraocular lens (IOL) calculation in pediatric cataract surgery is challenging due to the dynamic nature of pediatric ocular growth, difficulties in obtaining accurate measurements, the need for age-specific refractive targets, and the lack of pediatric-specific formulas. Unlike adult cataract surgery, where the goal of IOL calculation is to achieve an emmetropic visual outcome after surgery, the IOL power selection for pediatric cases focuses on ensuring optimal long-term visual development. The aim is to provide these young patients with the best possible vision as they grow, minimizing the risk of amblyopia or avoiding it altogether. Additionally, the risk of refractive surprises and the need for long-term management further complicate the process. Despite these challenges, advances in biometry, surgical techniques, and IOL design are helping to improve outcomes in pediatric cataract surgery.

This chapter provides an overview of the key factors that influence the determination of the postoperative refractive goal. These include IOL calculations (such as biometric measurements in pediatric cases and the choice of IOL calculation formulas), selecting the IOL power to achieve the best long-term visual outcomes, managing amblyopia and anisometropia (in both unilateral and bilateral cases), and understanding the dynamics of ocular growth in children.

All authors declare no financial interest.

F. M. Manurung (✉)
JEC Eye Hospitals & Clinics, Jakarta, Indonesia

H. P. Wreksoatmodjo
IEC Eye Care, Jakarta, Indonesia

G. Pardianto (ed.), *Intraocular Lens (IOL) Power Calculation*,
https://doi.org/10.1007/978-981-92-1223-1_5

5.2 Ocular Growth and Development

The unique dynamics of ocular growth and development in children must be thoroughly understood before performing biometric measurements, selecting the appropriate IOL formula, and determining the IOL power to ensure optimal long-term visual outcomes in adulthood.

A. *Axial length changes*: Children's eyes experience rapid growth, particularly during the first few years of life. The axial length (AL) increases significantly during infancy and continues to change until adolescence, directly influencing the refractive power of the eye. This ongoing growth presents challenges in predicting the final refractive outcome following IOL implantation. Understanding the stages of axial length elongation in relation to the timing of surgery is crucial [1]. These phases of growth can be described as follows.

    1. *Rapid growth in early childhood*: The most rapid increase in AL occurs during the first 2 years of life. At birth, the average AL is approximately 16–17 mm. By the age of 2, it increases to about 20–21 mm, accounting for a significant proportion of the total growth during this period.
    2. *Slower growth in later childhood*: After the age of 2, the rate of axial elongation slows but continues steadily throughout childhood. By the age of 5, the AL reaches approximately 22 mm, and by adolescence, it reaches the adult range of 23–24 mm.

    The rate of axial elongation at each stage requires careful consideration when determining the postoperative refractive target. If surgery is performed on a patient younger than 2 years old, the myopic shift will be more significant compared to a patient operated on at 5 years old. In a 2-year-old, approximately 6–7 mm of elongation occurs before reaching adulthood, which corresponds to a myopic shift of about −15 to −18 D or Diopters (assuming a 1 mm shift leads to a 2.5 D change). In contrast, for a 5-year-old, the myopic shift is likely to be much smaller, around −5 to −7 D.

B. *Corneal and lens changes*: The cornea and lens also undergo significant changes in curvature and power during growth, affecting the overall refractive status, thus complicating the calculation of the appropriate IOL power [2].

    1. *Steeper cornea at birth*: At birth, the cornea is relatively steep, with an average keratometry (K) value of approximately 51–52 D. This steep curvature contributes to the high refractive power of the small infant eye.
    2. *Rapid flattening in early childhood*: The cornea undergoes rapid flattening during the first 2 years of life, with the most significant changes occurring in the first 6–12 months. By the age of 2, the average keratometric (K) value decreases to about 44–45 D.
    3. *Gradual flattening in later childhood*: After the age of 2, the rate of corneal flattening slows but continues gradually throughout childhood and adolescence. By adulthood, the average K value stabilizes at around 42–44 D.

To perform biometric measurements for IOL calculation, both K value and AL are required. Measuring corneal curvature in children can be challenging and often needs to be done under general anaesthesia. During an examination under anaesthesia (EUA), if the K value cannot be obtained with a handheld keratometer—due to factors such as pressure from the speculum—or if a handheld keratometer is unavailable, the following guidelines can be used:

- For infants under 6 months of age: Use a K value of 48 D.
- For children between 6 months and 2 years: Use a K value of 45–46 D.
- For children over 2 years: Use a K value of 44 D.

C. *Anterior chamber depth changes*: The anterior chamber undergoes significant changes as the eye grows and develops.

1. *Shallow anterior chamber at birth*: At birth, the anterior chamber is relatively shallow, with an average depth of approximately 2.0–2.5 mm. This shallow anterior chamber depth (ACD) is a result of the smaller size of the eye and the relatively larger lens in infants.
2. *Rapid deepening in early childhood*: The anterior chamber deepens rapidly during the first few years of life as the eye grows. By the age of 2, the ACD increases to about 2.8–3.2 mm.
3. *Gradual deepening in later childhood*: After the age of 2, the rate of ACD deepening slows but continues gradually throughout childhood and adolescence. By adulthood, the average ACD stabilizes at around 3.0–3.5 mm.

The ACD must be considered before IOL implantation to avoid the risk of the IOL pushing the iris forward, which could potentially induce angle-closure glaucoma.

D. *White-to-white (WTW) distance*: Also known as the corneal diameter, which is the horizontal measurement of the cornea from one limbus to the other.

1. *Smaller corneal diameter at birth*: At birth, the average WTW distance is approximately 9.5–10.5 mm. The cornea is relatively small, reflecting the overall smaller size of the infant eye.
2. *Rapid growth in early childhood*: The WTW distance increases rapidly during the first two years of life, with the most significant growth occurring in the first 6–12 months. By the age of 2, the average WTW distance reaches about 11.0–11.5 mm.
3. *Gradual growth in later childhood*: After the age of 2, the rate of WTW growth slows but continues gradually throughout childhood and adolescence. By adulthood, the average WTW distance stabilizes at around 11.5–12.5 mm.

It is well-established that the capsular bag of the crystalline lens is typically larger than the WTW diameter of the cornea, with an average difference of about 1 mm. Most IOLs used in pediatric cataract surgery are designed for adult cataract surgery, with an average maximum compressed diameter of 9.5 mm. To properly accommodate an adult IOL, the minimum diameter of the pediatric capsular bag should be at least 9.5 mm. A smaller capsular bag (less than 9.5 mm) can make it challenging to insert the IOL. Attempting to force an "in-the-bag" implantation in such cases could cause the IOL to bulge forward, potentially leading to pupillary block and/or angle-closure glaucoma, especially if the anterior chamber is shallow. To prevent these serious complications, IOL implantation should be avoided in pediatric cases where the WTW diameter is less than 9.0–9.5 mm.

5.3 Difficulties in Accurate Biometry

Accurate biometry measurement in pediatric cataract surgery is particularly challenging due to the unique anatomical and physiological features of children's eyes, as well as the practical difficulties in obtaining precise measurements. Unlike adult eyes, pediatric eyes are still growing and developing, which complicates the process of obtaining accurate data. These challenges can significantly affect the precision of IOL power calculations, potentially leading to refractive surprises and long-term visual issues if not carefully managed. However, by employing specialized techniques, pediatric-specific formulas, and diligent postoperative monitoring, clinicians can enhance biometry accuracy and improve visual outcomes for children undergoing cataract surgery.

Obtaining accurate measurements of AL, keratometry (corneal curvature), and ACD in children is challenging due to factors such as poor cooperation, nystagmus, or dense cataracts. For very young or uncooperative children, EUA or general anaesthesia is essential. Additionally, the small size of pediatric eyes, the difficulty in measuring keratometry, even with a handheld keratometer, and the potential inaccuracy of standard biometry devices for children further complicate the process. These factors make accurate biometry in pediatric cataract cases more complex.

Immersion A-scan is often preferred over contact methods to prevent corneal indentation [3, 4], but it requires specialized equipment (such as a Praeger shell) and a skilled operator, which may not always be available in the operating theatre. Optical biometry devices (e.g., IOL Master (Carl Zeiss Meditec, Dublin, CA), Lenstar (Haag-Streit, Köniz, Switzerland), Aladin (Topcon, Tokyo, Japan)) are typically more effective for older, cooperative children or those with less dense cataracts [5]. However, in cases of dense pediatric cataracts, nystagmus, or strabismus with unstable fixation, optical biometry may face challenges in delivering accurate measurements.

5.4 Postoperative Refractive Goals

Unlike adults, where the target of refractive surgery is often emmetropia (zero refractive error), children require a hyperopic target to account for the myopic shift that will occur as the eye grows. Determining the appropriate amount of hyperopia is challenging and varies with age due to the differences in growth and changes in both the anterior and posterior segments of the eye. As a result, the target refraction needs to be adjusted based on the child's age. Younger children typically require more hyperopia, as they are likely to experience a greater myopic shift as they grow [6]. Since the rate of axial growth varies among children, it is difficult to predict how much the eye will change postoperatively, which can lead to significant long-term refractive surprises [7]. These surprises may necessitate additional interventions, such as glasses, contact lenses, or even IOL exchange.

The primary goal of refractive correction in pediatric cataract surgery is to prevent amblyopia, which can arise from significant refractive errors or anisometropia. Achieving proper refractive outcomes is crucial for supporting normal visual development during the critical period of visual plasticity in childhood. Refractive goals must also consider the future growth of the eye to reduce the need for frequent changes in glasses or the risk of requiring secondary surgical interventions. Below are general guidelines for age-specific refractive goals:

A. *Infants (0–2 years)*: The target refraction for infants undergoing cataract surgery should be +6.0 to +8.0 D of hyperopia. This approach takes into account the rapid growth of infants' eyes, allowing for the expected axial elongation and myopic shift as the child matures. Overcorrection is essential to prevent significant myopia in adulthood, ensuring better long-term visual outcomes.
B. *Toddlers (2–6 years)*: For toddlers, the target refraction should be +3.0 to +6.0 D of hyperopia. Although the rate of axial growth begins to slow during this stage, it remains substantial, which is why a moderate degree of hyperopia is aimed for. The exact target will vary depending on the child's age and anticipated growth patterns, taking into account the individual's development and future changes in eye size.
C. *Older children (6–12 years)*: For older children, the target refraction should be +1.0 to +3.0 D of hyperopia, or in some cases, emmetropia (zero refractive error). By this age, axial growth has slowed significantly, and the eye is approaching its adult size. In many cases, targeting emmetropia may be appropriate to reduce the child's reliance on glasses and provide a more stable long-term refractive outcome.
D. *Adolescents (12+ years)*: The target refraction for this group is typically emmetropia or slight myopia (−0.5 to −1.0 D). By this stage, the eye has nearly reached its adult size, with minimal growth expected. In some cases, slight myopia may be preferred to account for any residual growth and to ensure optimal long-term visual outcomes.

To better understand and achieve more precise targeting of the postoperative refractive outcome based on the child's age at the time of surgery, we can refer to Tables 5.1, 5.2, and 5.3.

In the context of logarithmic eye growth, the rate of refractive growth (RRG) parameter quantifies the rate of change in refractive error (e.g., myopia or hyperopia) over time. This parameter is modelled using a logarithmic function.

In pediatric cataract surgery, the rate of refractive growth 2 (RRG2) parameter is used in IOL power calculations to account for the rapid, age-dependent axial elongation and refractive changes that occur in a child's eye post-surgery [9]. Unlike adults, children's eyes grow logarithmically, rendering standard adult IOL formulas (e.g., Sanders-Retzlaff-Kraff/Theoretical (SRK/T), Holladay) inadequate in predicting long-term refractive outcomes. By incorporating RRG2, the calculation models future eye growth, thereby optimizing IOL power selection.

Table 5.1 Recommended postoperative refractive goals based on age [8]

Recommended postoperative refractive goals for children aged 1 to 8 years, from various authors			
	Postoperative goal (D)		
Age at surgery (year)	Enyedi et al. (1998)	Plager et al. (2002)	Trivedi and Wilson (2009)
1	+6		+6
2	+5		+5
3	+4	+5	
4	+3	+4	+4
5	+2	+3	+3
6	+1	+2.25	+2
7	0	+1.5	+1.5
8	−1 to −2	+1	+1
10		+0.5	+0.5
>14			0

Table 5.2 Recommended postoperative refractive goals based on age for unilateral cataracts [8]

Management of unilateral cataracts			
Age at surgery (year)	Management	Initial refractive goal if IOL is implanted (D)	Likely refraction at age 20 years (D)
<0.5	Aphakia	–	+11
0.1–1	Aphakia or pseudophakia	+9 to +6	–3.4 to −4.9
1	IOL	+5	–4.9
2	IOL	+4	–3.4
4	IOL	+2.5	–2.7
8	IOL	+1.25	–1.5

Note, these goals are illustration only: We do not have science to suggest that one goal is better than another. "Likely refraction at age 20 years" is the mean based on the reanalysis of the refractive growth 2 (RRG2) model of refractive growth; many children will have a greater or lesser refractive error at this age

Table 5.3 Recommended postoperative refractive goals based on age for bilateral cataracts [8]

Management of bilateral cataract			
Age at surgery (year)	Management	Initial refractive goal if IOL is implanted (D)	Likely refraction at age 20 years (D)
<0.5	Aphakia	–	+ 11
0.1–1	Aphakia	–	+11
1	Aphakia or pseudophakia	+7	–3.0
2	IOL	+5	–2.5
4	IOL	+3.5	–1.7
8	IOL	+2	–0.8

Note, these goals are illustration only: We do not have science to suggest that one goal is better than another. The lifelong safety of bilateral pseudophakia after cataract surgery in childhood is not yet determined; bilateral aphakia is generally well tolerated. "Likely refraction at age 20 years" is the mean based on the RRG2 model of refractive growth; many children will have a greater or lesser refractive error at this age

Although the validity of refractive residual gradient (RRG2) in infants and older children has not yet been established, long-term studies in infants who underwent surgery before 3 months have not been conducted. Furthermore, the results of older children are still controversial, indicating a relatively small myopic shift over a relatively short period of follow-up. Additionally, the standard deviation of RRG2 is approximately 45% of the value of RRG2, which limits the precision of future refraction predictions using RRG2.

Children undergoing bilateral cataract surgery are not at risk of anisometropia; it may be acceptable to leave them with a higher initial hyperopia compared to children with unilateral cataracts. Since IOL implantation carries a greater risk in infants, it is often recommended to keep infants with bilateral cataracts aphakic for the first 1 or 2 years.

Several additional factors must be considered in each case, including family circumstances, the ability to ensure proper follow-up, and the potential for alternative approaches, such as planning for the implantation of a secondary IOL in aphakic eyes.

5.5 Limited Pediatric-Specific Formulae

Pediatric IOL calculation requires specialized formulas and adjustments to account for the unique anatomical and physiological characteristics of children's eyes. Most standard IOL power calculation formulas (e.g., SRK/T, Holladay 1, Hoffer Q) were developed for adult eyes and may not fully address the specific needs of pediatric eyes. Although some formulas have been adapted for children, there is no universally accepted formula for pediatric IOL calculation, resulting in variability in postoperative outcomes [10].

Several formulas are used to calculate IOL power in pediatric patients, each offering distinct advantages and limitations, as outlined below:

Holladay 2 formula: The Holladay 2 formula is an advanced formula that considers additional parameters such as AL, keratometry, ACD, lens thickness, and WTW distance. It can be adapted for pediatric eyes by inputting age-specific adjustments for ACD and lens position. The advantage is that this formula is more comprehensive and adaptable to pediatric eyes compared to simpler formulas.

Barrett Universal II formula: The Barrett Universal II formula is a newer, nonlinear formula that performs well across a wide range of AL and ages. It has been validated for use in pediatric eyes and is considered one of the most accurate formulas for children. This formula provides reliable results in both short and long eyes, making it suitable for the wide range of AL seen in pediatric patients.

SRK/T with pediatric adjustments: The SRK/T formula is a popular regression-based formula for IOL calculation. In children, the A-constant is often adjusted to account for the shallower anterior chamber and smaller eye size. It is simple to use and widely available, but requires careful adjustment for pediatric eyes.

Hoffer Q with pediatric adjustments: The Hoffer Q formula is optimized for short eyes, making it potentially useful in younger children with shorter AL. It is similar to SRK/T, the A-constant or surgeon factor may need adjustment for pediatric cases. This formula performs well in eyes with shorter axial lengths, which are common in infants and young children.

SRK/T, Holladay 1, and Hoffer Q are commonly used formulas for pediatric IOL power calculations, but they often require adjustments to accommodate the unique characteristics of pediatric eyes. Some formulas, such as Holladay 2 and Barrett Universal II, have been adapted or validated for use in children [8]. To account for future axial growth, many surgeons adjust the target refraction, typically aiming for a hyperopic outcome. These adjustments often involve modifying the A-constant or surgeon factor to better align with pediatric eye anatomy. In particular, the A-constant is frequently increased by 0.5–1.0 to account for the shallower anterior chamber and smaller eye size seen in children (Table 5.4).

Although newer formulas, such as Holladay 2 and Barrett Universal II, offer improved accuracy and are available on the market, they are not yet integrated into

Table 5.4 Formula with pediatric adaptation and its advantages [8]

Formula	Pediatric adaptation	Advantages
Holladay 2	Input age-specific adjustments for ACD and lens position	Comprehensive; accounts for multiple ocular parameters
Barrett Universal II	Validated for pediatric use; no major adjustments needed	Accurate across a wide range of axial lengths and ages
SRK/T	Increase A-constant by 0.5–1.0 for pediatric eyes	Simple and widely available
Hoffer Q	Increase A-constant or surgeon factor for pediatric eyes	Optimized for short eyes, common in infants and young children

most ultrasound (A-scan) biometry devices. Given that many pediatric patients are young children or uncooperative, optical biometry is often not feasible. As a result, SRK/T and Hoffer Q formulas (with necessary adjustments) remain the most commonly used formulas in the operating theatre for pediatric cases.

5.6 Risk of Refractive Surprises

Refractive surprises in pediatric cataract IOL calculations present a major challenge due to the ongoing growth and development of the eye. These unexpected outcomes can result in amblyopia and may necessitate further interventions, such as glasses, contact lenses, or even secondary surgical procedures such as IOL exchange. Additionally, uncorrected refractive errors can significantly impact a child's quality of life.

Refractive surprises can be caused by several factors, including rapid ocular growth, changes in corneal curvature, inaccurate biometry, and the limitations of IOL formulas. Surgical factors also play a role, such as variations in IOL position (effective lens position or ELP), which can be influenced by differences in the size and elasticity of the capsular bag in children. Additionally, the availability of appropriate IOL powers may contribute to these unexpected outcomes [11].

Capsular bag contraction is another potential cause of postoperative refractive changes. In pediatric patients, the capsular bag is more elastic and prone to contraction, which can impact the IOL's position and ultimately affect the refractive outcome. Additionally, postoperative inflammation or the development of posterior capsule opacification (PCO) can further alter the refractive result, leading to changes in visual outcomes.

5.7 Summary of Risks and Mitigation Strategies (Table 5.5)

Table 5.5 Risk factor and mitigation strategy [8]

Risk factor	Mitigation strategy
Rapid ocular growth	Target age-appropriate hyperopia; monitor AL changes postoperatively
Changes in corneal Curvature	Use accurate keratometry measurements; account for corneal flattening in calculations
Inaccurate biometry	Use immersion ultrasound or optical biometry; take multiple measurements
Limitations of IOL formulas	Use pediatric-specific formulas (e.g., Holladay 2, Barrett Universal II)
Surgical factors	Ensure proper IOL positioning; consider IOL exchange if necessary
Postoperative changes	Monitor for capsular bag contraction and PCO; treat inflammation promptly

5.8 Future Directions

Advances in biometry and imaging techniques are expected to enhance the accuracy of IOL calculations in pediatric eyes. The development of IOLs specifically designed for pediatric patients may improve outcomes. Therefore, ongoing research and long-term studies are essential to refine IOL calculation strategies and improve visual outcomes in children.

Advancements in biometry and imaging technologies are anticipated to improve the accuracy of IOL calculations for pediatric eyes. The development of IOLs tailored specifically for children could also lead to better visual outcomes. Therefore, ongoing research and long-term studies are crucial to refine IOL calculation methods and optimize visual results for pediatric patients.

5.9 Conclusion

IOL calculation in pediatric cataract surgery is a complex process that requires a deep understanding of the unique anatomical and physiological characteristics of children's eyes. There is currently no standardized approach to IOL calculation for children, and practices can vary significantly among surgeons. This lack of consensus presents a challenge in achieving consistent and predictable outcomes. Accurate preoperative measurements, careful selection of the appropriate formula, and meticulous postoperative management are crucial for optimizing visual outcomes. As technology and surgical techniques continue to advance, the ability to predict and manage refractive outcomes in pediatric cataract patients is expected to improve, leading to better long-term visual prognosis for these young patients.

References

1. Bach A, Villegas VM, Gold AS, Shi W, Murray TG. Axial length development in children. Int J Ophthalmol. 2019;12(5):815–9. https://doi.org/10.18240/ijo.2019.05.18. PMID: 31131242; PMCID: PMC6520278.
2. Bluestein E, Wilson M, Wang X, et al. Dimensions of the pediatric crystalline lens: Implications for intraocular lenses in children. J Pediatr Opthalmol Strabismus. 1996;33(1):18–20.
3. Trivedi R, Wilson M. Prediction error after pediatric cataract surgery with intraocular lens implantation: contact versus immersion A-scan biometry. J Cataract Refract Surg. 2011;37:501–5.
4. Ben-Zion I, Neely D, Plager D, et al. Accuracy of IOL calculations in children: a comparison of immersion versus contact A-scan biometry. J AAPOS. 2008;12:440–4.
5. Lenhart P, Hutchinson A, Lynn M, et al. Partial coherence interferometry versus immersion ultrasonography for axial length measurement in children. J Cataract Refract Surg. 2010;36:21000–2104.

6. Plager D, Kipfer H, Sprunger D, et al. Refractive change in pediatric pseudophakia: 6-year follow up. J Cataract Refract Surg. 2002;28(5):810–5.
7. Mezer E, Rootman D, Abdolell M, et al. Early postoperative refractive outcomes of pediatric intraocular lens implantation. J Cataract Refract Surg. 2004;30(3):603–10.
8. Trivedi R, Wilson M, Reardon W. Accuracy of the Holladay 2 intraocular lens formula for pediatric eyes in the absence of preoperative refraction. J Cataract Refract Surg. 2011;37(7):1239–43.
9. Mc Clatchey S, Hofmeister E. The optics of aphakic and pseudophakic eyes in childhood. Surv Ophthalmol. 2010;55(2):174–82.
10. Wilson M Jr, Bartholomew L, Trivedi R. Pediatric cataract surgery and intraocular lens implantation: practice styles and preferences of the 2001 ASCRS and AAPOS memberships. J Cataract Refract Surg. 2003;29(9):1811–20.
11. Indaram M, VanderVeen D. Postoperative refractive errors following pediatric cataract extraction with intraocular lens implantation. Semin Ophthalmol. 2018;33(1):51–8.

Chapter 6
Intraocular Lens Power Calculation for Postkeratoplasty

Sharita Rosalyne Siregar

6.1 Introduction

Keratoplasty, including penetrating keratoplasty (PK), deep anterior lamellar keratoplasty (DALK), and endothelial keratoplasty (EK), remains a vital therapeutic option for corneal pathologies. As many of these patients eventually develop cataract or require simultaneous cataract surgery, accurate IOL power calculation becomes essential for optimal visual outcomes. However, postkeratoplasty corneal alterations pose significant challenges to conventional IOL power prediction formulas.

6.2 Challenges in Postkeratoplasty IOL Calculation

The altered corneal structure following keratoplasty leads to changes in anterior and posterior corneal curvature, irregular astigmatism, and variable refractive indices, complicating both keratometric and biometric measurements. These abnormalities may result from:

- Graft-host junction healing irregularities
- Corneal ectasia or steepening

Author declares no financial interest.
Author declares that the table belongs to author

S. R. Siregar (✉)
JEC Eye Hospitals & Clinics, Jakarta, Indonesia

G. Pardianto (ed.), *Intraocular Lens (IOL) Power Calculation*,
https://doi.org/10.1007/978-981-92-1223-1_6

- Posterior corneal surface deviations
- Suture-induced astigmatism or long-term remodeling

Furthermore, the potential for progressive changes in corneal curvature over time can lead to unexpected refractive errors postoperatively, especially hyperopic surprises in cases where standard keratometric indices are relied upon without posterior surface assessment.

6.3 Keratometry (K) and Corneal Power (CP) Assessment

Conventional keratometry or automated keratometers often overestimate corneal power in postkeratoplasty eyes by assuming a fixed anterior–posterior curvature ratio. In reality, this ratio is altered after keratoplasty, particularly in PK and DALK eyes.

To address this, advanced corneal imaging techniques are preferred:

- Scheimpflug imaging (e.g., Pentacam AXL (Oculus Optikgeräte, Wetzlar, Germany)) and anterior segment OCT provide total corneal power measurements, incorporating posterior curvature.
- True net power (TNP) and total corneal refractive power (TCRP) values derived from these devices can better represent the actual corneal refractive status.

Several studies advocate for the use of these parameters in IOL calculations to reduce prediction error and improve refractive accuracy [1, 2].

6.4 Biometry and Axial Length (AL) Considerations

AL measurement using optical biometry (e.g., IOLMaster (Carl Zeiss Meditec, Jena, Germany), Lenstar (Haag-Streit, Köniz, Switzerland)) remains reliable in most postkeratoplasty eyes unless significant corneal opacity persists. In such cases, immersion ultrasound biometry may be necessary. It is important to ensure correct fixation and avoid alignment errors, especially in eyes with irregular corneal optics.

6.5 Formula Selection

In postkeratoplasty eyes, standard third- or fourth-generation formulas often yield less predictable results due to their dependence on inaccurate keratometric inputs (Table 6.1). Consider the following approaches:

Table 6.1 IOL formulas suitable for postkeratoplasty patient

Formula	Type	Best use case
Sanders-Retzlaff-Kraff/ Theoretical (SRK/T)	Third-generation	Basic use; limited accuracy postkeratoplasty
Hoffer Q	Third-generation	Short eyes; not ideal for irregular corneas
Holladay 1/2	Third/ fourth-gen	Requires accurate anterior chamber depth (ACD) and keratometry
BUII	AI/Theoretical	Highly accurate with abnormal corneas
Kane Formula	AI/Theoretical	Performs well with irregular corneas
PEARL-DGS	AI-Based	Designed for postrefractive surgery eyes
Barrett True-K (PK)	Modified	For postkeratoplasty keratometry
Ray-Tracing (OKULIX, etc.)	Physical modeling	Uses corneal tomography for higher accuracy

1. *Standard IOL Formulas (with Modified Inputs)*
    - Use TNP or TCRP instead of standard K-values.
    - Avoid default keratometric index (1.3375) for post-PK or DALK patients.
2. *Ray-Tracing Methods*

Ray-tracing IOL calculation platforms (e.g., OKULIX, PhacoOptics) simulate light propagation using anterior and posterior corneal topography and measured axial length. These are theoretically more accurate and less reliant on empirical formulas [3].

3. *AI (Artificial Intelligence)-Based and New-Generation Formulas*

Formulas such as Barrett Universal II (BUII), Kane, or postoperative spherical equivalent prediction using artificial intelligence and linear algorithms by Guillaume Debellemanière, Damien Gatinel, and Alain Saad (PEARL-DGS) incorporate AI and theoretical modeling, offering improved performance in atypical eyes. Barrett True-K (postkeratoplasty version) can be used where available.

4. *Manual Optimization and Historical Methods*

In cases of sequential cataract surgery postkeratoplasty, previous manifest refraction or historical K-values (prekeratoplasty or stable postop period) may assist in refining IOL power estimation. However, their reliability is limited in eyes with ongoing corneal changes.

6.6 Simultaneous Versus Sequential Surgery

In combined triple procedures (PK + cataract extraction + IOL implantation), the unpredictability of final corneal curvature makes precise IOL power prediction difficult. Under these circumstances, a slightly myopic target may help reduce postoperative refractive surprises. For sequential surgeries, deferring cataract extraction until the corneal graft stabilizes is preferred [4, 5].

6.7 Toric IOL Considerations

Toric IOL implantation is controversial postkeratoplasty due to variable and often irregular astigmatism. In selected cases with stable, regular astigmatism and clear corneal topography, toric IOLs may provide good outcomes. However, postoperative rotation and residual irregularity must be anticipated.

6.8 Postoperative Outcomes and Optimization

Patients should be counseled about the possibility of residual refractive errors and the potential need for spectacles, contact lenses, or further corneal refractive procedures (e.g., PRK or arcuate keratotomy). A thoroughly informed consent process is crucial.

6.9 Conclusion

Accurate IOL power calculation in postkeratoplasty patients remains a complex process due to altered corneal anatomy and optical irregularity. Employing advanced imaging technologies, newer-generation formulas, and individualized approaches can significantly enhance refractive predictability and visual rehabilitation. Continued research and refinement of IOL power calculation methods in these eyes are essential to improving long-term outcomes.

References

1. Savini G, Barboni P, Carbonelli M, Ducoli P, Hoffer KJ. Intraocular lens power calculation after myopic excimer laser surgery: selecting the best method using available clinical data. J Cataract Refract Surg. 2015;41(9):1880–8. https://doi.org/10.1016/j.jcrs.2015.10.026.
2. Aramberri J. Intraocular lens power calculation after corneal refractive surgery: double-K method. J Cataract Refract Surg. 2003;29(11):2063–8. https://doi.org/10.1016/s0886-3350(03)00957-x.
3. Borasio E. IOL power calculation in keratoplasty. In: Aramberri J, Hoffer KJ, Olsen T, Savini G, Shammas HJ, editors. Intraocular lens calculations. Essentials in ophthalmology. Cham: Springer; 2024. p. 963–72. https://doi.org/10.1007/978-3-031-50666-6_69.
4. Oie Y, Nishida K. Triple procedure: cataract extraction, intraocular lens implantation, and corneal graft. Curr Opin Ophthalmol. 2017;28(1):63–6. https://doi.org/10.1097/ICU.0000000000000337.
5. Hayashi K, Hayashi H. Visual outcomes after simultaneous versus sequential triple procedure. Br J Ophthalmol. 2003;87(9):1050–2. https://doi.org/10.1097/01.ico.0000230496.22520.93.

Chapter 7
Intraocular Lens Power Calculations After Refractive Surgery

Eric R. Chen, Sanchay Gupta, Li Wang, and Douglas D. Koch

7.1 Introduction

While nowadays corneal refractive surgery (CRS) offers excellent and outstanding visual results, it also introduces significant challenges in the precise calculation of the power of intraocular lens (IOL) power [1]. This chapter provides a concise examination of the challenges associated with IOL power calculation in eyes with CRS, alongside a discussion of potential mitigations. It further explores the practical implementation and current technological landscape for managing these complex cases, encompassing web-integrated calculators, optical coherence tomography (OCT)-derived formulas, real-time intraoperative biometry, and postoperative lens adjustment or refinement strategies.

7.2 Problems Induced by CRS

The two main origins of inaccuracy in IOL power estimation for eyes following previous refractive surgery consist of imprecise power of the cornea measurements derived from topography or tomography and the erroneous prediction of the effective lens position (ELP) by different IOL calculation formulas.

All authors declare no financial interest.

E. R. Chen · S. Gupta · L. Wang · D. D. Koch (✉)
Department of Ophthalmology, Cullen Eye Institute, Baylor College of Medicine, Houston, TX, USA
e-mail: dkoch@bcm.edu

G. Pardianto (ed.), *Intraocular Lens (IOL) Power Calculation*,
https://doi.org/10.1007/978-981-92-1223-1_7

- Standard keratometry and simulated keratometry readings only assess small paracentral zones of the cornea, failing to account for the more significant central alterations caused by ablation. These techniques solely measure the anterior corneal surface and estimate the posterior corneal curvature, both of which are altered by CRS.
- Complicating this is that the relationship of the anterior and posterior corneal curvatures has been altered, such that anterior corneal measurements are not reliable for predicting posterior power of the cornea.
- Many vergence IOL calculation formulas utilize measured power of the cornea as a key factor to predict ELP. Following myopic laser in situ keratomileusis (LASIK) and photorefractive keratectomy (PRK), flattened keratometric (K) values cause an erroneously predicted shallow or anteriorly displaced ELP, resulting in the selection of inaccurate IOL power and the characteristic postoperative hyperopic surprise.
  - Variations in the magnitude of ELP-related errors are contingent upon the individual formula, the volume of refractive treatment, and the patient's axial length (AL) [2, 3].

7.3 Strategies to Problems Induced by CRS

Various methods have been developed to enhance precision of IOL power calculation in eyes after CRS (Table 7.1). These methods can be categorized into three groups:

1. Utilizing pre-LASIK/PRK alongside post-LASIK/PRK refractive data, only with no use of current corneal measurements
2. Application of contemporary corneal measurements in conjunction with regression formulas derived from LASIK/PRK-induced refractive changes to adjust either parameter:
   (a) Measured anterior power of the cornea or
   (b) Calculated IOL power
3. Utilizing solely current measurements to:
   (a) Adjust the measured anterior power of the cornea through the application of regression-based formulas
   (b) Estimate posterior curvature with biometric parameters
   (c) Perform direct assessments of both anterior and posterior corneal curvature

Table 7.1 Methods for IOL power calculation in eyes following CRS

Method	Strength	Weakness	Technique
Ignore current corneal measurements and use pre-LASIK/PRK data	Reliable if accurate pre-LASIK/PRK data available	Dependent on the accuracy of pre-LASIK/PRK data One-to-one diopter error if any historical data incorrect Difficult to get historical data Less accurate compared to other methods	Clinical History Feiz-Mannis Corneal Bypass
Use current corneal measurements and modify them	Avoid one-to-one error found in approaches relying entirely on historical data	Amount of refractive correction required for modification based on ΔMR	Adjusted EffRP Adjusted Atlas Values Adjusted K Adjusted Keratometry Adjusted ACCP Wang-Koch-Maloney Shammas Method Haigis-L Galilei TCP Pearl-DGS
Use current corneal measurements to calculate and modify IOL power	Avoid one-to-one error found in approaches relying entirely on historical data	Requires amount of refractive correction (ΔMR)	Masket formula Modified Masket formula
Measure actual anterior and posterior corneal curvatures to calculate true TCP	No prior data needed True TCP calculated	Certain adjustments to TCP still needed to achieve accurate IOL power calculation	Slit-scanning system Scheimpflug imaging devices OCT systems EVO Hoffer QST

7.3.1 *Pre-LASIK/PRK Data Only*

IOL power is determined using the pre-LASIK keratometry and manifest refraction, the manifest refraction (MR) acquired prior to the onset of refractive alterations induced by cataracts, and the surgically induced change in MR (ΔMR). These methods include the Clinical History Method [4], the Feiz-Mannis Method [5], and the Corneal Bypass Method [6]. Due to uncertainties of the accuracy of historical data, including refractions prior to cataract development, outcomes have been inconsistent and subsequently have fallen out of favor compared to other approaches [7].

7.3.2 Modification of Current Biometric Measurements Derived from Regression Formulas for Refractive Changes Induced by LASIK/PRK

7.3.2.1 Modification to Measured Anterior Power of the Cornea

These methods adjust current power of the cornea measurements using regression analysis based on refraction changes induced by refractive surgery. By relying on current corneal data during surgical evaluation, this avoids the errors of relying solely on historical data. However, all these formulas require accurate refraction data prior to cataract development and results vary contingent upon the reliability of those data.

- *Barrett True-K Formula:* True-K is determined by refining measured K-values based on the degree of refractive change induced by previous CRS, which is incorporated into the Barrett Universal formula. Further iterations and its application can be seen in the sections below.

The values generated from the following formulas can be utilized in the ASCRS online IOL power calculator tool for eyes with prior refractive surgery discussed later.

- *Adjusted values taken from the Atlas topographer (Carl Zeiss AG, Oberkochen, Germany):*
  - *Adjusted Atlas Ring Values:* The average value of the 0-, 1-, 2-, and 3-mm annular rings (AnnCP) taken from the Atlas topographer is adjusted by a fraction of the ΔMR.

    Adjusted AnnCP in post*myopic* LASIK/PRK = AnnCP – 0.2 × (ΔMR)
    Adjusted AnnCP in post*hyperopic* LASIK/PRK = AnnCP + 0.191 × (ΔMR) – 0.396
  - *Adjusted Atlas Zone Value:* The 4-mm zone value obtained from the Atlas 9000 topographer is modified by subtracting 0.2 × (ΔMR).
- *Adjusted average central power of the cornea (ACCP) from TMS topographer (Tomey, Nagoya, Japan)*
  - *Adjusted ACCP*: The ACCP from the TMS topographer is the measured power of the cornea within the central 3-mm zone and is adjusted to predict refractive power of the cornea after myopic LASIK: [8]

    Adjusted ACCP in post*myopic* LASIK/PRK = ACCP – 0.16 × (ΔMR)

7.3.2.2 Modification to Calculated IOL Power

- *Masket Formula* [9]: IOL power is adjusted by using IOLMaster's keratometry readings with the SRK/T formula:
  - IOL adjustment = ([ΔMR] × 0.326) + 0.101
- *Modified Masket Formula*: Modification by Hill for IOL adjustment as below (presented at ASCRS 2006):
  - IOL adjustment = ([ΔMR] × 0.4385) + 0.0295

7.3.3 Current Corneal Measurements Only

7.3.3.1 Modification to Measured Anterior Power of the Cornea Based on Regression Formulas

- *Wang-Koch-Maloney:* The Atlas 4-mm zone value obtained from the Atlas topographer is converted to anterior power of the cornea:
  - Adjusted corneal power = (Atlas 4-mm zone × 1.114) − 5.59
- *Shammas Method:* Modifies the postrefractive power of the cornea by adjusting the measured post-LASIK/PRK keratometry readings (Kpost) [10]:
  - Adjusted corneal power = 1.14 × Kpost − 6.8
- *Haigis-L:* The IOL power is determined using the Haigis formula with the corrected corneal radius obtained from data from the IOLMaster input into the regression equation below [11]:
  - Corrected corneal radius = 331.5/(−5.1625 × post-LASIK corneal radius from IOLMaster + 82.2603 – 0.35)
- *Galilei Total Corneal Power (TCP) Method:* The power of the cornea in myopic LASIK eyes is adjusted utilizing a regression equation based on the TCP obtained from the Galilei:
  - Adjusted corneal power in myopic LASIK eyes = 1.057 × TCP – 1.8348

7.3.3.2 Estimation of Posterior Corneal Curvature (PEARL-DGS Formula)

One method to enhance accuracy of IOL calculation is utilizing machine learning models to predict the posterior corneal radius and the theoretical internal lens position. The Postoperative spherical equivalent prediction using ARtificial Intelligence and Linear algorithms by Guillaume Debellemanière, Damien Gatinel, and Alain

Saad (PEARL-DGS) formula is an open-source model based on the thick IOL calculation formulas and can be utilized in either postmyopic/hyperopic laser vision correction (LVC) or post-RK (Radial Keratotomy) eyes [12]. It can be utilized directly on https://iolsolver.com.

7.3.3.3 Directly Measure Anterior and Posterior Corneal Curvature

Scheimpflug imaging devices and OCT systems are the main technologies that allow for anterior and posterior corneal surface measurement, with the Pentacam (Oculus Optikgeräte, Wetzlar, Germany) and Galilei (Ziemer, Biel, Switzerland) Scheimpflug imaging devices showing reliable, reproducible measurements of the posterior cornea [13–15]. The total corneal power (TCP) can then be determined once both the anterior and posterior corneal curvatures are measured using two methods: the Gaussian optics thick lens formula and the ray tracing method [16].

While devices can provide TCP values with measurement of the posterior corneal surface, adjustments are still required to achieve accurate IOL power calculation in eyes with prior CRS. More researches are required to integrate these data to improve accuracy in power of the cornea measurements and develop new calculations in these circumstances.

- *OCT-based IOL power calculation:* OCT is a noncontact and noninvasive imaging technology that is able to measure both anterior and posterior power of the corneas with high axial resolution [17]. The net power of the cornea (NCP) is determined using the RTVue (Optovue Inc, Fremont, CA) and then modified to generate the effective power of the cornea (ECP) for an OCT-based IOL power calculation [18]:
  - ECP in post*myopic* LASIK/PRK = 1.0208 × NCP − 1.6622
  - ECP in post*hyperopic* LASIK/PRK = 1.11 × NCP − 5.736

The OCT-based IOL formula uses five preoperative biometric measurements: AL, anterior chamber depth (ACD), NCP, posterior power of the cornea, and central corneal thickness (CCT) from the OCT, which have been integrated into the American Society of Cataract and Refractive Surgery (ASCRS) postrefractive IOL calculator, detailed below.

- *Emmetropia Verifying Optical (EVO) Formula*: Based on the thick lens formula, the axial length is modified by the measured corneal curvatures, taking into account the optical dimensions of the eye based on the theory of emmetropization [19]. Posterior curvature is obtained from either optical biometry, OCT, or tomographer. This formula can be utilized directly on evoiolcalculator.com for postmyopic LASIK/PRK only, or for postmyopic or hyperopic LASIK/PRK on the European Society of Cataract and Refractive Surgeons (ESCRS) website, as detailed below.

- *Hoffer Q/Giacomo Savini/Leonardo Taroni (Hoffer QST) Formula*: The Hoffer Q formula was modified with artificial intelligence (AI) to generate a nonlinear regression model and to modify AL based on several biometric data, including posterior curvature measurements directly in the Hoffer QST formula [20]. This formula can be utilized for postmyopic LASIK/PRK only and is available to use on hofferqst.com or the ESCRS calculator, as below.

7.4 Tools for IOL Power Calculation

7.4.1 Web-Based Postrefractive IOL Calculator at ASCRS.org

Performing calculations using the various methods discussed in the last section can be complex and time-consuming. To streamline this process, Hill, Wang, and Koch published a web-based or online IOL power calculator in 2007 (www.ascrs.org), which is regularly updated and is utilized over a million times per year. The calculator consists of three modules: (1) prior myopic LASIK/PRK, (2) prior hyperopic LASIK/PRK, and (3) prior refractive keratoRK (https://iolcalc.ascrs.org/). After selecting the type of prior CRS, users can input pre- and post-LASIK/PRK data along with biometric measurements and then click "Calculate" to view the results at the bottom (https://iolcalc.ascrs.org/wbfrmCalculator.aspx). The calculator categorizes some different calculation methods into two groups depending on the availability of historical data: (1) methods using ΔMR and corneal measurements at the time of cataract surgery (shown on the bottom left), and (2) methods using no prior data (shown on the bottom right). The IOL power is determined using the double-K Holladay 1 formula, Shammas-PL, or Haigis-L method. In the double-K Holladay 1 formula, pre-LASIK/PRK keratometry values are utilized to estimate the ELP. If pre-LASIK/PRK keratometry is not available, a value of 43.86 D is utilized. In addition to presenting the average and range of IOL powers from all available methods, the average IOL power is also listed for methods using ΔMR only and methods using no prior data.

In post-RK eyes, unlike eyes that have undergone LASIK/PRK, posterior corneal curvature is also altered, typically increasing the Gullstrand ratio (ratio of the radii of posterior to anterior curvature). Due to the significant variability in the power of the cornea in post-RK eyes, we recommend using an average power of the cornea measurement over the central 2–4 mm. The ASCRS postrefractive surgery calculator allows users to input the average power of the corneas from the Atlas for the 1-, 2-, 3-, and 4-mm annular rings, the Atlas 4-mm zone value, the effective refractive power (EffRP) from the EyeSys, and the TCP from the Galilei. Other topographers that provide the average power of the cornea over the central 2–4 mm may also be suitable. Compensation for potential miscalculation in ELP is still required by utilizing the double-K version of some IOL formulas (the ASCRS online calculator uses the double-K Holladay 1 formula).

7.4.2 Web-Based Postrefractive IOL Calculator at ESCRS.org

Another useful online tool for calculation in post-LASIK/PRK eyes is available on the ESCRS website and can be accessed at iolcalculator.escrs.org [21]. It features an IOL calculator that incorporates advanced formulas such as the Barrett True K, EVO, and Hoffer QST. The Hoffer QST only works for eyes with prior myopic-LASIK/PRK. At the top of the online tool, the user can toggle which calculators they wish to use. Users should select the "Post LASIK/PRK" option, indicate whether the patient previously underwent myopic or hyperopic laser correction, and enter biometric data (https://iolcalculator.escrs.org/). The Barrett, EVO, and Hoffer A-constants will auto-populate after the user inputs the desired IOL implant under the "Manufacturer" and "Select IOL" sections. After clicking on the "Calculate" button, the screen advances to another page with a table summarizing predicted residual spherical equivalents at different IOL powers for each of the formulas (https://iolcalculator.escrs.org/). One limitation of this calculator is that it does not have an option for post-RK eyes.

7.4.3 Barrett True-K and True-K No History Formulas

The Barrett formulas are available through the Post-Refractive IOL Calculator at https://iolcalc.ascrs.org/ or the Asia Pacific Association of Cataract and Refractive Surgery (APACRS) website at https://calc.apacrs.org/TRueKToric105/truektoric.aspx. The No History formula can also be utilized when the value of refractive correction is not ready and available. For IOL power calculation, the Barrett Universal II (BUII) formula is utilized, but details regarding the design of the True-K and BUII formulas are not published [22, 23].

7.4.4 OCT-Based IOL Formula

The OCT-based IOL formula is available for download at www.coollab.net. It is also integrated into the ASCRS IOL calculator, allowing users to conduct and review all of their calculations on a single platform.

7.5 Intraoperative Measurements

Intraoperative refractive biometry (IRB) describes the process of performing aphakic retinoscopy in the operating room after cataract extraction to calculate IOL power [24]. The Optiwave Refractive Analysis (ORA) System (WaveTec Vision,

Aliso Viejo, CA) uses the aphakic spherical equivalent and preoperative AL and Ks to predict the ELP and calculate the IOL power. Note that the ELP from this system is an estimate, and therefore prone to errors introduced by variables such as intraocular pressure, patient fixation, and surface/corneal factors.

7.6 Comparative Data for the Modern Formulas Incorporating Intraoperative Measurements

Key findings across a number of studies comparing various formulas and approaches to postrefractive IOL calculations are summarized below:

- Wang et al. presented higher IOL predictive accuracy in No History methods in comparison with methods requiring pre-refractive data [7].
- For postmyopic refractive patients, a large meta-analysis demonstrated higher predictive accuracy when utilizing the ASCRS average compared to Shammas-PL, Haigis-L, and Wang-Koch-Maloney [25]. The OCT-based IOL formula has also been revealed to produce equal or even higher predictive accuracy than the Shammas, Haigis-L, and Wang-Koch-Maloney formulas in postmyopic eyes [25–29].
- For posthyperopic refractive patients, two small-sample studies discovered no significant difference in mean absolute IOL prediction errors for the formulas compared [30, 31]. Studies looking at outcomes in this patient population are currently limited, and currently the data suggest that the currently available tools are comparable.
- Post-RK eyes pose a unique challenge due to variability in anterior and posterior corneal curvature. The literature recommends setting a target of −0.75 to −1.00 in IOL power calculations in these eyes, given the gradual hyperopic shift that occurs in 20% to 50% of RK eyes [32–34].
- When compared to several other formulas, the Barrett True-K formula resulted in a smaller median absolute refraction prediction error and a larger proportion of eyes within ±0.50 D of predicted error [25, 35].
- A modified version of the OCT-based IOL formula has been presented to reduce hyperopic surprises in post-RK eyes [36].
- Ianchulev et al. demonstrated greater predictive accuracy of the ORA when compared with the Shammas and Haigis-L methods [37]. Another smaller study demonstrated no significant difference between OCT, ORA, and Haigis-L, lending additional support to newer methods of ORA and OCT [38].
- Kenny et al. found that newer formulas using both anterior and posterior corneal measurements, such as the Barrett True-K TK and EVO formulas, demonstrated comparable performance to existing formulas, such as the Haigis-L, Shammas, and Barrett True-K No History in eyes with prior myopic LVC [39].

7.7 Premium IOL Use in Postrefractive Patients

Global adoption of presbyopia-correcting lenses such as bifocal, trifocal, and extended depth of focus (EDOF) IOLs is on the rise. For many patients seeking independence from glasses, these IOLs offer a promising alternative. However, refractive accuracy and overall vision quality represent important limitations. Patients with these IOLs may frequently experience glare, halos, spiderwebs, and starbursts, as well as a decline in contrast sensitivity. There is currently a paucity of data looking at multifocal IOLs in postrefractive patients. Several authors have previously reported success rates ranging from 47.6% to 100% in post-CRS eyes using the Barrett True-K No History formula (defined as a final refraction within 0.5D of target refraction) [40–43]. However, additional work is needed to characterize corneal higher-order aberrations and visual outcomes with premium IOLs in order to help guide patient selection and expectation setting.

7.7.1 Postoperative IOL Adjustment

One category of premium lens that bears particular promise in the field of post-CRS IOL calculations is the light-adjustable lens (LAL; RxSight, Inc, Aliso Viejo, CA). This lens allows residual spherical and cylindrical errors to be adjusted after the postoperative refraction has stabilized, rendering it particularly useful in patients with a history of refractive surgery, where IOL calculations are often less predictable. The lens is composed of photosensitive silicone macromers that can be selectively polymerized using ultraviolet light from the light delivery device to reshape the optic (LDD (light delivery device); RxSight, Inc, Aliso Viejo, CA). According to the label by the United States Food and Drug Administration (US FDA), the IOL has a dioptric range from 10.0 to 30.0 diopters and can be utilized to make spherical adjustments in 0.25 diopter (D)increments up to ±2.0 D and cylindrical adjustments anywhere from −0.5 D to −3.0 D. The lens can undergo up to three adjustments and up to two lockins. In clinical practice, the first treatment is typically performed ≥3 weeks post surgery (8 weeks in eyes with prior RK), and additional treatments or lockins are performed on a weekly basis thereafter (every 2 weeks in eyes with prior RK).

There is a growing body of evidence to suggest that LAL technology may be beneficial in postrefractive surgery patients. Brierley analyzed whether postoperative refractive power correction of a LAL improves refractive outcomes in patients who have been subjected to prior LASIK or PRK [44]. In 34 eyes of 21 patients with a history of myopic CRS, the final manifest refraction spherical equivalent relative to target refraction was within ±0.25 D in 74% of eyes, within ±0.50 D in 97% of eyes, and within ±1.00 D in 100% of eyes. Mean absolute error (MAE) was 0.19 D ± 0.20 D. In a separate analysis looking at 12-month outcomes, Moshirfar et al. reported an uncorrected distance visual acuity (UDVA) of 20/25 or better in 53% of eyes with prior CRS [45]. In an analysis of our in-house data, which expands on early results previously reported by Kozhaya et al., refractive outcomes with second-generation LAL (equipped with enhanced ultraviolet (UV) absorbers) in patients with a history of RK, myopic LASIK/PRK, or no prior CRS were compared to target refractions [46]. This analysis showed that second-generation LAL achieved final postoperative refractions within ±0.25 D of target refraction in 60% and ±0.5 D in 93% of post-LASIK/PRK eyes ($n = 57$). These findings closely approximated refractive correction accuracy using second-generation LAL in normal eyes without a history of CRS (64% and 96%, respectively; $n = 28$). Meanwhile, in post-RK eyes, 52% achieved a final postoperative refraction within ±0.25 D of target, and 84% were within ±0.5 D. These data suggest that the LAL may help reduce reliance on preoperative IOL power calculations and increase postsurgical refractive precision.

While IOL exchange is certainly another approved option for postoperative adjustment, the appeal of the LAL lies in its easy adjustability. Other intraocular lens (IOL) technologies that are not yet FDA approved, such as the Juvene fluid-filled accommodating IOL (Juvene; LensGen, Irvine, CA) and the OmniVu modular shape-changing lens system (OmniVu; Atia Vision, Campbell, CA), similarly aim to achieve the "holy grail" in our field—namely, providing adjustable and easily exchangeable IOLs that can adapt to patients' changing visual needs, correct residual higher order aberrations, and compensate for aging corneal changes [47]. Nguyen et al. are also exploring the use of femtosecond (femto) laser technology for in vivo IOL power adjustments, which may enable noninvasive addition or removal of toricity or multifocality to IOLs [48]. However, the long-term effectiveness of these new advances remains to be seen.

7.8 Conclusion

While the accuracy of IOL power calculations in eyes with prior CRS has significantly improved in the past few years, refractive surprises still manifest, particularly in eyes with radial keratotomy. In modern practice, multiple formulas are utilized, with greater reliance on those incorporating current data, such as corneal topography/tomography. Fortunately, formula development is constantly ongoing, and new models are being developed. We ultimately recommend a cautious approach that employs multiple IOL calculation methods, particularly newer formulas like the Barrett and EVO, and bases power selection on the consensus among them (Table 7.2) [2, 3, 49]. At present, the most accurate results appear to be a combination of modern postrefractive formulas and postoperative adjustments with LAL, but this approach has obvious limitations, including limited lens and patient selection. More work is needed in the measurement of the power of the cornea, predicting ELP, and calculating the IOL power.

Table 7.2 Authors' strategy for IOL power calculation in eyes following CRS

Preoperative measurements	OCT scans Galilei measurement IOLMaster Lenstar
Patient consultation	Warn patients of IOL power calculation inaccuracy and possible additional surgery, with its associated cost
IOL power calculation	Enter all available data and run IOL calculator at ASCRS, which includes OCT-based IOL power and Barrett True-K formulas
IOL power selection	Rely more on methods that use current data from ASCRS IOL calculator Select the IOL power based on the consensus of multiple methods from ASCRS calculator
Postoperative IOL adjustment	If utilizing LAL lens, adjust power of lens to desired refraction and lock in configuration once desired refraction is reached

References

1. Koch DD, Liu JF, Hyde LL, Rock RL, Emery JM. Refractive complications of cataract surgery after radial keratotomy. Am J Ophthalmol. 1989;108(6):676–82. https://doi.org/10.1016/0002-9394(89)90860-x.
2. Koch DD, Wang L. Calculating IOL power in eyes that have had refractive surgery. J Cataract Refract Surg. 2003;29(11):2039–42. https://doi.org/10.1016/j.jcrs.2003.10.009.
3. Koch DD, Wang L, Booth M. Intraocular lens calculations after LASIK. In: LASIK-advances, controversies and custom. Slack Inc; 2004. p. 259–67.
4. Holladay J. Consultations in refractive surgery. Refract Corneal Surg. 1989;5(3):202–3.
5. Feiz V, Mannis MJ, Garcia-Ferrer F, et al. Intraocular lens power calculation after laser in situ keratomileusis for myopia and hyperopia: a standardized approach. Cornea. 2001;20(8):792–7. https://doi.org/10.1097/00003226-200111000-00003.
6. Walter KA, Gagnon MR, Hoopes PC, Dickinson PJ. Accurate intraocular lens power calculation after myopic laser in situ keratomileusis, bypassing power of the cornea. J Cataract Refract Surg. 2006;32(3):425–9. https://doi.org/10.1016/j.jcrs.2005.12.140.
7. Wang L, Hill WE, Koch DD. Evaluation of intraocular lens power prediction methods using the American Society of Cataract and Refractive Surgeons Post-Keratorefractive Intraocular Lens Power Calculator. J Cataract Refract Surg. 2010;36(9):1466–73. https://doi.org/10.1016/j.jcrs.2010.03.044.
8. Awwad ST, Manasseh C, Bowman RW, et al. Intraocular lens power calculation after myopic laser in situ keratomileusis: estimating the corneal refractive power. J Cataract Refract Surg. 2008;34(7):1070–6. https://doi.org/10.1016/j.jcrs.2008.03.020.
9. Masket S, Masket SE. Simple regression formula for intraocular lens power adjustment in eyes requiring cataract surgery after excimer laser photoablation. J Cataract Refract Surg. 2006;32(3):430–4. https://doi.org/10.1016/j.jcrs.2005.12.106.
10. Shammas HJ, Shammas MC, Garabet A, Kim JH, Shammas A, LaBree L. Correcting the power of the cornea measurements for intraocular lens power calculations after myopic laser in situ keratomileusis. Am J Ophthalmol. 2003;136(3):426–32. https://doi.org/10.1016/s0002-9394(03)00275-7.
11. Haigis W. Intraocular lens calculation after refractive surgery for myopia: Haigis-L formula. J Cataract Refract Surg. 2008;34(10):1658–63. https://doi.org/10.1016/j.jcrs.2008.06.029.
12. Debellemanière G, Dubois M, Gauvin M, et al. The PEARL-DGS formula: the development of an open-source machine learning–based thick IOL calculation formula. Am J Ophthalmol. 2021;232:58–69. https://doi.org/10.1016/j.ajo.2021.05.004.

13. Wang L, Shirayama M, Koch DD. Repeatability of power of the cornea and wavefront aberration measurements with a dual-Scheimpflug Placido corneal topographer. J Cataract Refract Surg. 2010;36(3):425–30. https://doi.org/10.1016/j.jcrs.2009.09.034.
14. Ciolino JB, Belin MW. Changes in the posterior cornea after laser in situ keratomileusis and photorefractive keratectomy. J Cataract Refract Surg. 2006;32(9):1426–31. https://doi.org/10.1016/j.jcrs.2006.03.037.
15. Jain R, Dilraj G, Grewal SPS. Repeatability of corneal parameters with Pentacam after laser in situ keratomileusis. Indian J Ophthalmol. 2007;55(5):341.
16. Wang L, Mahmoud AM, Anderson BL, Koch DD, Roberts CJ. Total corneal power estimation: ray tracing method versus gaussian optics formula. Invest Ophthalmol Vis Sci. 2011;52(3):1716–22. https://doi.org/10.1167/iovs.09-4982.
17. Khurana RN, Li Y, Tang M, Lai MM, Huang D. High-speed optical coherence tomography of corneal opacities. Ophthalmology. 2007;114(7):1278–85. https://doi.org/10.1016/j.ophtha.2006.10.033.
18. Tang M, Li Y, Huang D. An intraocular Lens power calculation formula based on optical coherence tomography: a pilot study. J Refract Surg Thorofare NJ 1995. 2010;26(6):430–7. https://doi.org/10.3928/1081597X-20090710-02.
19. EVO Formula. Accessed 17 Mar 2025. https://www.evoiolcalculator.com/.
20. Hoffer KJ. Hoffer formulas. In: Aramberri J, Hoffer KJ, Olsen T, Savini G, Shammas HJ, editors. Intraocular lens calculations. Springer International Publishing; 2024. p. 649–60. https://doi.org/10.1007/978-3-031-50666-6_43.
21. IOL Calculator. Accessed 17 Mar 2025. https://iolcalculator.escrs.org/.
22. Barrett GD. Intraocular lens calculation formulas for new intraocular lens implants. J Cataract Refract Surg. 1987;13(4):389–96. https://doi.org/10.1016/s0886-3350(87)80037-8.
23. Barrett GD. An improved universal theoretical formula for intraocular lens power prediction. J Cataract Refract Surg. 1993;19(6):713–20. https://doi.org/10.1016/s0886-3350(13)80339-2.
24. Ianchulev T, Salz J, Hoffer K, Albini T, Hsu H, Labree L. Intraoperative optical refractive biometry for intraocular lens power estimation without axial length and keratometry measurements. J Cataract Refract Surg. 2005;31(8):1530–6. https://doi.org/10.1016/j.jcrs.2005.01.035.
25. Li H, Nan L, Li J, Song H. Accuracy of intraocular lens power calculation formulae after laser refractive surgery in myopic eyes: a meta-analysis. Eye Vis. 2020;7:37. https://doi.org/10.1186/s40662-020-00188-1.
26. Tang M, Chen A, Li Y, Huang D. Power of the cornea measurement with Fourier-domain optical coherence tomography. J Cataract Refract Surg. 2010;36(12):2115–22. https://doi.org/10.1016/j.jcrs.2010.07.018.
27. Tang M, Wang L, Koch DD, Li Y, Huang D. Intraocular lens power calculation after previous myopic laser vision correction based on power of the cornea measured by Fourier-domain optical coherence tomography. J Cataract Refract Surg. 2012;38(4):589–94. https://doi.org/10.1016/j.jcrs.2011.11.025.
28. Huang D, Tang M, Wang L, et al. Optical coherence tomography-based power of the cornea measurement and intraocular lens power calculation following laser vision correction (an American Ophthalmological Society thesis). Trans Am Ophthalmol Soc. 2013;111:34–45.
29. Wang L, Tang M, Huang D, Weikert MP, Koch DD. Comparison of newer intraocular lens power calculation methods for eyes after corneal refractive surgery. Ophthalmology. 2015;122(12):2443–9. https://doi.org/10.1016/j.ophtha.2015.08.037.
30. Hamill EB, Wang L, Chopra HK, Hill W, Koch DD. Intraocular lens power calculations in eyes with previous hyperopic laser in situ keratomileusis or photorefractive keratectomy. J Cataract Refract Surg. 2017;43(2):189–94. https://doi.org/10.1016/j.jcrs.2016.11.041.
31. Francone A, Lemanski N, Charles M, et al. Retrospective comparative analysis of intraocular lens calculation formulas after hyperopic refractive surgery. PLoS One. 2019;14(11):e0224981. https://doi.org/10.1371/journal.pone.0224981.

32. Arrowsmith PN, Marks RG. Visual, refractive, and keratometric results of radial keratotomy. Five-year follow-up. Arch Ophthalmol Chic Ill 1960. 1989;107(4):506–11. https://doi.org/10.1001/archopht.1989.01070010520023.
33. Deitz MR, Sanders DR, Raanan MG, DeLuca M. Long-term (5- to 12-year) follow-up of metal-blade radial keratotomy procedures. Arch Ophthalmol Chic Ill 1960. 1994;112(5):614–20. https://doi.org/10.1001/archopht.1994.01090170058022.
34. Waring GO, Lynn MJ, Gelender H, et al. Results of the prospective evaluation of radial keratotomy (PERK) study one year after surgery. Ophthalmology. 1985;92(2):177–98, 307. https://doi.org/10.1016/s0161-6420(85)34054-x.
35. Abulafia A, Hill WE, Koch DD, Wang L, Barrett GD. Accuracy of the Barrett true-K formula for intraocular lens power prediction after laser in situ keratomileusis or photorefractive keratectomy for myopia. J Cataract Refract Surg. 2016;42(3):363–9. https://doi.org/10.1016/j.jcrs.2015.11.039.
36. Waisbren E, Wang L, Weikert MP, Koch DD. Using optical coherence tomography for IOL power calculations in eyes with prior ablative corneal surgery. In: Bissen-Miyajima H, Koch DD, Weikert MP, editors. Cataract surgery: maximizing outcomes through research. Springer Japan; 2014. p. 47–57. https://doi.org/10.1007/978-4-431-54538-5_5.
37. Ianchulev T, Hoffer KJ, Yoo SH, et al. Intraoperative refractive biometry for predicting intraocular lens power calculation after prior myopic refractive surgery. Ophthalmology. 2014;121(1):56–60. https://doi.org/10.1016/j.ophtha.2013.08.041.
38. Fram NR, Masket S, Wang L. Comparison of intraoperative aberrometry, OCT-based IOL formula, Haigis-L, and Masket formulae for IOL power calculation after laser vision correction. Ophthalmology. 2015;122(6):1096–101. https://doi.org/10.1016/j.ophtha.2015.01.027.
39. Kenny PI, Kozhaya K, Truong P, Wang L, Koch DD, Weikert MP. Performance of IOL calculation formulas that use measured posterior power of the cornea in eyes following myopic laser vision correction. J Cataract Refract Surg. 2024;50(1):7. https://doi.org/10.1097/j.jcrs.0000000000001300.
40. Fisher B, Potvin R. Clinical outcomes with distance-dominant multifocal and monofocal intraocular lenses in post-LASIK cataract surgery planned using an intraoperative aberrometer. Clin Experiment Ophthalmol. 2018;46(6):630–6. https://doi.org/10.1111/ceo.13153.
41. Vrijman V, Abulafia A, van der Linden JW, van der Meulen IJE, Mourits MP, Lapid-Gortzak R. Evaluation of different IOL calculation formulas of the ASCRS calculator in eyes after corneal refractive laser surgery for myopia with multifocal IOL implantation. J Refract Surg Thorofare NJ 1995. 2019;35(1):54–9. https://doi.org/10.3928/1081597X-20181119-01.
42. Palomino-Bautista C, Carmona-González D, Sánchez-Jean R, et al. Refractive predictability and visual outcomes of an extended range of vision intraocular lens in eyes with previous myopic laser in situ keratomileusis. Eur J Ophthalmol. 2019;29(6):593–9. https://doi.org/10.1177/1120672118804950.
43. Li QM, Wang F, Wu ZM, et al. Trifocal diffractive intraocular lens implantation in patients after previous corneal refractive laser surgery for myopia. BMC Ophthalmol. 2020;20(1):293. https://doi.org/10.1186/s12886-020-01556-0.
44. Brierley L. Refractive results after implantation of a light-adjustable intraocular lens in postrefractive surgery cataract patients. Ophthalmology. 2013;120(10):1968–72. https://doi.org/10.1016/j.ophtha.2013.03.010.
45. Moshirfar M, Henrie MK, Payne CJ, Hansen AM, Ronquillo YC, Hoopes PC. Comparing visual outcomes of light adjustable intraocular lenses in patients with and without prior history of corneal refractive surgery. J Refract Surg Thorofare NJ 1995. 2023;39(5):311–8. https://doi.org/10.3928/1081597X-20230222-01.
46. Kozhaya K, Wang L, Weikert MP, Koch DD. Early outcomes of second-generation light-adjustable lenses in eyes with and without corneal refractive surgery. J Cataract Refract Surg. 2023;49(11):1180. https://doi.org/10.1097/j.jcrs.0000000000001282.

47. Kennedy S, Werner L, Bontu S, et al. Explantation/exchange of the components of a new fluid-filled, modular, accommodating IOL. J Cataract Refract Surg. 2021;47(2):238–44. https://doi.org/10.1097/j.jcrs.0000000000000367.
48. Nguyen J, Werner L, Ludlow J, et al. Intraocular lens power adjustment by a femtosecond laser: in vitro evaluation of power change, modulation transfer function, light transmission, and light scattering in a blue light-filtering lens. J Cataract Refract Surg. 2018;44(2):226–30. https://doi.org/10.1016/j.jcrs.2017.09.036.
49. Randleman JB, Foster JB, Loupe DN, Song CD, Stulting RD. Intraocular lens power calculations after refractive surgery: consensus-K technique. J Cataract Refract Surg. 2007;33(11):1892–8. https://doi.org/10.1016/j.jcrs.2007.06.045.

Chapter 8
Optimizing IOL Power Calculation in Glaucoma: Challenges and Strategies for Precision Surgery

Emma Rusmayani

8.1 Introduction

Cataract surgery is one of the most frequently performed eye surgeries and of the various methods of surgical approaches in glaucoma patients with cataracts, particularly those diagnosed with lens-induced glaucoma or primary angle-closure glaucoma. Cataract surgery in glaucoma patients enhances visual acuity and reduces intraocular pressure (IOP), whether performed independently or in conjunction with glaucoma surgeries like trabeculectomy or microinvasive glaucoma surgeries (MIGS) [1, 2].

The management of glaucoma patients undergoing cataract surgery involves an intricate relationship between surgical treatments and the preexisting risks associated with both conditions. Difficulties arising from intraocular lens (IOL) implantation and calculation of power, as it demands a comprehensive evaluation relating to anatomical and physiological dynamics seen in glaucoma. Implementation of meticulous preoperative planning, careful intraoperative procedures, and vigilant postoperative monitoring can lead to optimized surgical outcomes and better quality of life for glaucoma patients undergoing cataract surgery. This article addresses the specific challenges related to IOL calculation in glaucoma patients undergoing cataract surgery, conveying anatomical changes, corneal biomechanics, intraocular spikes, and the long-term effects due to chronic use of antiglaucoma medications. Practical recommendations for optimizing biometry, selecting suitable formulas, and management of complex cases, including pseudoexfoliation syndrome, are presented, supported by current literatures.

Author declares no financial interest and the table belongs to the author.

E. Rusmayani (✉)
JEC Eye Hospitals & Clinics, Jakarta, Indonesia

G. Pardianto (ed.), *Intraocular Lens (IOL) Power Calculation*,
https://doi.org/10.1007/978-981-92-1223-1_8

8.2 Factors Affecting IOL Calculation in Glaucoma Patients

8.2.1 Axial Length (AL) Variability

Glaucoma patients, especially those with pseudoexfoliation (PEX) and angle-closure subtypes, often exhibit different AL due to anatomical changes caused by raised IOP [3]. Differences in AL also have implications for the formulas used. Formulas such as the Sanders-Retzlaff-Kraff/Theoretical (SRK/T) and Haigis formulas consider AL differently, which may provide varying refractive predictions between formulas [4]. AL relating to anatomical changes and formulas used for calculation must be carefully thought of, as these factors can lead to significant discrepancies between calculated and required lens power.

Accurate measurements of AL are an important element of precise IOL power calculation. Inaccurate measurement can cause significant differences between calculated and actual required lens power, leading to poor refractive outcomes. One study noted that an increase of 1 millimeter (mm) measured AL can produce different results in calculated lens power as much as 2.5 diopters (D) [5]. Traditional measurement techniques may be insufficient to produce accurate results in AL measurements and can lead to poor refractive outcomes. Studies have demonstrated that 54% of errors in refractive outcomes are related to inaccuracies in AL measurements [6]. Newer technologies, such as swept-source optical coherence tomography (SS-OCT) and partial coherence interferometry (PCI), may provide better AL accuracy compared to older measurement techniques [7].

8.2.2 Corneal Biomechanics and Keratometry

Patients with glaucoma often exhibit changes in corneal biomechanics, including stiffness, elasticity, and viscoelasticity. These changes can be attributed to the IOP fluctuations, long-term use of glaucoma medication, and age-related changes [8–10]. These alterations may cause measurement inaccuracies in keratometry, leading to refractive errors in glaucoma patients undergoing cataract surgeries. A comprehensive and more thorough assessment of corneal biomechanical parameters in keratometry measurements is highly essential in glaucoma patients, compared to healthy patients, to ensure accurate IOL outcomes. The European Society of Cataract and Refractive Surgeons (ESCRS) Guideline for cataract surgery recommends devices such as IOL master 700 (Carl Zeiss Meditec, Dublin, CA) and Lenstar LS900 (Haag-Streit, Köniz, Switzerland) for a more accurate keratometric reading in patients exhibiting corneal irregularities (edema and scarring) and patients with prior trabeculectomy as it can avoid corneal indentation errors from contact ultrasound. Furthermore, various keratometric algorithms have been developed to provide better IOL calculations in patients with diverse clinical conditions [11, 12].

8.2.3 Effects of IOP Changes

Fluctuation in IOP has a great influence on IOL implantation and power calculations for glaucoma patients undergoing cataract surgery. Prolonged elevation of IOP causes changes in the corneal structure, such as increased stiffness and reduced corneal hysteresis (CH), and overall decrease in biomechanical stability [13]. Corneal changes related to pressure dynamics cause inaccuracy in keratometric measurements that could translate into poor postoperative visual outcomes. Following cataract surgery, a decrease in IOP was observed alongside a deepened anterior chamber depth (ACD). This alteration affected the effective lens position (ELP) and subsequently influenced IOL power. Multiple studies reported a positive correlation between reduced postop IOP and IOL power, demonstrating that a decrease of IOP more than 10 mmHg is seen with an increase of IOL power by approximately 0.5 diopters [14]. This correlation may suggest that preoperative IOL calculation may not be accurate to facilitate for postoperative anatomical changes. In addition, IOL implantation exhibits a risk of pressure-related complications such as pupillary block or aqueous misdirection that can lead to secondary glaucoma. These potential complications must be carefully considered in preoperative planning, as they necessitate adjustments to IOL power calculation due to possible changes in fluid dynamics after surgery and require vigilant monitoring during postoperative follow-ups [15, 16].

8.2.4 Types and Position of IOL

The choice of IOL types has an influence on IOL calculation and implantation in glaucoma patients with cataract. Various designs, such as toric, spherical, aspheric, and premium lenses, have different implications on visual acuity, and the process of selection requires great attention to accommodate for various clinical characteristics often associated with glaucoma [17]. Lens positioning also has an impact on postoperative visual outcomes. Posterior lenses typically lead to better outcomes compared to anterior chamber lenses due to the higher risk of increased postoperative IOP associated with anterior chamber lenses [18]. Pressure-related complications may occur due to interactions between lens configuration and the type of preexisting glaucoma. Different types of lenses provide varying benefits; however, they may complicate postoperative IOP management, especially in patients with narrow angles or advanced glaucoma. Therefore, the selection of lens types in glaucoma patients is limited and requires careful consideration, as they can significantly influence both visual acuity and IOP after surgery. Long-term monitoring of glaucoma patients after cataract surgery is highly crucial, especially with lens types that may increase the risk of glaucoma progression [19].

8.2.5 Long-Term Use of Antiglaucoma Medications and Previous Filtering Surgery

In glaucoma patients undergoing cataract surgery, it is important to consider the effects of long-term use of glaucoma medications on the IOL power calculation indirectly. Patients prescribed with prostaglandin analogs, including latanoprost and bimatoprost, may have a notable reduction in central corneal thickness (CCT). Changes in the CCT may result in inaccurate measurements, leading to subsequent errors in IOL power calculations. Individuals on prostaglandin analogs often demonstrate reduced corneal hysteresis, making devices such as Corvis ST (Oculus Optikgeräte, Wetzlar, Germany), or Ocular Response Analyzer (ORA) System (WaveTec Vision, Aliso Viejo, CA) essential for corneal biomechanical assessment. Moreover, prostaglandin analogs induce an inflammatory response that impacts corneal clarity, thereby indirectly influencing IOL calculation even further [20, 21]. Another medication of interest is acetazolamide, influencing IOL power calculation through its effects on aqueous humor dynamics. Acute administration of acetazolamide induces a diuretic effect that causes temporary shifts in intraocular components, affecting ACD and potentially leading to different results in AL measurements for IOL implantation [22]. Patients' histories of previous filtering surgeries, such as trabeculectomy or tube shunt surgery, must also be taken into account, as these surgeries cause postsurgical changes in ocular dimensions [23]. In conclusion, long-term use of antiglaucoma medications and a previous history of filtering surgery induce changes in ACD and AL. Considerations for these biometric changes are crucial in order to optimize visual outcomes in glaucoma patients undergoing cataract surgery.

8.3 Optimizing IOL Calculation in Glaucoma Patients

8.3.1 Choosing Appropriate Biometry Method

The selection of the appropriate biometry method is essential for optimizing IOL calculations in patients with glaucoma. Unique ocular characteristics in glaucoma necessitate careful considerations in selecting biometry techniques, as it can significantly affect IOL implantation. Optical biometry is generally preferred in today's modern-day approach, as it has been shown to produce more precise measurements compared to traditional ultrasound techniques, especially when considering crucial parameters such as AL and corneal power. However, in specific cases, such as patients with dense media opacities, the application of optical methods may be challenging to perform; therefore, immersion ultrasound biometry can serve as an alternative [8, 24, 25].

Table 8.1 Recommendation of IOL power calculation formula based on AL and anterior segment anatomy

Formulas	Short AL approach	Long AL approach
SRK/T	Not used in short AL	Wang-Koh AL adjustment
Holladay 1	Optimized lens constant	Wang-Koh AL adjustment
Hoffer Q	Optimized lens constant	Typically not used in Long AL
Holladay 2	Optimized lens constant	Holladay 2 AL adjustment
Haigis	Optimized a0, a1, a2	Optimized a0, a1, a2 and Wang-Koh AL adjustment
Olsen		Requires LT and ACD

8.3.2 *Selecting the Suitable IOL Formula*

Formulas used to calculate IOL power must account for the unique glaucoma ocular characteristics in AL, ACD, and angle, as well as the form and severity of glaucoma [26]. Among the available IOL calculation formulas, the Haigis, SRK/T, and Barrett Universal II (BUII) formulas have proven effective in glaucoma patients. According to the 2023 ESCRS Guideline for cataract surgery, eyes with atypical anterior segment anatomy would benefit from formulas such as the BUII. In contrast, the SRK/T is commonly used for patients with normal anterior segment anatomy but tends to be less accurate in patients with significant ACD variation. The Haigis Formula is advised for eyes with prior glaucoma surgeries, including trabeculectomy and tube shunts, due to its reliance on ACDs and lack of corneal curvature assumptions. In addition to considering anterior segment anatomy, it is also crucial to account for the variability of AL when selecting IOL formula for glaucoma patients. Adjustments are required for the Holladay I and II, Haigis, and SRK/T formula when managing glaucoma patients with high to extreme axial myope and AL greater than 25.00 mm [27–29]. IOL power calculation formula can be considered and selected based on AL and anterior segment anatomy (Table 8.1) [30].

8.3.3 *Intraoperative Considerations*

Cataract surgery in patients with glaucoma requires thorough preoperative planning and careful intraoperative execution, especially regarding the accurate placement of the IOL. These precautions are highly necessary to reduce potential complications such as posterior capsule opacification and secondary glaucoma that could occur due to incorrect lens placement [31]. Furthermore, combining cataract surgery with procedures such as goniosynechialysis can help mitigate risks of postoperative IOP spikes and improve overall surgical and visual outcomes in difficult cases, such as angle-closure glaucoma [32].

8.3.4 Accounting for Postoperative Anterior Chamber Changes

Post implantation of IOL in glaucoma patients, major changes are expected in the anterior chamber, including depth, angle of anterior chamber, and IOP. Studies have reported that cataract extraction generally results in a deepened ACD, especially in patients diagnosed with primary angle-closure glaucoma [33]. Changes in anterior chamber angle can also be expected; one study noted a potential increase of as much as 10° postoperatively [34]. Anticipating these changes and adjusting IOL power calculations to account for potential hyperopic and myopic shifts can provide benefits of improving visual acuity.

8.3.5 Special Considerations: PEX

IOL implantation in patients exhibiting PEX requires careful selection of appropriate IOL formulas as individuals with PEX may have higher mean absolute errors, and traditional formulas may not accurately predict the ELP. Studies suggest that employing advanced formulas, such as the Barrett or the Holladay 2 formula, may offer better predictive accuracy in this population [35]. Consideration regarding surgical techniques is essential to accommodate potential anatomical challenges. In PEX cases where standard IOL implantation is deemed challenging due to zonular instability, alternative fixation techniques, such as scleral-fixated IOLs, or the use of capsular tension rings may be employed to facilitate stability and minimize the risk of displacement [36]. In addition, patients with PEX often require a combined approach, such as phacotrabeculectomy, to treat both cataracts and the underlying glaucoma, which has been proven to effectively control pressure and restore vision. Careful postoperative monitoring is also highly crucial due to increased risk of post-surgical complications, including high IOP, inflammation, and lens displacement. Regular follow-ups and prescription of anti-inflammatory medications can be employed to minimize these risks [37, 38].

8.3.6 Special Considerations: Uveitic and Neovascular Glaucoma (NVG)

Uveitis-induced Inflammation and retinal ischemia seen in neovascular glaucoma may result in alterations within the corneal shape and ACD, resulting in a significant impact On AL measurements and keratometry readings, which are essential for precise IOL power calculations. These conditions can also result in anterior segment complications, such as synechiae, which may impact the mobility and positioning of the IOL. The compromised position of the IOL may result in additional refractive errors, as the power of the IOL is greatly influenced by its relative position to the retina. Challenges also arise due to limited availability of the formulas that can be used. Traditional formulas such as SRK/T or Hoffer Q may not be able to provide accurate results if not adjusted for the anatomical changes [39].

Uveitic and neovascular glaucoma pose challenges for cataract surgeries; however, various strategies can be implemented to ensure success. Maintaining a stable ocular environment through inflammation control is a vital requirement for uveitic patients undergoing cataract surgery. This is achieved via the administration of anti-inflammatory medications, particularly corticosteroids, for a minimum of 3 months before surgery [40]. For NVG, patients must be assessed for retinal health and the degree of ischemia and neovascularization prior to surgery. Imaging modalities such as optical coherence tomography and fluorescein angiography can provide valuable insights regarding the retinal status. Full attention must also be directed to the type of IOL given. Uveitic patients may benefit more from the use of hydrophilic acrylic lenses, as these lenses present a reduced risk of causing postoperative inflammation in comparison to hydrophobic lenses. The IOL provided must closely match the length and the anatomical profile of the patient's eye to minimize potential physical interaction with the iris and surrounding structures, thereby reducing the risk of subsequent inflammation. The surgical technique utilized must be precise, minimizing ocular trauma [39]. Postoperatively, careful monitoring is essential, with particular attention to IOP spikes and signs of complications. In summary, managing inflammation, recognizing preexisting pathological changes, meticulous surgical planning, and monitoring of possible postoperative complications are crucial for uveitic and neovascular glaucoma patients undergoing cataract surgery.

8.3.7 Special Considerations: Pediatric Glaucoma

Pediatric cataract patients with concurrent glaucoma frequently exhibit altered ocular anatomy, such as buphthalmos, resulting in enlarged ocular dimensions and changes in corneal curvature. These changes affect AL measurements, resulting in inaccuracies in IOL power calculations and subsequent postoperative refractive errors [41]. Several studies have reported significant improvements in accuracy with the use of Holladay II formula for buphthalmic eyes, with adjustments made for altered ACD and posterior corneal curvature for better estimates of ELP [42]. Progressive axial elongation is frequently observed in individuals with congenital glaucoma, making frequent and comprehensive assessment of AL necessary. In addition, biometric measurements should be conducted immediately prior to surgery to ensure a measurement that accurately represents the current profile of the eye. The Implementation of advanced measurement techniques, such as swept-source optical coherence tomography, greatly enhances accuracy in measuring AL, corneal topography, and ACD [43].

Special care must also be taken during selection of IOL types for pediatric patients, especially regarding stability. Single-piece IOLs are recommended for their superior stability, particularly in pediatric patients undergoing surgery at a young age. Hydrogel or acrylic IOLs are also generally preferred for children due to their superior biocompatibility, allowing for reduced risk of immune rejection [44]. In buphthalmic eyes, posterior chamber fixation for the IOL would be beneficial as other fixation methods have been associated with a higher tendency for decentration and tilt [45].

8.3.8 Special Considerations: Postfiltering Surgery

Cataract surgery in glaucoma patients with a previous history of filtering surgeries, such as trabeculectomy, necessitates careful considerations for accurate IOL calculations. It is well advised to wait 2 to 3 months after trabeculectomy before calculating IOL power calculations. The rationale for this time frame is to allow stabilization of IOP and ACD, which may have been altered and still undergoing changes due to the filtering surgery [34]. Anatomical changes must also be taken into account during the calculation as they can directly affect the ELP and the subsequent refractive outcomes. Ignoring the biomechanical changes commonly seen after filtering surgeries can lead to increased incidence of refractive surprises postoperatively, including hyperopic and myopic errors [34].

8.4 Employment of Artificial Intelligence for IOL Formula

Newer studies demonstrated potential benefits of using the newer generation of IOL formulas that incorporate artificial intelligence (AI). Traditional IOL formulas may demonstrate adequate results in typical eyes; however, their accuracy decreases when biometric parameters are significantly different from normal ranges. This presents a challenge, especially in the management of cataracts with concurrent glaucoma, which often features great AL variability, changes in corneal biomechanics, and ACD fluctuations. Newer AI-driven formulas, including Hill-Radial Basis Function (RBF) 3.0 and Kane, demonstrated superior predictive accuracy attributed to their incorporation of extensive datasets and various biomechanical parameters [46].

The primary advantage of AI-driven formulas over traditional methods is the incorporation of machine learning. This incorporation facilitates the processing of large datasets from various ocular conditions and anatomical variations. The Hill-RBF 3.0 employs an artificial intelligence-enhanced pattern recognition feature to analyze over 20 biometric parameters, which facilitates more precise IOL power prediction calculations. The calculation results from Hill-RBF 3.0 demonstrate superior performance compared to the Barrett Universal II in eyes with a previous history of glaucoma surgeries (MAE: ±0.38 D (Hill) vs. ±0.52 D (Barrett)) [47, 48].

The use of artificial intelligence also allows for the incorporation of deep learning capabilities. AI models can be trained using data obtained from supporting devices, such as the Corvis ST and Optical Biometer ORA. Advanced algorithms can be developed with a superior predictive capability integrating a larger and more unique biomechanical dataset, such as including CH, corneal stiffness, and IOP-induced corneal deformation patterns, in contrast to static-based data from traditional formulas [49, 50].

The new generation of AI-driven formulas will consider preoperative trends to significantly improve predictive analysis for postoperative IOP outcomes, benefiting patients with glaucoma and PEX. The deep learning models integrated into the calculation can effectively utilize preoperative data regarding IOP, including preoperative IOP trends and the effect of medication histories, such as prostaglandin-analog corneal thinning, to optimize IOL power calculation to better anticipate ELP and minimize myopic/hyperopic errors [51, 52].

8.5 Conclusion

Accurate IOL power calculation in glaucoma patients presents significant challenges due to the complex implications of anatomical variability, history of medical and surgical treatments, and alteration of corneal biomechanics. Precise calculation necessitates a comprehensive and individualized assessment, requiring appropriate biometric methods, careful selection of formula, and a complete understanding of changes associated with glaucoma. The rising utilization of artificial intelligence and its incorporation in IOL calculation formulas offer superior accuracy, particularly in complex cases. The integration of data-driven algorithms, advanced biometric technologies, and traditional clinical insights will greatly improve visual outcomes and long-term quality of life for glaucoma patients undergoing cataract surgery.

References

1. Tabatabaei SA, Samadi M, Soleimani M, Fonoodi H, Ghods S, Inanloo B. Accuracy of different lens power calculation formulas in patients with phacomorphic glaucoma. Taiwan J Ophthalmol. 2022;12(2):164–9. Published 2022 Apr 13. https://doi.org/10.4103/tjo.tjo_1_22.
2. Roy A, Almeida A, Rao A. Outcomes of "complex" cataract surgeries performed by long-term glaucoma fellows in a tertiary eye centre from Eastern India. Clin Ophthalmol. 2023;17:1315–21. https://doi.org/10.2147/OPTH.S405772.
3. Kabata Y, Oki T, Nakano T. Comparison of refractive prediction error by axial length in flanged intrascleral intraocular lens fixation. Clin Ophthalmol. 2024;18:895–900. Published 2024 Mar 21. https://doi.org/10.2147/OPTH.S455178.
4. Tamaoki A, Kojima T, Hasegawa A, et al. Clinical evaluation of a new swept-source optical coherence biometer that uses individual refractive indices to measure axial length in cataract patients. Ophthalmic Res. 2019;62(1):11–23. https://doi.org/10.1159/000496690.
5. Nakhli FR, Emarah K, Jeddawi L. Accuracy of formulae for secondary intraocular lens power calculations in pediatric aphakia. J Curr Ophthalmol. 2017;29(3):199–203. Published 2017 Jun 13. https://doi.org/10.1016/j.joco.2017.05.007.

6. Carr F, Gangwani V. Refractive surprise after cataract surgery secondary to smeared optics of swept-source optical coherence tomography biometer: a case report. BMC Ophthalmol. 2020;20(1):352. Published 2020 Aug 28. https://doi.org/10.1186/s12886-020-01629-0.
7. Patel SS, Sahu RK, Chandrakar AK, et al. Comparative study of manual versus automated biometry on refractive outcome of cataract surgery. J Evolution Med Dent Sci. 2018;7(45):4893–489. https://doi.org/10.14260/jemds/2018/1089.
8. Brazuna R, Alonso RS, Salomão MQ, Fernandes BF, Ambrósio R. Ocular Biomechanics and Glaucoma. Vision. 2023;7(2):36. https://doi.org/10.3390/vision7020036.
9. Silva N, Ferreira A, Baptista PM, Figueiredo A, Reis R, Sampaio I, et al. Corneal biomechanics for ocular hypertension, primary open-angle glaucoma, and amyloidotic glaucoma: a comparative study by Corvis ST. Clin Ophthalmol. 2022;16:71–83. https://doi.org/10.2147/OPTH.S350029.
10. Zarei R, Zamani MH, Eslami Y, Fakhraei G, Tabatabaei M, Esfandiari AR. Comparing corneal biomechanics and IOP between healthy individuals and glaucoma subtypes: a cross-sectional study. Ann Med Surg. 2022;82:104677. https://doi.org/10.1016/j.amsu.2022.104677.
11. Camps V, Piñero D, Caravaca E, De Fez D. Preliminary validation of an optimized algorithm for IOL power calculation in keratoconus. Indian J Ophthalmol. 2017;65(8):690–9. https://doi.org/10.4103/ijo.IJO_274_16.
12. Piñero DP, Camps VJ, Caravaca-Arens E, de Fez D, Blanes-Mompó FJ. Algorithm for correcting the keratometric error in the estimation of the corneal power in keratoconus eyes after accelerated corneal collagen crosslinking. J Ophthalmol. 2017;2017:8529489. https://doi.org/10.1155/2017/8529489.
13. Hayakawa Y, Inada T. Background of MIGS-adapted patients for cataract surgery in glaucoma. 2024;13(18):5378. Published 2024 Sep 11. https://doi.org/10.3390/jcm13185378.
14. Shin JH, Kim SH, Oh SH, Lee KM. Factors associated with refractive prediction error after phacotrabeculectomy. 2023;12(17):5706. Published 2023 Sep 1. https://doi.org/10.3390/jcm12175706.
15. Nagata M, Matsushima H, Senoo T. A case of pigment dispersion syndrome after placement of sulcus IOL with 7-mm optic diameter after posterior capsule rupture. Case Rep Ophthalmol. 2022;13(3):1003–9. https://doi.org/10.1159/000527750.
16. Moinul P, Hutnik C. Aqueous misdirection syndrome: an interesting case presentation. Clin Ophthalmol. 2015:183–6. https://doi.org/10.2147/OPTH.S75698.
17. Hua N, Ning Y, Zheng H, Zhao L, Qian X, Wormington C, et al. Recurrent dislocation of binocular crystal lenses in a patient with cystathionine beta-synthase deficiency. BMC Ophthalmol. 2021;21(1):212. https://doi.org/10.1186/s12886-021-01974-8.
18. Gatzioufas Z, Kopsidas K, Gyongyossy B, Moschos M, Seitz B. Late-onset anterior dislocation of a posterior chamber IOL in a patient with Pseudoexfoliation syndrome. Case Rep Ophthalmol. 2011;2(1):1–4. https://doi.org/10.1159/000323861.
19. Abbas I, Ahmed AM, Dayal SM, Sirhindi GA. Frequency of pseudophakic glaucoma in patients with cataract surgery. Pak J Med Health Sci. 2021;15(5):1151–3. https://doi.org/10.53350/pjmhs211551151.
20. Wu N, Chen Y, Yang Y, Sun X. The changes of corneal biomechanical properties with long-term treatment of prostaglandin analogue measured by Corvis ST. BMC Ophthalmol. 2020;20(1):422. https://doi.org/10.1186/s12886-020-01693-6.
21. Gozawa M, Takamura Y, Iwasaki K, Arimura S, Inatani M. Conjunctival structure of glaucomatous eyes treated with anti-glaucoma eye drops: a cross-sectional study using anterior segment optical coherence tomography. BMC Ophthalmol. 2020;20(1):244. https://doi.org/10.1186/s12886-020-01518-6.
22. Christine RN, Respatika HD, Simanjuntak G. Oral acetazolamide administration to control IOP on first day post phacoemulsification surgery: is it necessary ? Ophthalmol Indones. 2019;43(2):118.
23. Pakravan M, Alvani A, Esfandiari H, Ghahari E, Yaseri M. Post-trabeculectomy ocular biometric changes. Clin Exp Optom. 2017;100(2):128–32. https://doi.org/10.1111/cxo.12477.

24. Chandran P, Sneha C, Subramanian S, Raman GV. Comparison between ocular biometry parameters in patients with unilateral congenital glaucoma. Indian J Ophthalmol. 2023;71(8):2962–6. https://doi.org/10.4103/IJO.IJO_122_23.
25. Dhawlikar NS, Dai YL, Hughes KV, Rao NK. IOL power calculation in special situations. In: Pardianto G, editor. The intraocular lens power calculation. Medan: Anak Sudarti Foundation; 2022. p. 43–73.
26. Ji Z, Ma J, Sun Z, Zhang M. Comparison of two formulas for calculating IOL in patients with angle-closure glaucoma. Medicine. 2024;103(45):e40387. https://doi.org/10.1097/MD.0000000000040387.
27. Glisic S, Jovanovic M, Gakovic A, Dacic-Krnjaja B. Cataract surgery and IOL power calculation in a patient with anterior megalophthalmos with normal sized crystalline lens: case report. SANAMED. 2015;10(3):209–13. https://doi.org/10.5937/sanamed1503209G.
28. Hoffer KJ, Savini G. Update on IOL power calculation study protocols. Ophthalmology. 2021;128(11):e115–20. https://doi.org/10.1016/j.ophtha.2020.07.005.
29. Lee JY, Lai JM, Lam R, Wong BT, Yick DF, Tse RK. Retrospective analysis of the risk factors for developing phacomorphic glaucoma. Indian J Ophthalmol. 2011;59(6):471. https://doi.org/10.4103/0301-4738.86316.
30. Haigis W. IOL power calculation formulas. East Valley Ophthalmology. Available from: https://doctor-hill.com/iol-power-calculations/formulas/.
31. Khokhar S, Pillay G, Sen S, Agarwal E. Clinical spectrum and surgical outcomes in spherophakia: a prospective interventional study. Eye. 2018;32(3):527–36. https://doi.org/10.1038/eye.2017.229.
32. Sitoula RP, Sarkar I, Nayak D, Singh SK. Lens induced glaucoma: an experience in tertiary eye care center in eastern Nepal. Nepal J Ophthalmol. 2017;8(2):161–6. https://doi.org/10.3126/nepjoph.v8i2.17006.
33. Wang J, Du E, Tang J. The treatment of malignant glaucoma in nanophthalmos: a case report. BMC Ophthalmol. 2018;18(1):54. https://doi.org/10.1186/s12886-018-0714-5.
34. Ciftci S, Simsek. Evaluation of ultrasonic biomicroscopy results in anterior eye segment before and after cataract surgery. Clin Ophthalmol. 2012:1931. https://doi.org/10.2147/OPTH.S37614.
35. Tekcan H, Mangan MS, İmamoğlu S, Alpogan O. Refractive outcomes of uneventful cataract surgery in pseudoexfoliation syndrome and pseudoexfoliation glaucoma. Korean J Ophthalmol. 2022;36(3):226–35. https://doi.org/10.3341/kjo.2021.0183.
36. Bansal A, Malik KPS, Malik VK, Jain K. Phaco-nucleotomy techniques in management of pseudoexfoliation syndrome. Nepal J Ophthalmol. 2017;8(2):144–50. https://doi.org/10.3126/nepjoph.v8i2.17003.
37. Thevi T, Abas AL. Intraoperative and postoperative complications of cataract surgery in eyes with pseudoexfoliation—an 8-year analysis. Oman J Ophthalmol. 2019;12(3):160–5. https://doi.org/10.4103/ojo.OJO_238_2018.
38. Kareem A, Neamah GA. Corneal endotheliopathy in pseudoexfoliation syndrome. Iraqi J Med Sci. 2018;16(1):57–65.
39. Rodriguez-Garcia A, Foster CS. Cataract surgery in patients with uveitis: preoperative and surgical considerations. In: Difficulties in cataract surgery. InTech; 2018. https://doi.org/10.5772/intechopen.71031.
40. Mamani Maquera DJ, Pantoja Dávalos N, Catacora Contreras M. Uveitis - Glaucoma - Hyphema syndrome: clinical case. Rev Fac Med Hum. 2023;23(3).
41. Shuaib A, Elhusseiny AM, Hassanein D, Zedan RH, Elhilali H. Predictive value of IOL power calculation formulae in children. Clin Ophthalmol. 2021;15:2527–36. https://doi.org/10.2147/OPTH.S316697.
42. Jasman AA, Shaharuddin B, Noor RAM, Ismail S, Ghani ZA, Embong Z. Prediction error and accuracy of IOL power calculation in pediatric patient comparing SRK II and pediatric IOL calculator. BMC Ophthalmol. 2010;10(1):20. https://doi.org/10.1186/1471-2415-10-20.

43. Zhao QH. Commentary review: challenges of IOL implantation for congenital cataract infants. Int J Ophthalmol. 2021;14(6):923–30. https://doi.org/10.18240/ijo.2021.06.19.
44. Kleinmann G, Zaugg B, Apple DJ, Bleik J. Pediatric cataract surgery with hydrophilic acrylic IOL. J Am Assoc Pediatr Ophthalmol Strabismus. 2013;17(4):367–70. https://doi.org/10.1016/j.jaapos.2013.04.007.
45. Coh P, Moghimi S, Chen RI, Hsu CH, Masís Solano M, Porco T, et al. Lens position parameters as predictors of IOP reduction after cataract surgery in glaucomatous versus nonglaucomatous eyes. Invest Ophthalmol Vis Sci. 2016;57(6):2593. https://doi.org/10.1167/iovs.16-19384.
46. Stopyra W, Cooke DL, Grzybowski A. A review of IOL power calculation formulas based on artificial intelligence. J Clin Med. 2024;13(2):498. https://doi.org/10.3390/jcm13020498.
47. Tsessler M, Cohen S, Wang L, Koch DD, Zadok D, Abulafia A. Evaluating the prediction accuracy of the Hill-RBF 3.0 formula using a heteroscedastic statistical method. J Cataract Refract Surg. 2022;48(1):37–43. https://doi.org/10.1097/j.jcrs.0000000000000702.
48. Eom Y, Bae SH, Yang SK, Kim DH, Song JS, Cooke DL. Modified IOL power selection method according to biometric subgroups Eom IOL power calculator. Sci Rep. 2024;14(1):4228. https://doi.org/10.1038/s41598-024-54346-9.
49. Moshirfar M, Durnford KM, Jensen JL, Beesley DP, Peterson TS, Darquea IM, et al. Accuracy of six IOL power calculations in eyes with AL greater than 28.0 mm. J Clin Med. 2022;11(19):5947. https://doi.org/10.3390/jcm11195947.
50. Stopyra W, Voytsekhivskyy O, Grzybowski A. Prediction of seven artificial intelligence-based IOL power calculation formulas in medium-long Caucasian eyes. Life. 2025;15(1):45. https://doi.org/10.3390/life15010045.
51. Han T, Shi W, Chen Y, Shen Y, Xu Y, Zhou X. Predictive models for IOPs measured with NCT, GAT, and ORA among patients undergoing SMILE. Front Bioeng Biotechnol. 2022;10:1030458. https://doi.org/10.3389/fbioe.2022.1030458.
52. Vallée R, Meduri E, Vallée JN, Lallouette A, Haffane Z, Paillard A, et al. Predictive biomarkers of intra-ocular pressure decrease after cataract surgery associated with trabecular washout in patients with pseudo exfoliative glaucoma. Sci Rep. 2024;14(1):13567. https://doi.org/10.1038/s41598-024-53893-5.

Chapter 9
IOL Calculation in Vitrectomized Eyes

Muhammad Bayu Sasongko and Rinanto Prabowo

9.1 Introduction

Pars plana vitrectomy (PPV) is a surgical technique used to treat posterior segment disorders such as retinal detachment, macular hole, or vitreous opacity [1–3]. In the last decade, advancement in surgical techniques, instrumentation, and ophthalmic anaesthesia has changed the surgical threshold and expanded the indications of PPV [1, 4, 5]. Therefore, PPV has become a more and more common surgical procedure performed in various settings, from tertiary eye care to day surgery clinic [1].

Cataract is one of the most common sequelae of PPV, occurring in up to 80% of individuals with a history of PPV within 2 years [6–8]. Evidence suggested that during PPV, various factors that disrupt crystalline lens physiology, including light toxicity, fluid turbulence in the vitreous cavity, mechanical trauma/ lens touch, and use of gas or silicon oil as intraocular tamponade, may increase postoperative oxygen tension and oxidation of lens protein, hence accelerate the formation of cataract [7–10]. Moreover, due to the abovementioned pathological mechanisms, post-PPV-induced cataract has a relatively harder nucleus compared to age-related cataract [7–10].

In this modern era of cataract surgery, the desired outcome of cataract surgery is to obtain optimal, spectacle-free refractive outcomes [10, 11]. Unfortunately, cataract surgery in individuals with vitrectomized eye has higher risks of surgical

All authors declare no financial interest.

M. B. Sasongko (✉)
Department of Ophthalmology, Faculty of Medicine, Public Health, and Nursing, Universitas Gadjah Mada, Yogyakarta, Indonesia
e-mail: mb.sasongko@ugm.ac.id

R. Prabowo
Dr. Yap Eye Hospital, Yogyakarta, Indonesia

G. Pardianto (ed.), *Intraocular Lens (IOL) Power Calculation*,
https://doi.org/10.1007/978-981-92-1223-1_9

complications, mainly because lack of vitreous support may cause unexpectedly deep and unstable anterior chamber and unstable capsular bag due to zonular injury during PPV [6, 10–13]. More importantly, the other challenge for cataract surgery in eyes previously undergone PPV is to accurately predict postoperative refractive outcomes [10, 11, 14–16]. Previous evidence has documented that around 20% of cataract surgery in vitrectomized eyes had postoperative refractive surprises for several reasons. First, substitution of vitreous with aqueous humour results in changes in refractive index of the posterior segment, which affects the accuracy of focal point and axial length (AL) measurement; and second, increased mobility of the posterior capsule leads to less stable intraocular lens (IOL) and IOL movement after surgery [10, 11, 14–16].

To date, there are different IOL calculation methods suitable for various eye conditions, allowing more accurate postoperative refractive prediction. Few studies have also investigated and refined IOL calculation methods for eyes with previous PPV. However, there has been lack of compelling evidence that provides a comprehensive overview of the available methods for IOL measurement in vitrectomized eyes. This chapter will review and compare the most recent IOL calculation methods for vitrectomized eyes available from studies published within the last 5 years.

9.2 Studies Evaluating Various Intraocular Lens Calculation Methods in Vitrectomized Eyes

9.2.1 Lamson and Colleagues, Journal of Cataract and Refractive Surgery *2019 [14]*

In this study, Lamson and colleagues retrospectively reviewed refractive outcomes of patients who underwent phacoemulsification with previous PPV in the same eye. A total of 61 eyes without any exposure to refractive surgery, silicon oil tamponade, and other factors that prevented accurate IOL calculation were included in the analysis. All subjects had uncomplicated phacoemulsification with in-the-bag IOL placement. The authors presented comparisons of preoperative predicted refractive measures to postoperative ones using various IOL calculation formulas.

The study shows that Holladay 2 provided the most consistent accuracy, with nearly 30% of eyes were within ±0.25 D residual refractive outcomes, over 60% of eyes within ±0.50 D and 85% within ±1.00 D, while Hill-RBF also performed well at broader ranges, achieving 82% within ±1.00 D. Traditional formulas such as Holladay 1, SRK/T, and Barrett yielded moderate accuracy, with about three-quarters of eyes within ±1.00 D but fewer than 30% within ±0.25 D. Ladas was less reliable overall, with the lowest proportion within ±0.50 D (45.9%). Application of the WKA improved broad tolerance accuracy (up to 92.9% within ±1.00 D for

WKA Holladay 1) but substantially reduced precision at tighter ranges. Overall, Holladay 2 emerged as the best-balanced formula, combining low prediction error with strong performance across all D ranges.

9.2.2 *Tan and Colleagues,* American Journal of Ophthalmology *2020 [15]*

This study by Tan and colleagues was a retrospective evaluation of 111 vitrectomized eyes (111 patients) that subsequently underwent uncomplicated cataract surgery with implantation of an enVista MX60 IOL (Bausch Health Companies Inc., Rochester, NY). They compared the predictive performance of several modern IOL formulas—BUII, Emmetropia Verifying Optical (EVO), Kane, and LSF—against traditional formulas (Haigis, Hoffer Q, Holladay 1, and SRK/T) incorporating Wang-Koch axial length adjustments (WK) where appropriate.

The study presents mean of difference prediction error between postoperative refractive outcome and preoperative prediction refractive outcome in eyes with AL shorter and longer than 26 mm. For eyes with AL < 26 mm, all formulas showed that 80–86% of eyes had residual refractive outcome within ±0.75 D of predicted refraction. Among them, the Kane formula achieved the highest proportion of residual refraction within ±0.25 D (36.5%), closely followed by LSF (34.6%). Traditional formulas such as Haigis and SRK/T performed comparably, but Holladay 1 and Hoffer Q were the two lowest, with fewer eyes within ±0.25 D and ±0.50 D. Overall, the new generation formulas (Kane, EVO, BUII) demonstrated slightly better accuracy and tighter prediction compared to older formulas.

In eyes with AL ≥ 26 mm, predictive accuracy dropped across all formulas, with only 60–76% of eyes having residual refractive outcome within ±0.75 D. In this group, after first linear AL adjustment using Wang-Koch method, Haigis (Haigis-WK1) and Holladay 1 (Holladay 1-WK1) showed improved performance up to 75.8% within ±0.75 D, similar to Haigis alone. Among new formulas, EVO and BUII maintained good performance (72.7% and 69.7% within ±0.75 D), while LSF had the highest proportion within ±0.25 D (42.4%) but lower consistency at wider ranges. Traditional formulas without WK adjustment (Hoffer Q, Holladay 1, SRK/T) performed the worst, with fewer than 61% of eyes within ±0.75 D.

9.2.3 *Xu and Colleagues,* Current Eye Research *2021 [16]*

This study by Xu and colleagues compared postoperative refractive outcomes in vitrectomized versus nonvitrectomized eyes. A total of 193 eyes in each group were matched for AL and cataract severity. Both new-generation IOL power formulas (BUII, Kane, LSF) and traditional vergence formulas (SRK/T, Holladay 1, Hoffer Q, Haigis) were evaluated, with and without the WK.

The study shows that vitrectomized eyes had lower accuracy when compared to nonvitrectomized eyes. Vitrectomized eyes had mean prediction error values around 0.66–0.74 D, whereas nonvitrectomized eyes were closer to 0.41–0.51 D, reflecting a modest hyperopic shift and greater variability after vitrectomy. BUII and Kane formula consistently achieve the highest percentages in both vitrectomized and non-vitrectomized eyes, with the highest percentages of residual refractive error within ±0.25 D.

9.2.4 *Zhang and Colleagues,* American Journal of Ophthalmology *2024 [10]*

This study by Zhang et al. developed and validated the Ensemble Artificial Intelligence-Based Thick Intraocular Lens Calculation Formula for Vitrectomized Eyes (LISA-PPV) formula, an ensemble artificial intelligence–based IOL calculation method specifically designed for eyes that had undergone pars plana vitrectomy, where standard formulas often yield less predictable refractive outcomes. By integrating multiple modern formulas and adjusting for unique biometric changes in vitrectomized eyes, LISA-PPV aimed to reduce systematic errors and improve refractive precision.

This study shows that in eyes with an AL less than 26 mm, most IOL power calculation formulas achieved good refractive predictability, with around 80% of eyes falling within ±1.00 D of the predicted refraction. Among them, the LISA-PPV formula performed best, reaching the highest proportion of residual refractive outcome, 27.6% within ±0.25 D, 57% within ±0.50 D, and 82.9% within ±1.00 D. Other formulas such as Hill-RBF and LSF also showed comparable performance, while PEARL-DGS lagged behind, with the lowest proportion of eyes within ±0.25 D and ±0.50 D.

In eyes with longer AL (≥26 mm), refractive accuracy declined across all formulas, with only 65–78% of eyes reaching ±1.00 D. Despite this general reduction, LISA-PPV again provided the best results (28% within ±0.25 D, 57% within ±0.50 D, and 78.1% within ±1.00 D), outperforming commonly used formulas such as BUII, EVO, Kane, and Hoffer-QST, which clustered around 71.9%. PEARL-DGS once more showed the weakest performance, with just 65.6% of eyes within ±1.00 D.

9.3 Summary and Clinical Implications

In summary, the performance of IOL power calculation formulas in vitrectomized eyes shows a consistent pattern: Newer-generation formulas are generally superior to traditional formulas, and the accuracy of all formulas is lower in highly myopic eyes (AL $\geq$ 26 mm). A study by Zhang et al. demonstrated that the LISA-PPV formula provided the most reliable results across both normal and long eyes, with the highest proportion of eyes having residual refractive outcomes within ±0.25 D and ±0.50 D.

Practically, it is evident that no single formula is perfect, but surgeons can optimize outcomes in vitrectomized eyes by tailoring formula choice to AL. For eyes < 26 mm, new-generation formulas such as Kane, EVO, BUII, and LISA-PPV or Holladay 2 provide the best precision. For highly myopic eyes ≥ 26 mm, refractive predictability declines across all formulas, but LISA-PPV remains consistently strong, while WK-adjusted traditional formulas (Haigis-WK, Holladay 1-WK, SRK/T-WK) can achieve results comparable to newer methods. Patients should be counselled that despite improved formula design, refractive error variability remains higher after vitrectomy, especially in long eyes, and that formula selection, favouring LISA-PPV, Kane, or Holladay 2 with WK in high myopia may help minimize refractive surprises.

References

1. Recchia FM, Scott IU, Brown GC, Brown MM, Ho AC, Ip MS. Small-gauge pars plana vitrectomy: a report by the American Academy of Ophthalmology. Ophthalmology. 2010;117(9):1851–7. https://doi.org/10.1016/j.ophtha.2010.06.014.
2. Do DV, Gichuhi S, Vedula SS, Hawkins BS. Surgery for postvitrectomy cataract. Cochrane Database Syst Rev. 2018;1(1):CD006366. Published 2018 Jan 10. https://doi.org/10.1002/14651858.CD006366.pub4.
3. Soliman MK, Hardin JS, Jawed F, et al. A database study of visual outcomes and intraoperative complications of postvitrectomy cataract surgery. Ophthalmology. 2018;125(11):1683–91. https://doi.org/10.1016/j.ophtha.2018.05.027.
4. Chen SN, Chen SJ, Wu TT, Wu WC, Yang CH, Yang CM. Refining vitrectomy for proliferative diabetic retinopathy. Graefes Arch Clin Exp Ophthalmol. 2023;261(12):3659–70. https://doi.org/10.1007/s00417-023-06134-w.
5. Thompson JT. Advantages and limitations of small gauge vitrectomy. Surv Ophthalmol. 2011;56(2):162–72. https://doi.org/10.1016/j.survophthal.2010.08.003.
6. Shousha MA, Yoo SH. Cataract surgery after pars plana vitrectomy. Curr Opin Ophthalmol. 2010;21(1):45–9. https://doi.org/10.1097/ICU.0b013e32833303bf.
7. Hernandez-Bogantes E, Abdala-Figuerola A, Olivo-Payne A, Quiros F, Wu L. Cataract following pars plana vitrectomy: a review. Semin Ophthalmol. 2021;36(8):824–31. https://doi.org/10.1080/08820538.2021.1924799.
8. Kataria AS, Thompson JT. Cataract formation and progression in patients less than 50 years of age after vitrectomy. Ophthalmol Retina. 2017;1(2):149–53. https://doi.org/10.1016/j.oret.2016.09.007.
9. Yee KMP, Tan S, Lesnik Oberstein SY, et al. Incidence of cataract surgery after vitrectomy for vitreous opacities. Ophthalmol Retina. 2017;1(2):154–7. https://doi.org/10.1016/j.oret.2016.11.012.
10. Zhang J, Jin A, Han X, et al. The LISA-PPV formula: an ensemble artificial intelligence-based thick intraocular lens calculation formula for vitrectomized eyes. Am J Ophthalmol. 2024;262:237–45. https://doi.org/10.1016/j.ajo.2024.02.037.
11. Zhang J, Han X, Chen X, et al. Choice of intraocular lens calculation formula for cataract patients with prior pars plana vitrectomy. J Cataract Refract Surg. 2023;49(9):956–63. https://doi.org/10.1097/j.jcrs.0000000000001253.

12. Braunstein RE, Airiani S. Cataract surgery results after pars plana vitrectomy. Curr Opin Ophthalmol. 2003;14(3):150–4. https://doi.org/10.1097/00055735-200306000-00007.
13. Rey A, Jürgens I, Maseras X, Dyrda A, Pera P, Morilla A. Visual outcome and complications of cataract extraction after pars plana vitrectomy. Clin Ophthalmol. 2018;12:989–94. Published 2018 May 25. https://doi.org/10.2147/OPTH.S161223.
14. Lamson TL, Song J, Abazari A, Weissbart SB. Refractive outcomes of phacoemulsification after pars plana vitrectomy using traditional and new intraocular lens calculation formulas. J Cataract Refract Surg. 2019;45(3):293–7. https://doi.org/10.1016/j.jcrs.2018.10.032.
15. Tan X, Zhang J, Zhu Y, et al. Accuracy of new generation intraocular lens calculation formulas in vitrectomized eyes. Am J Ophthalmol. 2020;217:81–90. https://doi.org/10.1016/j.ajo.2020.04.035.
16. Xu Y, Liu L, Li J, et al. Refractive outcomes and anterior chamber depth after cataract surgery in eyes with and without previous pars Plana vitrectomy. Curr Eye Res. 2021;46(9):1333–40. https://doi.org/10.1080/02713683.2021.1887271.

Chapter 10
Intraocular Lens Power Calculation in Uveitic Cataract

Muhammad Edrial, Jessica Zarwan, Faraby Martha, and Febrina Art

10.1 Introduction

Cataract formation represents the most prevalent secondary complication in patients with chronic or recurrent uveitis. This lens opacification is driven by a synergistic interplay between persistent intraocular inflammatory mediators and the long-term administration of corticosteroid therapy. The resulting disruption of lens fiber homeostasis necessitates a specialized surgical approach to mitigate preoperative and postoperative inflammatory risks [1–4]. The main signs and symptoms include blurred vision, photophobia, and pain when active inflammation occurs. Complications of this cataract include posterior synechiae, capsular opacities, and possible postoperative inflammation [2].

The uveitic cataract population is epidemiologically distinct, characterized by its younger age distribution and a high frequency of sight-threatening comorbidities. Unlike routine age-related cases, these patients require a multidisciplinary approach to manage the sequelae of chronic inflammation. Recognizing these baseline differences is paramount for establishing realistic refractive goals and long-term functional outcomes [3]. The surgical management of uveitic cataracts is fundamentally

All authors declare no financial interest.
Authors declare that all figures belong to the authors.

M. Edrial (✉)
IEC Eye Care, Jakarta, Indonesia

J. Zarwan · F. Martha
Cipto Mangunkusumo Hospital, Jakarta, Indonesia

Universitas Indonesia, Jakarta, Indonesia

F. Art
Universitas Sriwijaya, Palembang, Indonesia

G. Pardianto (ed.), *Intraocular Lens (IOL) Power Calculation*,
https://doi.org/10.1007/978-981-92-1223-1_10

different from that of senile cataracts due to unique intraoperative challenges and postoperative risks. Because inflammatory sequelae are markedly nonuniform across the spectrum of uveitis, a syndrome-specific analysis is essential. Evaluating each entity separately allows for a more precise understanding of potential ocular morbidities and a more realistic estimation of the visual prognosis [5–7].

The incidence of uveitic cataracts ranges from 25% to 50% in patients with chronic uveitis, depending on the etiology and duration of inflammation. It can appear in any form of uveitis, most common in anterior and intermediate uveitis [6, 7]. The incidence of cataract formation exhibits significant variability across different uveitic phenotypes. Longitudinal data indicate a prevalence of approximately 50% in patients with juvenile idiopathic arthritis (JIA)-associated uveitis and posterior uveitis. In contrast, this figure rises to 75% in cases of chronic anterior uveitis, suggesting that sustained proximity of inflammatory mediators to the lens, combined with chronic corticosteroid exposure, significantly heightens the risk of lenticular opacification [8–16]. Lenticular opacification is a primary driver of vision loss in the uveitic population, accounting for approximately 40% of the visual impairment observed in these patients. Consequently, it has emerged as the most frequent indication for surgical intervention within the spectrum of intraocular inflammatory diseases. Addressing this complication is paramount, as timely phacoemulsification often facilitates not only visual rehabilitation but also improved visualization of the posterior segment for ongoing disease monitoring [1, 2]. Uveitic cataracts represent approximately 1.2% of the global cataract surgical workload, yet they demand a disproportionately high level of technical precision. These cases are more surgically demanding than routine age-related procedures. Consequently, specialized perioperative management is essential to mitigate the heightened risk of inflammatory exacerbation [1].

Surgical intervention in uveitic eyes is inherently complex, necessitated by anatomical distortions such as pupillary rigidity and extensive posterior synechiae. The primary objective of a successful procedure is to minimize a broad spectrum of inflammatory sequelae. This includes preventing fibrinoid reactions within the anterior chamber, peripheral anterior synechiae (PAS), and iris bombé. Furthermore, meticulous surgical technique is required to reduce the incidence of anterior capsular fibrosis, IOL deposits, and vision-threatening conditions such as secondary glaucoma, hypotony, cystoid macular edema (CME), and accelerated posterior capsular opacification (PCO) [1, 2]. To avoid cataract surgery complications in uveitic cataracts, it is important to control the preoperative inflammation pre- and postoperatively [2, 3]. Achieving optimal outcomes in uveitic cataract surgery is strictly contingent upon a sustained period of ocular stability. Standard clinical protocols mandate that the eye remains entirely quiescent for a minimum of three months prior to surgical intervention. Furthermore, maintaining rigorous control of intraocular inflammation throughout the postoperative phase is essential to prevent the exacerbation of inflammatory sequelae and to ensure the long-term viability of the intraocular lens [1–4]. Preoperative treatment includes topical or systemic corticosteroids and intraocular pressure management [2]. In cases of noncomplicated uveitic cataracts, inflammatory control can typically be achieved through a regimen of potent topical corticosteroids. For these patients, the surgical trajectory aligns closely with routine phacoemulsification protocols, provided that the preoperative period of quiescence is strictly maintained. This subgroup often exhibits a more stable blood-aqueous barrier, allowing for favorable refractive outcomes with standard perioperative care [6]. A proactive approach to inflammatory control is adopted by administering topical corticosteroids (1% prednisolone acetate or 0.5% dexamethasone) starting one week before surgery. This preoperative dosing frequency of 4–6 times per day is critical for patients with a history of uveitis, as it primes the ocular tissues and reduces the propensity for intraoperative miosis and postoperative fibrinous reactions [5, 6]. For advanced uveitis requiring robust inflammatory suppression, the standard regimen includes high-dose oral corticosteroids (1 mg/kg/day) or intravenous pulse therapy. However, given the significant risk of systemic side effects associated with high-dose steroids, there is an increasing clinical consensus favoring the use of steroid-sparing immunomodulating drugs. These agents provide a viable pathway for long-term inflammation control while facilitating a gradual tapering of corticosteroids, thereby optimizing the patient's systemic safety profile [2, 3].

In addition to the intraoperative challenges, uveitic cataracts also pose challenges in the preoperative stage. Intraocular lens calculation has its difficulties in uveitic cataracts. This chapter will elaborate on preoperative planning, especially the IOL power calculation.

10.2 IOL Material Selection

The insertion of an IOL could initiate a complex milieu of biological responses, encompassing acute inflammation and a sustained foreign body reaction. These processes are further compounded by the activation of the complement and coagulation cascades, alongside a surgically induced disruption of the blood-aqueous barrier. This altered intraocular environment facilitates enhanced cellular adhesion and the aberrant proliferation of lens epithelial cells (LECs) across the IOL's anterior surface, ultimately culminating in anterior capsule phimosis, fibrotic transformation, and PCO [3]. The long-term ocular outcomes in uveitic eyes are influenced by IOL positioning and the biocompatibility of the implanted IOL, both of which can contribute to persistent intraocular inflammation. The gold standard for intraocular lens (IOL) implantation in uveitic patients is the secure placement of a posterior chamber IOL (PC-IOL) within the capsular bag. This "in-the-bag" configuration not only guarantees optimal centration and long-term stability but also functions as a critical barrier against mechanical uveal irritation. By sequestering the IOL from highly reactive vascular tissues, this approach mitigates the risk of a protracted breakdown of the blood-aqueous barrier, thereby preventing the initiation of a deleterious inflammatory cascade [7, 16–18].

The IOL material type used for uveitic cataracts must consider biocompatibility and inflammatory risk. Some material choices include:

- Hydrophobic acrylic: The best choice because it has a low affinity for inflammatory proteins and minimal cellular adhesion [19].
- Hydrophilic acrylic: Hydrophilic acrylic lenses offer an advantageous uveal profile but lack the robust capsular biocompatibility inherent in hydrophobic materials. This often translates to an increased risk of anterior and posterior capsular fibrosis. However, modern surgical experience shows that functional results remain high across all acrylic platforms when a square-edged optic is utilized. The mechanical barrier provided by the edge design appears to compensate for the hydrophilic material's susceptibility to LEC migration, ensuring sustained visual clarity in uveitic eyes [19].
- PMMA (polymethyl-methacrylate): Inert and stable but more prone to cellular adhesion. Less popular in uveitic patients due to the need for a large incision (5.5 mm or larger), which can be related to higher postoperative inflammation compared to small incision foldable IOL (2.8 mm or less) [19].
- Silicone: Less preferred due to its higher propensity to induce inflammation compared to alternative options. Additionally, its tendency to adhere to silicone oil may complicate future management in patients with uveitis [19].

Modern IOL technology has significantly reduced intraocular trauma by optimizing the interface between the implant and ocular tissues. A fundamental principle in uveitis management is that higher biocompatibility directly correlates with a diminished inflammatory cascade. This is a stark contrast to the first-generation PMMA lenses, which, despite their perceived inertness, frequently triggered complex immunological responses, including protein adsorption and subsequent activation of the complement system, leading to chronic low-grade inflammation [3].

To attenuate the host's immunological reaction, various surface modification techniques have been integrated into IOL design. These strategies primarily involve altering the lens's wettability, either by enhancing hydrophilicity—as seen in heparin-coated PMMA lenses—or by promoting hydrophobicity through surface passivation. These physicochemical alterations aim to minimize protein adsorption and subsequent cellular adhesion, thereby stabilizing the intraocular environment in highly reactive eyes [3]. Clinical evidence demonstrates that eyes implanted with either acrylic or heparin-surface-modified (HSM)-PMMA IOLs achieve significantly superior visual outcomes compared to those receiving unmodified PMMA or silicone lenses. The enhanced biocompability of acrylic and HSM-PMMA surfaces serves to suppress chronic inflammatory signaling, thereby reducing the incidence of vision-threatening complications such as cystoid macular edema and persistent vitreous haze, which are more frequently encountered with silicone-based or nonmodified polymers [20]. Heparin-surface-modified IOLs represent a strategic advancement in reducing the iatrogenic inflammatory burden associated with cataract surgery in uveitic patients. Unlike standard PMMA, the heparinized surface inhibits the activation of the complement and coagulation cascades upon contact with the aqueous humor. This improved biocompatibility profile is essential for eyes at risk for exuberant postoperative inflammation, as it stabilizes the intraocular environment and diminishes the requirement for aggressive systemic corticosteroid escalation [3]. The shift toward heparin-coated foldable IOLs in uveitis management is driven by their ability to minimize biomaterial-related morbidity. Heparin functionalization confers high hydrophilicity to the IOL optic, creating a hydration layer that discourages the attachment of inflammatory cells and plasma proteins. By reducing this "surface-associated" cellular activity, HSM technology effectively optimizes uveal biocompatibility. Although initial PMMA-based HSM lenses have fallen out of favor, the foldable variants remain a recommended option for mitigating exuberant postoperative inflammation and maintaining long-term ocular quiescence in patients with preexisting uveitis [3, 20]. However, long-term observations have indicated that HSM does not confer a significant advantage in the prevention of PCO.

Foldable IOL technology utilizes both hydrophobic and hydrophilic surface properties to achieve immunological passivity. Hydrophobic substrates are characterized by their inherent resistance to cellular docking, whereas hydrophilic modifications focus on the attenuation of electrostatic forces. These properties are critical for inhibiting the attraction of leukocytes and the proliferation of fibroblasts on the optic surface. Understanding these interfacial dynamics is paramount for surgeons, as the prevention of surface-associated cellular activation is a cornerstone in the successful management of complex cataract cases [3].

Silicone-based lenses demonstrate inferior uveal and capsular biocompatibility relative to PMMA, HSM, and hydrogel materials. The implantation of silicone optics is associated with heightened anterior chamber cellular activity and a marked predisposition toward anterior capsular fibrosis. This fibrotic tendency often manifests as total capsulorhexis closure and enhanced PCO formation. Given these documented risks, the use of silicone IOLs is generally cautioned against in eyes predisposed to inflammation, where acrylic or heparinized materials offer a more stable and predictable postoperative course [19].

Surgical success in high-risk eyes is contingent upon preventing the sequelae of aggressive capsular fibrosis. While centripetal contraction can compromise zonular stability and lead to lens displacement, the use of IOLs with rigid PMMA haptics offers a robust mechanical barrier against such distortions. Unlike Prolene haptics, which may lack sufficient radial stiffness, PMMA components maintain the circularity of the capsular bag. Additionally, the implantation of a capsular tension ring serves as a vital stabilizing element, distributing contractile stress and preserving the integrity of the zonular apparatus. Other essential considerations related to IOL implantation [3]:

- Hydrophobic acrylic IOL demonstrates excellent uveal tolerance, specifically by mitigating the formation of posterior synechiae. Comparative longitudinal data indicate that these polymers elicit a significantly reduced inflammatory response during the critical early postoperative phase (days 1, 4, 7, and 15) when compared to silicone-based optics. This diminished cellular activity in the anterior chamber is paramount for preventing the early-stage exudative complications that frequently compromise refractive outcomes in uveitic cohorts [3, 20].

- HSM-modified polymers offer a biologically inert interface that reduces the rate of chronic postoperative uveitis. This is further enhanced by incorporating angulated haptics, which facilitate a posterior displacement of the optic within the capsular bag. This anatomical clearance is vital for preventing mechanical "chafing" of the posterior iris, a known precursor to pigment dispersion and sustained intraocular inflammation [3].
- Primary IOL implantation has shown limited efficacy in controlling the intense inflammatory sequelae of Behçet's disease and juvenile rheumatoid uveitis. Given the high propensity for postoperative complications—including hypotony and dense secondary membranes—aphakia should be seriously considered as the primary surgical plan. This conservative approach is particularly vital for younger patients, as it minimizes the risk of irreversible structural damage and allows for a more flexible secondary rehabilitation strategy once sustained clinical quiescence is achieved through aggressive immunomodulation [3].

10.3 Factors Related to IOL Calculation [21]

Biometry is the method of applying mathematics to calculate the ideal intraocular lens power. IOL calculation in uveitic cataracts is different from normal eyes. Some factors that affect IOL calculation in uveitic cataracts [21–28]:

- ACD (anterior chamber depth) changes: Inflammation can cause a reduction or increase in anterior chamber depth (normal value 3.0–3.5 mm; it can be reduced due to anterior synechiae or increased due to hypotonus).
- K (keratometry reading) changes: Chronic inflammation can change the shape of the cornea, usually adding irregularity and astigmatism.
- AL (axial length) changes: Fibrosis can cause differences in biometric accuracy, with normal values ranging from 22 to 25 mm.
- LT (lens thickness) changes: Increased lens thickness due to inflammation or nuclear sclerosis (normal values around 4–5 mm, but can increase to 5.5–6 mm in denser lenses). Lens thickness measurement values sometimes can be lower in patients with active uveitis [27].

Preoperative planning for uveitic cataracts is inherently complex due to coexisting ocular comorbidities. Calcific band-shaped keratopathy often renders standard keratometry unreliable, while extensive posterior synechiae can lead to a shallowing or irregular deepening of the anterior chamber, confounding ACD-based IOL formulas. Additionally, macular pathology such as epiretinal membranes and the anatomical shifts associated with hypotony can falsely alter axial length measurements. Recognizing these confounding factors is essential for clinicians to manage patient expectations regarding postoperative refractive outcomes [22]. In eyes with complex structural alterations, Immersion Amplitude Mode Scan (A-scan) biometry offers superior reliability for the simultaneous determination of ACD and AL. By utilizing a fluid-filled coupling medium, the immersion technique eliminates corneal compression—a common source of error in contact biometry—thereby ensuring more accurate refractive predictions. Furthermore, the integration of anterior segment optical coherence tomography (AS-OCT) has emerged as a high-resolution adjunct, providing micron-scale precision in ACD mapping that is essential for modern IOL power calculation formulas [21].

The corneal endothelium in eyes with chronic uveitis is uniquely susceptible to injury through multiple pathological mechanisms. The presence of preexisting endothelial compromise significantly elevates the surgical risk, particularly when phacoemulsification is further complicated by posterior synechiae, persistent miosis, and zonular instability. These anatomical hurdles necessitate prolonged intraocular manipulation and increased ultrasonic energy, which may synergistically exacerbate endothelial cell loss and predispose the patient to postoperative bullous keratopathy [21, 24].

10.4 Effects of Velocity in Aqueous, Lens, and Vitreous

In an ultrasonographic examination, the eye is divided into four components with different velocities of sound waves. The cornea is 1641 m/s, the anterior chamber is 1532 m/s, the lens is 1641 m/s, and the vitreous cavity is 1532 m/s, respectively. In normal phakic eyes, the average velocity is 1555 m/s. Velocity of sound is 980 m/s for 1000 centistokes (cSt) silicone oil, 1040 m/s for 5000 cSt, 2718 m/s for PMMA, and 2120 m/s for acrylic [23–26]. In uveitis, increased aqueous viscosity and changes in the refractive index of the lens due to inflammation can cause errors in biometry calculations.

10.5 Choosing the Right IOL Formula

There is no consensus on the most accurate formula for uveitic cataracts. However, several recommended formulas can be used for uveitic cataracts:

- Haigis: Suitable for a wide range of ACD, with adjustable a0, a1, and a2 parameters.
- Hoffer Q: For short AL (<22 mm), taking LT into account more specifically.
- Barrett Universal II (BUII): Modern and accurate in various eye conditions with adaptive algorithms for ACD and LT.

10.6 IOL Examination Modality

- Amplitude/Brightness Mode Scan/Display (A/B Scan)

A/B scan is used when the ocular media is too cloudy for optical biometry. Ultrasound biometry is clinically executed through two primary techniques: applanation (contact) and immersion. In the applanation approach, the transducer probe is placed in direct contact with the corneal surface, utilizing the natural precorneal tear film as the acoustic coupling agent. Conversely, the immersion technique employs a saline-filled scleral shell to house the A-scan probe, thereby preventing direct corneal contact. This fluid-filled interface ensures that the ultrasound waves transition through a consistent medium, which is critical for achieving high-resolution axial measurements without iatrogenic anatomical distortion. Thus, saline is in between the cornea and the probe. Immersion technique is recommended over applanation because it provides more accurate axial length results [22–26].

A/B Scan usage guide [24–28]:

(a) A-Scan mode:

- Used to measure the AL (Fig. 10.1).
- Immersion technique is recommended to avoid corneal compression that can cause measurement errors.
- The velocity can be adjusted accordingly.
  - Cornea: 1641 m/s
  - Aqueous humor: 1532 m/s
  - Lens: 1641–1660 m/s, precise biometry in cataractous eyes requires an understanding of how lens morphology affects sound conduction. Because ultrasound travels slower in hydrated tissues, intumescent cataracts demonstrate a reduced velocity (1590 m/s) compared to the standard lens. In contrast, posterior capsular and advanced nuclear sclerotic cataracts typically demonstrate higher acoustic impedance and faster sound transmission, with nuclear sclerosis averaging 1641 m/s. Failure to adjust the biometer's velocity constants for these specific lens types can lead to a "pseudo-elongation" or "pseudo-shortening" of the measured AL.
    Vitreous humor: 1530 m/s
- Take at least five measurements, and take the average for more accurate results [29].

(b) Brightness mode scan/display (B-scan) mode (Fig. 10.2):

- Used to assess the condition of the retina if there is significant media opacity.
- Make sure there is no macular edema or epiretinal membrane that can affect the IOL calculation results.
- Compare the results with optical coherence tomography (OCT) to confirm the retina's condition [30].

(c) Critical points in using A/B scan [29, 30].

- Comparative measurement of both eyes in every patient to ensure internal validation.
- Indications for biometric remeasurement:
  1. Interocular AL difference > 0.03 mm between eyes.
  2. AL outliers <22 mm or > 25 mm.

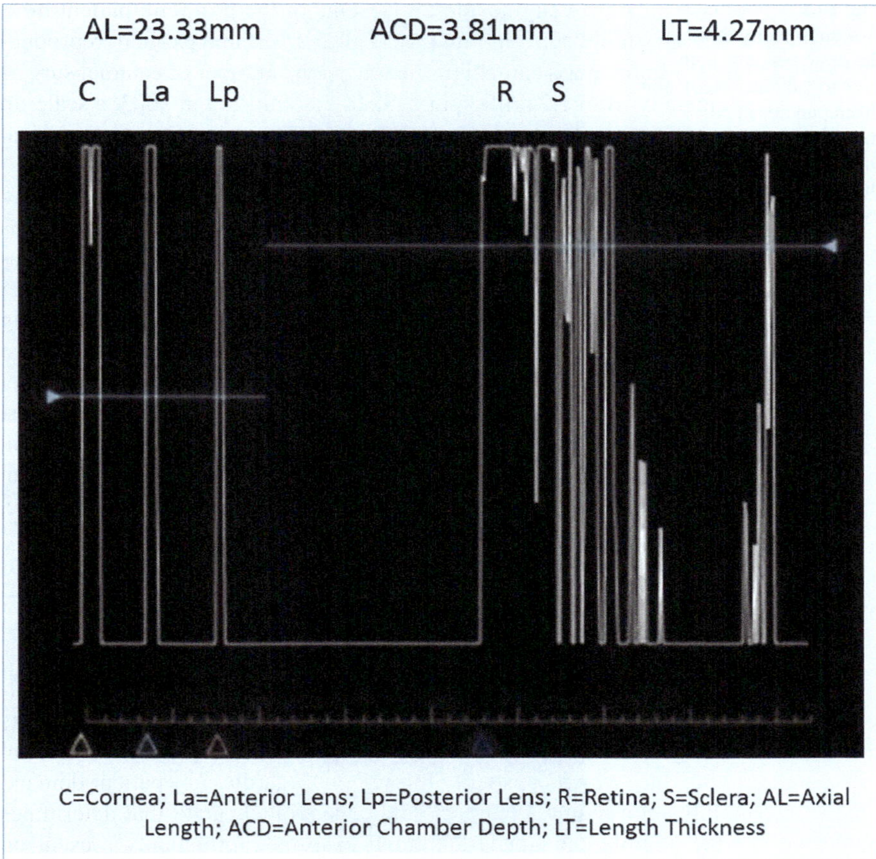

Fig. 10.1 Display of various echospikes from an A-scan biometry

3. Lack of correlation with clinical refractive history.
4. Optimal biometry requires steeply ascending, high-amplitude echoes that lack "stair-stepped" artifacts. Proper axial alignment is confirmed when the retinal and scleral spikes exhibit comparable magnitudes, ideally maintaining a height differential within an 80% tolerance.
5. Fixation and patient cooperation issues.
6. Interocular average K difference ≥ 1.0 D.
7. High measurement variability (SD > 0.05 mm)
8. B-scan documentation of AL disparity.

- *Partial Coherence Interferometry and Swept-Source OCT*
  Partial coherence interferometry (PCI) and swept-source optical coherence tomography (SS-OCT) are other examination modalities that can be used in media that are not too cloudy. However, SS-OCT can give precise eye measure-

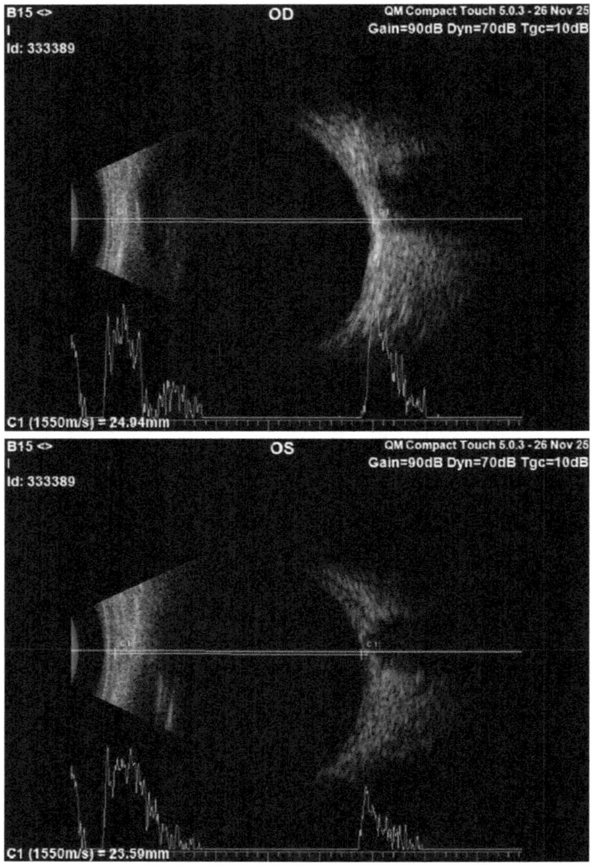

Fig. 10.2 Comparative B-scan imaging through the optic nerve of both eyes to validate interocular discrepancies in AL measurements (drawing the black line to document differences of AL between eyes)

ments with more difficult media, such as fibrosis or synechiae. In addition, SS-OCT is also better at detecting the ACD and LT variability that often occurs in uveitis patients, thus helping select a more optimal IOL formula [24–28].

- *Other Examination Tools*
  - Pentacam: To verify corneal shape and topography.
  - OCT: To assess the condition of the retina before surgery.
  - Scheimpflug Imaging: Helps evaluate lens opacity

Pearls and Tips

- Ensure that inflammation is controlled before surgery.
- Check media transparency: Use PCI or SS- OCT to measure the IOL calculation parameter. If there is significant opacity, consider immersion USG biometry.
- Adjust the IOL formula based on biometric parameters and eye condition.
- Choose an IOL with a biocompatible material such as hydrophobic acrylic.

References

1. Chan NS, Ti SE, Chee SP. Decision-making and management of uveitic cataract. Indian J Ophthalmol. 2017;65(12):1329–39. https://doi.org/10.4103/ijo.IJO_740_17. PMID: 29208813; PMCID: PMC5742961.
2. Chen JL, Bhat P, Lobo-Chan AM. Perioperative management of uveitic cataracts. Adv Ophthalmol Optom. 2019;4:325–39. https://doi.org/10.1016/j.yaoo.2019.04.014.
3. Rodriguez-Garcia A, Foster CS. Cataract surgery in patients with uveitis: preoperative and surgical considerations [Internet]. Difficulties in cataract surgery. INTECH; 2018. Available from: https://doi.org/10.5772/intechopen.71031
4. Sen HN, Abreu FM, Louis TA, et al. Cataract surgery outcomes in uveitis: the multicenter uveitis steroid treatment trial. Ophthalmology. 2016;123(1):183–90. https://doi.org/10.1016/j.ophtha.2015.09.022.
5. Baheti U, Siddique SS, Foster CS. Cataract surgery in patients with a history of uveitis. Saudi J Ophthalmol. 2012;26(1):55–60. https://doi.org/10.1016/j.sjopt.2011.10.003.
6. Chipont E, Alio JL. Cataract surgery in the patients with uveitis. In: Agarwal A, Agarwal A, Jacob S, editors. Phacoemulsification. 4th ed. Jaypee Brothers Medical Publishers; 2012. p. 407–12.
7. Hooper PL, Rao NA, Smith RE. Cataract extraction in uveitis patients. Surv Ophthalmol. 1990;35(2):120–44. https://doi.org/10.1016/0039-6257(90)90068-7.
8. Heger H, Drolsum L, Haaskjold E. Cataract surgery with implantation of IOL in patients with uveitis. Acta Ophthalmol. 1994;72:478–82. https://doi.org/10.1111/j.1755-3768.1994.tb02801.x.
9. Foster RE, Lowder CY, Meisler DM, et al. Extracapsular cataract extraction and posterior chamber intraocular lens implantation in uveitis patients. Ophthalmology. 1992;99:1234–41. https://doi.org/10.1016/s0161-6420(92)31818-4.
10. Krishna R, Meisler DM, Lowder CY, et al. Long term follow-up of extracapsular cataract extraction and posterior chamber intraocular lens implantation in patients with uveitis. Ophthalmology. 1998;105:1765–9. https://doi.org/10.1016/S0161-6420(98)99051-0.
11. Okhravi N, Lightman SL, Towler HM. Assessment of visual outcome after cataract surgery in patients with uveitis. Ophthalmology. 1999;106:710–22. https://doi.org/10.1016/S0161-6420(99)90155-0.
12. Rauz S, Stavrou P, Murray PI. Evaluation of foldable intraocular lenses in patients with uveitis. Ophthalmology. 2000;107:909–19. https://doi.org/10.1016/s0161-6420(00)00056-7.
13. Estafanous MF, Lowder CY, Meisler DM, et al. Phacoemulsification cataract extraction and posterior chamber lens implantation in patients with uveitis. Am J Ophthalmol. 2001;131:620–5. https://doi.org/10.1016/s0002-9394(00)00909-0.

14. Suresh PS, Jones NP. Phacoemulsification with intraocular lens implantation in patients with uveitis. Eye. 2001;15:621–8. https://doi.org/10.1038/eye.2001.197.
15. Meacock WR, Spalton DJ, Bender L, et al. Steroid prophylaxis in eyes with uveitis undergoing phacoemulsification. Br J Ophthalmol. 2004;88:1122–4. https://doi.org/10.1136/bjo.2003.032482.
16. Buratto L, Brint SF, Caretti L. Chapter 11: Cataract surgery in patients with uveitis. In: Buratto L, Brint SF, Caretti L, editors. Cataract surgery in complicated cases. USA: SLACK Incorporated; 2013. p. 121–9. https://doi.org/10.1201/9781003522904.
17. Van Gelder RN, Leveque TK. Cataract surgery in the setting of uveitis. Curr Opin Ophthalmol. 2009;20(1):42–5. https://doi.org/10.1097/ICU.0b013e32831b9b22.
18. Harapriya A, Anthony E. Managing cataract surgery in patients with uveitis. Community Eye Health. 2019;31(104):82–3. PMCID: PMC6390518 PMID: 31086436
19. Luo C, Wang H, Chen X, et al. Recent advances of intraocular lens materials and surface modification in cataract surgery. Front Bioeng Biotechnol. 2022;10:913383. https://doi.org/10.3389/fbioe.2022.913383.
20. Mehta S, Linton MM, Kempen JH. Outcomes of cataract surgery in patients with uveitis: a systematic review and meta-analysis. Am J Ophthalmol. 2014;158(4):676–692.e7. https://doi.org/10.1016/j.ajo.2014.06.018.
21. Chan NSW, Chee SP. Cataract surgery in uveitis. In: Pardianto G, Tassignon MJ, editors. Innovation in cataract surgery. Singapore: Springer; 2024. p. 205–17.
22. Leung TG, Lindsley K, Kuo IC. Types of intraocular lenses for cataract surgery in eyes with uveitis. Cochrane Database Syst Rev. 2014;3(3):CD007284. Published 2014 Mar 4. https://doi.org/10.1002/14651858.CD007284.pub2
23. Phatak S, Lowder C, Pavesio C. Controversies in intraocular lens implantation in pediatric uveitis. J Ophthalmic Inflamm Infect. 2016;6(1):12. https://doi.org/10.1186/s12348-016-0079-y.
24. Güell JL, Moura-Coelho N. Cataract surgery in uveitis. In: Pardianto G, Tassignon MJ, editors. Innovation in cataract surgery. Singapore: Springer; 2024. p. 247–70.
25. Aramberri J, Hoffer KJ, Olsen T, Savini G, Shammas HJ, editors. Intraocular lens calculations. Cham: Springer; 2024. https://doi.org/10.1007/978-3-031-50666-6.
26. Pardianto G, Tassignon M-J, editors. Innovation in cataract surgery. Singapore: Springer; 2024. https://doi.org/10.1007/978-981-97-5192-1.
27. Sakallioğlu AK, Alacamli G, Sattarpanah S, Guclu H. Evaluation of the structural changes of uveitis patients by optical biometry. Rom J Ophthalmol. 2023;67(3):238–43. https://doi.org/10.22336/rjo.2023.40.
28. Sen S, Tripathy K. Ultrasound Biometry. [Updated 2024 Jan 11]. In: StatPearls [Internet]. Treasure Island: StatPearls Publishing; 2025 Jan-. Available from: https://www.ncbi.nlm.nih.gov/books/NBK599551/
29. Prager TC. Chapter 8: Immersion using the prager shell. In: Hoffer KJ, editor. IOL power. USA: SLACK Incorporated; 2011. p. 53–62. https://doi.org/10.1201/9781003524687.
30. Shammas HJ. Chapter 5: A-scan biometry: Immersion technique. In: Hoffer KJ, editor. IOL power. USA: SLACK Incorporated; 2011. p. 25–8. https://doi.org/10.1201/9781003524687.

Chapter 11
Calculation for Premium and Special Selected Intraocular Lenses (IOLs)

Rinanto Prabowo, Rio Rhendy, Ricky E. Rooroh, and Jessica Zarwan

11.1 Introduction

Cataract surgery has evolved from a simple procedure that restores vision to a highly sophisticated refractive surgery, where patient expectations for spectacle independence have increased significantly. The choice of intraocular lens design for cataract surgery is a critical decision that can significantly impact postoperative visual outcomes. Premium intraocular lenses (IOLs) refer to advanced lens technologies designed to correct presbyopia, astigmatism, and near and intermediate vision, providing patients with superior postoperative visual outcomes [1]. These include multifocal, trifocal, extended-depth-of-focus (EDOF), toric, accommodating, light-adjustable, and refractive-diffractive IOLs [2]. The selection and calculation of premium and specially selected IOLs require a precise understanding of corneal biomechanics, anterior chamber depth (ACD), and postoperative refractive target adjustments [3]. Errors in measurements and calculations can lead to suboptimal results, often resulting in expensive corrective procedures such as laser vision correction or IOL exchange [4, 5].

This chapter will discuss the crucial considerations for selecting and calculating premium and special IOLs. It will cover key biometric assessments, advanced

All authors declare no financial interest.

R. Prabowo (✉)
YAP Eye Hospital, Yogyakarta, Indonesia

R. Rhendy · J. Zarwan
Cipto Mangunkusumo Hospital, Jakarta, Indonesia

Universitas Indonesia, Jakarta, Indonesia

R. E. Rooroh
KMN Eye Care, Jakarta, Indonesia

G. Pardianto (ed.), *Intraocular Lens (IOL) Power Calculation*,
https://doi.org/10.1007/978-981-92-1223-1_11

calculation formulas, and strategies for optimizing outcomes in challenging cases. Furthermore, intraoperative refinements and postoperative management approaches will be reviewed to minimize refractive surprises and enhance patient satisfaction.

11.2 Preoperative Assessment

11.2.1 Key Biometric Parameters

Accurate preoperative measurements are essential for selecting the appropriate premium IOL and ensuring optimal postoperative refractive outcomes. The following biometric parameters play a crucial role.

Axial Length (AL) Measurement
AL is one of the most critical parameters in IOL power calculation, measuring the distance between the anterior cornea and the retinal pigment epithelium of the retina. Errors in its measurement can lead to significant refractive surprises, especially in very long eyes (>26 mm) or very short (<22 mm) [6]. Two main types of instruments are used to measure the AL: optical biometry and A-scan ultrasound (applanation ultrasound). The most accurate method for AL measurement is optical biometry based on the principle of partial coherence interferometry (PCI), such as the IOL Master 500 (Carl Zeiss Meditec, Dublin, CA) or Lenstar LS-900 (Haag-Streit, Köniz, Switzerland) [7, 8, 9]. The advantage of PCI is that this noncontact method neither requires local anesthesia nor represents a risk of infection. In addition, the method precludes an additional source of error in AL measurement caused by the indentation of the cornea. Moreover, pupil dilation is unnecessary in optical biometry using PCI, which has a high longitudinal and transversal resolution. The main drawback of optical biometry is its limited usability in cases of fixation problems or advanced cataract. In cases where optical biometry is not possible due to dense cataracts, ultrasound A-scan biometry can be used, although it is less precise [10, 11, 12]. Measurement of AL constitutes the largest source of error in IOL power calculation. An error of 0.1 mm in AL can cause an error of 0.3 Diopters (D) in IOL power, highlighting the need for precise techniques. Measurement accuracy is considered satisfactory if there is no more fluctuation than 0.15 mm in the same eye and 0.3 mm between the fellow eyes [10, 11, 12, 13].

Another modality uses swept-source optical coherence tomography (SS-OCT)–based biometers. These devices offer improved AL measurements by acquiring data along six axes, enhancing tissue penetration and enabling faster data acquisition. The superior light penetration capabilities and extended scanning range of SS-OCT in imaging posterior segment structures contribute to a higher success rate in AL measurements. This, in turn, is associated with reduced refractive prediction errors, making SS-OCT particularly advantageous for enhancing the accuracy of refractive outcomes. The high acquisition speed of SS-OCT enables the capture of two- and three-dimensional data within hundredths of a millisecond, offering high lateral and axial resolution (approximately 5 μm), while minimizing motion artifacts resulting from patient eye movements. Additionally, SS-OCT employs an invisible light source, which enhances patient comfort and improves the signal-to-noise ratio. The IOLMaster 700 (Carl Zeiss Meditec, Dublin, CA), the first biometer based on SS-OCT technology, acquires multiple biometric parameters—including AL, ACD, lens thickness (LT), and central corneal thickness (CCT)—in a single acquisition aligned with the eye's visual axis. It also allows for visualization of the foveal contour, facilitating confirmation of proper fixation during measurement [14].

Keratometry and Corneal Topography
Keratometry (K-values) is essential for determining corneal curvature, which directly impacts IOL power calculation and the selection of toric IOLs. Scheimpflug tomography offer improved accuracy by assessing both anterior and posterior corneal surfaces and global pachymetry in noncontact manner [15], whereas Placido-based corneal topography only measures the anterior corneal surface [16]. The importance of posterior corneal astigmatism has been increasingly recognized, as neglecting it can lead to incorrect toric IOL power selection and residual astigmatism postoperatively [17, 18, 19]. In addition, topography helps detect corneal irregular astigmatism (higher-order aberrations [HOAs]) including spherical aberration and corneal shape abnormalities after corneal refractive surgery, which may influence IOL choice.

ACD and LT
ACD and LT are important for predicting effective lens position (ELP), which influences IOL power calculation [20]. ACD measurement is particularly relevant in patients receiving multifocal or accommodating IOLs, as variations in lens position can alter the expected refractive outcome. Shallow anterior chambers, often seen in hyperopic eyes, can affect the predictability of multifocal and EDOF IOLs, making accurate preoperative measurements essential [21]. Accurate assessment of ACD is essential to minimize the risk of suboptimal refractive outcomes, particularly in the context of intraocular lens power calculations and surgical planning. ACD can be measured through a range of clinical modalities, including optical and ultrasonic pachymetry, optical low-coherence reflectometry (OLCR) biometry, PCI, scanning slit videokeratography (Orbscan (Bausch and Lomb Inc., Rochester, NY)), slit-scanning Scheimpflug imaging (Pentacam (Oculus Optikgeräte, Wetzlar, Germany)), dual Scheimpflug systems, anterior segment optical coherence tomography (AS-OCT), and magnetic resonance imaging. Both central ACD, defined as the distance between the anterior surface of the lens and the anterior corneal surface, and anatomical ACD, measured from the anterior lens surface to the posterior corneal surface, can be visualized and quantified through anterior segment imaging. Multiple comparative studies have evaluated the agreement and variability of ACD measurements across these technologies [14].

Pupil Size and Its Impact on Multifocal IOL Selection
Pupil size plays a crucial role in the success of multifocal IOLs. A small pupil may limit the function of diffractive multifocal IOLs, potentially reducing the range of

clear vision. Conversely, larger pupils can increase photic phenomena such as glare and halos, which are more pronounced with diffractive IOLs [22]. Assessing pupil size under different lighting conditions (mesopic and scotopic) allows for better patient selection and counselling, helping minimize postoperative dissatisfaction.

11.2.2 Challenges in Postrefractive Surgery Eyes

Patients with a history of corneal refractive surgery, such as laser in situ keratomileusis (LASIK), photorefractive keratectomy (PRK), or radial keratotomy (RK), present additional complexities in IOL power calculations. Since these procedures alter the corneal curvature, standard keratometry readings may no longer provide accurate corneal power estimates.

One major issue is inaccurate corneal power estimation, where conventional keratometry often underestimates the true corneal power, leading to errors in IOL power selection (Shammas, 2018). Specialized formulas such as the Barrett True K, Haigis-L, and Shammas-PL have been developed to improve accuracy in these cases [23]. Another challenge is altered ELP prediction, as postrefractive corneas behave differently compared to normal corneas, further complicating the selection of an appropriate IOL power [24].

Moreover, higher-order aberrations are more common in postrefractive surgery patients, potentially impacting vision quality. Wavefront aberrometer-guided IOL selection may be beneficial in these cases to reduce visual distortions and optimize postoperative clarity.

11.3 IOL Power Calculation Methods

11.3.1 Standard IOL Calculation Formulas

11.3.1.1 SKR/T Formula

The SRK/T (Sanders, Retzlaff, Kraff/Theoretical) formula is a third-generation theoretical formula designed to improve accuracy in longer eyes. It is expressed as:

$$P = A - 2.5L - 0.9K$$

where:

P= IOL power
A= A-constant (manufacturer-provided lens factor)
L= Axial length (in mm)
K= Average keratometry reading (in D (diopters))

SRK/T incorporates a theoretical model for predicting ELP based on AL and corneal curvature, making it more accurate for longer eyes (>24.5 mm).

11.3.1.2 Hoffer Q Formula

The Hoffer Q formula is best suited for shorter AL (<22 mm). It refines ELP estimation using a quadratic term:

$$P = A - 0.4(ACD) - 2.5L - 0.9K$$

where:

ACD= anterior chamber depth

Hoffer Q improves upon the SKR/T formula by better modelling ELP in short eyes [25].

11.3.1.3 Holladay 1 and 2 Formulas

The Holladay 1 formula refines ELP prediction by incorporating a surgeon factor (SF) based on historical outcomes:

$$P = A - SF - 2.5L - 0.9K$$

The Holladay 2 formula is an enhancement that incorporates more biometric variables, including white-to-white (WTW) distance, LT, and preoperative refraction, making it more accurate in both long and short eyes [26].

11.3.1.4 Haigis Formula

The Haigis formula uses three constants (a0, a1, a2) for more precise ELP estimation. It is given by:

$$P = a0 - (a1 \times ACD) - (a2 \times L)$$

where:

$a0$, $a1$, $a2$ are empirically derived lens constants.

The formula is particularly useful in postrefractive surgery eyes where standard ELP assumptions may not hold [27].

11.3.2 Advanced Formulas for Premium IOLs

11.3.2.1 Barrett Universal II (BUII) Formula

The BUII formula is one of the most advanced formulas, incorporating lens position prediction using artificial intelligence. It considers: AL, keratometry (K), ACD, LT, and WTW distance. Unlike traditional formulas, BUII adjusts for anterior segment size variability, making it highly accurate for premium IOLs and postrefractive eyes [28].

11.3.2.2 Olsen Formula

The Olsen formula predicts ELP using ray tracing techniques and integrates LT for a more precise estimation:

$$P = A - 2.5L - 0.9K + LT$$

where *LT* represents lens thickness. This formula is particularly beneficial for eyes with abnormal anterior segment dimensions [29].

11.3.2.3 Hill-RBF Formula

The Hill-RBF (radial basis function) method is an AI-driven formula trained on real-world cataract surgery data. It predicts IOL power using a machine learning model rather than a purely mathematical formula. It is especially effective in outlier eyes, where traditional formulas are less accurate [30].

11.3.2.4 Kane Formula

The Kane formula is a fourth-generation formula that integrates: AL, K, ACD, LT, WTW, and mathematical modelling from artificial intelligence (AI) databases. Studies suggest that the Kane formula has among the lowest mean absolute errors across different eye types [31].

11.3.3 Toric IOL Calculations

11.3.3.1 Barrett Toric Calculator

For astigmatic patients, toric IOL power calculations must account for total corneal astigmatism, not just anterior corneal curvature. The Barrett Toric Calculator incorporates posterior astigmatism to improve accuracy: [32]

$$TCA = ACA + PCA$$

where TCA is total corneal astigmatism, ACA is anterior corneal astigmatism, and PCA is posterior corneal astigmatism. Misalignment of toric IOLs by even one degree reduces astigmatism correction effectiveness by 3.3% [33].

11.3.4 Special Considerations for Postrefractive Surgery Patients

Barrett True K Formula
This formula adjusts keratometry readings for postrefractive surgery patients using historical data and AI-based corrections. It refines corneal power estimations by correcting for preoperative refractive shifts [34].

Haigis-L Formula
A modification of the Haigis formula, Haigis-L uses different lens constants based on altered corneal power in post-LASIK and PRK eyes. It is particularly useful when preoperative refraction data are unavailable. This formula is part of the built-in IOLMaster software. Corneal power is calculated by inputting IOL-Master biometry, which is as follows: AL, ACD, and keratometry (corneal radii). This formula is a regression formula based on statistics. Accuracy may decrease if the eye is on the edge of normal distribution (high myopic or high hyperopic eyes). It is based on LASIK data and is only suitable for post-LVC cases, not post-RK cases [35].

Shammas-PL Formula
Designed specifically for postmyopic LASIK patients, Shammas-PL adjusts standard keratometry readings to account for the reduced central corneal power after laser ablation (Shammas, 2018). It is a "no-history" method, meaning it does not rely on presurgical data [36].

Intraoperative Aberrometer
For eyes with previous refractive surgery, an intraoperative aberrometer (e.g., Optiwave Refractive Analysis (ORA) System (WaveTec Vision, Aliso Viejo, CA)) provides real-time IOL power adjustments. This method measures aphakic refraction before IOL implantation, improving accuracy [37].

11.4 Intraoperative and Postoperative Considerations

Careful intraoperative planning and postoperative assessment are essential for optimizing premium IOL outcomes. Intraoperative aberrometer, proper IOL alignment, and effective management of residual refractive errors enhance patient satisfaction and visual performance.

11.4.1 Role of Intraoperative Aberrometer

Intraoperative aberrometer is a real-time measurement technique used to refine IOL power selection and astigmatism correction. Systems such as the ORA System and Holos Intraop (Clarity Medical Systems, Inc., Houston, TX) provide live feedback on aphakic and pseudophakic refractive error, allowing the surgeon to adjust IOL power or rotation before finalizing implantation. This method is particularly useful in postrefractive surgery patients and those receiving toric IOLs, as it minimizes residual refractive surprises [37].

11.4.2 Managing Residual Refractive Errors

Despite careful preoperative calculations, some patients may experience unexpected postoperative refractive errors. Strategies to manage these include: (1) Laser Vision Correction (PRK/LASIK): suitable for low residual refractive errors post-IOL implantation; (2) Piggyback IOLs: secondary IOLs can be implanted for significant errors; and (3) IOL exchange: indicated when there is a major power miscalculation or dissatisfaction with multifocal/EDOF lenses [38].

11.4.3 Rotational Stability of Toric IOLs

Toric IOL rotation can occur postoperatively due to capsular bag contraction or capsular phimosis. Methods to enhance rotational stability include: capsular tension rings for better centration, marking the eye at the slit lamp before surgery to reduce errors, and intraoperative alignment verification with aberrometry [39].

11.4.4 Enhancement Options for Multifocal and EDOF IOLs

Patients receiving multifocal or extended depth-of-focus IOLs may report halos, glare, or insufficient intermediate vision. Management options include: (1) neuroadaptation counselling: most patients adapt within 3–6 months; (2) pupil-modulating drops: pilocarpine 0.1% can improve focus; (3) laser vision correction: can refine residual ametropia; (4) IOL exchange: reserved for extreme dissatisfaction [40].

11.4.5 Angle Kappa

Angle Kappa is defined as the angle between visual axis and pupillary axis. It has significant clinical implications for refractive surgeons, particularly in hyperopic patients, who often exhibit a large angle kappa. Resulting in misalignment of the center of the pupil with the path of light directed toward the fovea. Photic phenomena, including glare and halos, have been observed in patients implanted with multifocal intraocular lenses (IOLs), particularly in association with a large angle kappa. This is attributed to fovea-centric light rays striking the edge of the diffractive rings, resulting in edge-related glare effects. In contrast, such visual disturbances are generally absent in patients with similar angle kappa values who receive monofocal IOLs, likely due to the minimal presence of concentric steps or ring structures on their surface. Although many patients with a large angle kappa remain asymptomatic, the statistically significant association suggests that preoperative assessment of angle kappa should be considered when planning multifocal IOL implantation [41]. However, in the more recent study by Liu et al. [42], involving patients with large-angle kappa who underwent bilateral multifocal IOL implantation, showed no correlation between angle kappa and patient-reported satisfaction with vision or photic phenomenon. It is known that angle kappa will diminish following cataract surgery, and the angle kappa in this study was only gathered before the cataract surgery, which may interfere with the result. Moreover, this study did not use a validated questionnaire, as one is not available yet.

11.4.6 Angle Alpha

Angle alpha is the angle between center of the limbus and visual axis. Angle kappa appears to have limited reliability as a predictive parameter for patient selection before multifocal intraocular lens implantation, particularly given that it tends to decrease significantly following surgery. In contrast, angle alpha—which remains relatively stable throughout the IOL implantation process—has been shown to substantially influence postoperative visual outcomes, including visual acuity and optical aberrations [43].

11.5 Conclusion

The selection and calculation of premium and special IOLs have evolved significantly with advancements in biometric measurements, mathematical formulas, and artificial intelligence-based prediction models. Ophthalmologists now have access to a range of sophisticated tools, including the BUII, Hill-RBF, Kane, and Olsen formulas, which integrate multiple biometric parameters for enhanced accuracy. These modern approaches have significantly improved refractive outcomes, particularly in complex cases such as postrefractive surgery patients and toric IOL recipients.

A meticulous preoperative assessment, incorporating high-precision measurements of AL, ACD, corneal curvature, and posterior corneal astigmatism, remains the cornerstone of successful IOL implantation. Intraoperative technologies, such as aberrometry, provide real-time refinements that further reduce refractive surprises. Postoperative strategies, including laser enhancements and IOL exchange, serve as corrective measures when residual refractive errors occur.

Despite these advancements, challenges remain in accurately predicting ELP, especially in eyes with extreme biometric variations. The integration of machine learning and artificial intelligence into IOL power calculations is a promising frontier that may further refine outcomes. Future innovations in personalized lens designs and real-time adaptive optics will likely continue to revolutionize cataract and refractive surgery.

In conclusion, precise IOL power calculation is crucial for achieving optimal visual outcomes and patient satisfaction. By leveraging state-of-the-art formulas, intraoperative refinements, and postoperative management strategies, ophthalmologists can enhance the predictability and success of premium IOL implantation. The continued evolution of IOL technologies and calculation methodologies will undoubtedly shape the future of cataract and refractive surgery, offering patients superior vision and improved quality of life.

References

1. Zvorničanin J, Zvorničanin E. Premium intraocular lenses: the past, present and future. J Curr Ophthalmol. 2018;30(4):287–96. https://doi.org/10.1016/j.joco.2018.04.003.
2. Xiao G, Sulewski ME, Woreta FA. Current advances and future of premium IOLs. Curr Surg Report. 2022;10(12):223–30. https://doi.org/10.1007/s40137-022-00333-w.
3. Gupta A, Singh P. Intraocular lens power calculation. In: StatPearls [Internet]. Treasure Island: StatPearls Publishing; 2025. [cited 2025 Mar 11]. Available from: http://www.ncbi.nlm.nih.gov/books/NBK589643/.
4. Olsen T. Sources of error in intraocular lens power calculation. J Cataract Refract Surg. 1992;18(2):125–9. https://doi.org/10.1016/s0886-3350(13)80917-0.
5. Shammas HJ, Shammas MC, Jivrajka RV, Cooke DL, Potvin R. Effects on IOL power calculation and expected clinical outcomes of axial length measurements based on multiple vs single refractive indices. Clin Ophthalmol. 2020;14:1511–9. https://doi.org/10.2147/OPTH.S256851.
6. Wang L, Shirayama M, Ma XJ, Kohnen T, Koch DD. Optimizing intraocular lens power calculations in eyes with axial lengths above 25.0 mm. J Cataract Refract Surg. 2011;37(11):2018–27. https://doi.org/10.1016/j.jcrs.2011.05.042.
7. Sheng H, Bottjer CA, Bullimore MA. Ocular component measurement using the Zeiss IOLMaster. Optom Vis Sci. 2004;81(1):27–34. https://doi.org/10.1097/00006324-200401000-00007.
8. Pongsachareonnont P, Tangjanyatam S. Accuracy of axial length measurements obtained by optical biometry and acoustic biometry in rhegmatogenous retinal detachment: a prospective study. Clin Ophthalmol. 2018;12:973–80. https://doi.org/10.2147/OPTH.S165875. eCollection 2018

9. McAlinden C, Wang Q, Pesudovs K, Yang X, Bao F, Yu A, et al. Axial length measurement failure rates with the IOLMaster and lenstar LS 900 in eyes with cataract. PLoS One. 2015;10(6):e0128929. https://doi.org/10.1371/journal.pone.0128929. eCollection 2015
10. Hart L. Biometry/axial length in ophthalmic ultrasound. J Diagnostic Med Sonogr. 1999;15(6):238–42.
11. Rose LT, Moshegov CN. Comparison of the Zeiss IOLMaster and applanation A-scan ultrasound: biometry for intraocular lens calculation. Clin Experiment Ophthalmol. 2003;31(2):121–4. https://doi.org/10.1046/j.1442-9071.2003.00617.x.
12. Srinivas SP, Young AL, Behndig A, Chang DF, Dhubhghaill SN, Eom Y, Fan AH, Findl O, Gundersen KG, Khanna RC, Kohnen T, Mah FS, Miller KM, Nanavaty MA, Nuijts R, Oshika T, Pardianto G, Reus NJ, Ruit S, Sharma N, Venkatesh R, Zhang M, Zheng K, Rao SK, Alió JL. Controversies, consensuses and guidelines on modern cataract surgery by the Academy of Asia-Pacific Professors of Ophthalmology (AAPPO). Asia Pac J Ophthalmol (Phila). 2025:100224. https://doi.org/10.1016/j.apjo.2025.100224. PMID: 40628343
13. Agarwal A. Premium IOL In: Agarwal A, Agarwal A, Jacob S. Phacoemulsification. 4th edn. Jaypee Brothers Medical Publishers; 2012. p. 407–412. https://doi.org/10.5005/jp/books/11485_36
14. Gupta V, Pal H, Sawhney S, Aggarwal A, Vanathi M, Luthra G. Optimization of biometry for best refractive outcome in cataract surgery. Indian J Ophthalmol. 2024;72(1):29–43. https://doi.org/10.4103/IJO.IJO_1219_23.
15. Belin MW, Ambrósio R. Scheimpflug imaging for keratoconus and ectatic disease. Indian J Ophthalmol. 2013;61(8):401–6. https://doi.org/10.4103/0301-4738.116059.
16. Martin R. Cornea and anterior eye assessment with placido-disc keratoscopy, slit scanning evaluation topography and scheimpflug imaging tomography. Indian J Ophthalmol. 2018;66(3):360–6. https://doi.org/10.4103/ijo.IJO_850_17.
17. Liu W, Yang L, Liu J. The impact of posterior corneal astigmatism on surgically induced astigmatism in cataract surgery. Int J Gen Med. 2022;15:8417–25. https://doi.org/10.2147/IJGM.S382774.
18. Moshirfar M. Importance of posterior corneal astigmatism in eyes with Keratoconus. J Ophthalmic Vis Res. 2018;13(1):1–2. https://doi.org/10.4103/jovr.jovr_271_17.
19. Koch DD, Ali SF, Weikert MP, Shirayama M, Jenkins R, Wang L. Contribution of posterior corneal astigmatism to total corneal astigmatism. J Cataract Refract Surg. 2012;38(12):2080–7. https://doi.org/10.1016/j.jcrs.2012.08.036.
20. Findl O, Hirnschall N, Kronschläger M. Anterior chamber depth and IOL calculations. In: Aramberri J, Hoffer KJ, Olsen T, Savini G, Shammas HJ, editors. Intraocular lens calculations [Internet]. Cham: Springer International Publishing; 2024. [cited 2025 Mar 17]. p. 537–50. https://doi.org/10.1007/978-3-031-50666-6_35.
21. Lee Y, Kim MK, Oh JY, Choi HJ, Yoon CH. Intraocular lens power calculation in eyes with a shallow anterior chamber depth and normal axial length. PLoS One. 2023;18(7):e0288554. https://doi.org/10.1371/journal.pone.0288554.
22. Ukai Y, Mito T, Nakatsugawa Y, Seki Y, Mita N, Shibuya E, et al. Risk factors for photic phenomena in two different multifocal diffractive intraocular lenses. Sci Rep. 2025;15(1):121. https://doi.org/10.1038/s41598-024-83838-x.
23. Christopher KL, Patnaik JL, Miller DC, Lynch AM, Taravella MJ, Davidson RS. Accuracy of intraoperative Aberrometry, Barrett True-K with and without posterior cornea measurements, Shammas-PL, and Haigis-L formulas after myopic refractive surgery. J Refract Surg. 2021;37(1):60–8. https://doi.org/10.3928/1081597X-20201030-02.
24. Wang XZ, Cui R, Song XD, Yun B, Qian J, Ding N. Comparison of the accuracy of intraocular lens power calculation formulas for eyes after corneal refractive surgery. Ann Transl Med. 2020;8(14):871. https://doi.org/10.21037/atm-20-4624.
25. Hoffer KJ. The Hoffer Q formula: a comparison of theoretic and regression formulas. J Cataract Refract Surg. 1993;19(6):700–12. https://doi.org/10.1016/s0886-3350(13)80338-0.

26. CookeDL,AramberriJ.Holladayformulas.In:AramberriJ,HofferKJ,OlsenT,SaviniG,Shammas HJ, editors. Intraocular lens calculations [Internet]. Cham: Springer International Publishing; 2024. [cited 2025 Mar 17]. p. 661–72. https://doi.org/10.1007/978-3-031-50666-6_44.
27. Haigis W, Hoffer KJ. The Haigis Formula. In: Aramberri J, Hoffer KJ, Olsen T, Savini G, Shammas HJ, editors. Intraocular lens calculations [Internet]. Cham: Springer International Publishing; 2024. [cited 2025 Mar 17]. p. 625–36. https://doi.org/10.1007/978-3-031-50666-6_41.
28. Barrett GD. Barrett formulas: strategies to improve IOL power prediction. In: Aramberri J, Hoffer KJ, Olsen T, Savini G, Shammas HJ, editors. Intraocular lens calculations [Internet]. Cham: Springer International Publishing; 2024. [cited 2025 Mar 17]. p. 577–92. https://doi.org/10.1007/978-3-031-50666-6_37.
29. Olsen T. The olsen formula. In: Aramberri J, Hoffer KJ, Olsen T, Savini G, Shammas HJ, editors. Intraocular lens calculations [Internet]. Cham: Springer International Publishing; 2024. [cited 2025 Mar 17]. p. 731–40. https://doi.org/10.1007/978-3-031-50666-6_50.
30. Roberts TV, Hodge C, Sutton G, Lawless M, Contributors to the Vision Eye Institute IOL Outcomes Registry. Comparison of Hill-radial basis function, Barrett Universal and current third generation formulas for the calculation of intraocular lens power during cataract surgery. Clin Experiment Ophthalmol. 2018;46(3):240–6. https://doi.org/10.1111/ceo.13034.
31. Kane JX. Kane formula. In: Aramberri J, Hoffer KJ, Olsen T, Savini G, Shammas HJ, editors. Intraocular lens calculations [Internet]. Cham: Springer International Publishing; 2024. [cited 2025 Mar 17]. p. 689–94. https://doi.org/10.1007/978-3-031-50666-6_46.
32. Abulafia A, Barrett GD, Kleinmann G, Ofir S, Levy A, Marcovich AL, et al. Prediction of refractive outcomes with toric intraocular lens implantation. J Cataract Refract Surg. 2015;41(5):936–44. https://doi.org/10.1016/j.jcrs.2014.08.036.
33. Titiyal JS, Kaur M, Jose CP, Falera R, Kinkar A, Bageshwar LM. Comparative evaluation of toric intraocular lens alignment and visual quality with image-guided surgery and conventional three-step manual marking. OPTH. 2018;12:747–53. https://doi.org/10.2147/OPTH.S164175.
34. Debellemanière G, Mechleb N, Bernier T, Ancel JM, Gauvin M, Wallerstein A, et al. The development of a thick-lens post–myopic laser vision correction intraocular lens calculation formula. Am J Ophthalmol. 2024;262:40–7. https://doi.org/10.1016/j.ajo.2023.09.023.
35. Pan X, Wang Y, Li Z, Ye Z. Intraocular lens power calculation in eyes after myopic laser refractive surgery and radial keratotomy: bayesian network meta-analysis. Am J Ophthalmol. 2024;262:48–61. https://doi.org/10.1016/j.ajo.2023.09.026.
36. Shammas HJ, Cooke DL, Riaz KM, Tonk R, Shammas MC, Bleeker A, et al. Updating the no-history method in intraocular lens power calculation after myopic laser vision correction. J Cataract Refract Surg. 2024;50(10):1026. https://doi.org/10.1097/j.jcrs.0000000000001508.
37. Kaufman AR, Pineda R. Intraoperative aberrometry: an update on applications and outcomes. Curr Opin Ophthalmol. 2023;34(1):48–57. https://doi.org/10.1097/ICU.0000000000000915.
38. Alio JL, Abdelghany AA, Fernández-Buenaga R. Management of residual refractive error after cataract surgery. Curr Opin Ophthalmol. 2014;25(4):291–7. https://doi.org/10.1097/ICU.000000000000006.
39. Singh A, Kapoor G, Baranwal VK, Kalra N. Rotational stability of Toric intraocular lenses. Med J Armed Force India. 2022;78(1):68–73. https://doi.org/10.1016/j.mjafi.2020.03.014. Epub 2020 Jul 9
40. Alio JL, Abdelghany AA, Fernández-Buenaga R. Enhancements after cataract surgery. Curr Opin Ophthalmol. 2015;26(1):50–5. https://doi.org/10.1097/ICU.0000000000000111.
41. Prakash G, Jacob S, Agarwal A. Angle Kappa: the angle to the mystery of multifocal IOLs. In: Agarwal A, Agarwal A, Jacob S, editors. Phacoemulsification. 4th ed. Jaypee Brothers Medical Publishers; 2012. p. 407–12. https://doi.org/10.5005/jp/books/11485_36.

42. Liu X, Hannan SJ, Schallhorn SC, Schallhorn JM. Angle Kappa is not correlated with patient-reported outcomes after multifocal lens implantation. Clin Ophthalmol. 2024;18:605–12. https://doi.org/10.2147/OPTH.S452147.
43. Cervantes-Coste G, Tapia A, Corredor-Ortega C, Osorio M, Valdez R, Massaro M, Velasco-Barona C, Gonzalez-Salinas R. The influence of angle alpha, angle kappa, and optical aberrations on visual outcomes after the implantation of a high-addition trifocal IOL. J Clin Med. 2022;11(3):896. https://doi.org/10.3390/jcm11030896.

Chapter 12
Optimizing IOL Power Calculation in High-Volume, Hospital-Based Cataract Surgery

Nashrul Ihsan and Rio Rhendy

12.1 Introduction

Biometry is a critical step in modern cataract and refractive surgery. Biometry for cataract surgery typically includes measuring axial length (AL), keratometry (K), anterior chamber depth (ACD), lens thickness (LT), and cornea diameter (WTW). These measurements feed into the IOL calculator/formulae that we needed for emetropia or another desired refraction. In high-volume cataract center, performing this examination accurately is important because of the large number of patients and often limited opportunities for postoperative refinements [1].

Unlike personalized cataract procedures in private clinics, high-volume hospital settings face multiple limitations: time pressure in preoperative assessment, variable operator skills (including resident/fellowship programs), limited access to premium biometers, and incomplete patient history. Despite these challenges, achieving optimal refractive results remains essential to reduce postoperative spectacle dependence and improve patient satisfaction [1–3].

This chapter provides a structured guide to intraocular lens (IOL) calculation tailored to high-throughput, hospital-based environments [4–6]. Topics include device selection, formula application, workflow optimization, artificial intelligence integration, and practical considerations in complex cases.

All authors declare no financial interest.

N. Ihsan (✉)
JEC Eye Hospitals & Clinics, Jakarta, Indonesia

R. Rhendy
Cipto Mangunkusumo Hospital, Jakarta, Indonesia

Universitas Indonesia, Jakarta, Indonesia

G. Pardianto (ed.), *Intraocular Lens (IOL) Power Calculation*,
https://doi.org/10.1007/978-981-92-1223-1_12

12.2 Fundamentals of IOL Calculation in High-Volume, Hospital-Based Cataract Surgery

In high-volume hospital cataract surgery, precision and reproducibility are paramount. IOL power calculation depends primarily on accurate axial length (AL) and keratometry (K) measurements. Additional parameters such as anterior chamber depth (ACD) and lens thickness (LT) enhance modern formula accuracy [1].

Optical biometers (e.g., IOLMaster 700, IOLMaster 500 (Carl Zeiss Meditec, Dublin, CA)) are preferred for their speed and accuracy, but immersion Amplitude mode-scan or A-scan (e.g., Aviso (Quantel Medical, France), and AL Scan (Nidek Co, Aichi, Japan)) remains essential for mature cataracts. Device selection is based on clarity of the visual axis, patient cooperation, and workflow efficiency. Training protocols emphasize accuracy, with regular calibration and supervision. Integration of biometric data into EMRs or surgical planning systems improves documentation, reduces error, and supports postoperative audits [1–3].

Common formulas include Sanders-Retzlaff-Kraff/Theoretical (SRK/T), Hoffer Q, Barrett Universal II (BUII), and Kane. Each has specific indications based on axial length, device type, and available data. Training staff in biometry acquisition, ensuring consistent calibration, and adopting evidence-based formula selection protocols are key to optimizing outcomes [1, 4, 6, 7].

12.3 Workflow Optimization

A well-established cataract center will inevitably attract a large number of patients. Real-world hospital settings face challenges, including device downtime, trainee variability, and complex pathology. Standardized workflows are crucial: technician-led biometry, resident validation, preop planning sessions, and written protocols for subluxated, pediatric, or traumatic eyes. Standardization of examinations and accuracy in diagnostic assessments must be ensured and regularly evaluated by the clinical staff. Therefore, comprehensive training is essential to understand the principles of proper examination techniques and to recognize potential pitfalls [2, 4].

This can be achieved through training provided by the respective machine technicians. The training should cover the fundamentals of ocular anatomy, principles of ultrasound use, proper examination positioning, interpretation of reliable biometry results, and the ability to assess special cases. Training may be conducted prior to the machine's arrival, during the machine demonstration, or repeated as needed—for instance, when new hospital staff members join or when significant refractive surprises are observed postoperatively. Such training must be continuous; therefore, most eye centers establish their own internal training modules [2, 5].

Special delegation may be assigned to staff working in the Cataract Diagnostic Center (CDC) or, if necessary, to hospital personnel dedicated exclusively to biometry. Such restricted delegation helps improve the consistency of biometry results, particularly with contact and immersion techniques. Dedicated biometry staff should also be capable of operating different types of biometry devices. More experienced staff members may serve as reviewers for questionable results, such as significant axial length discrepancies between fellow eyes or suspicious keratometry values in postlaser vision correction cases [4, 6].

Advanced biometry devices provide greater reliability and automated measurements, making training easier to extend to a broader group of hospital staff. Optical biometry and swept-source biometry generally offer higher reliability compared to immersion and contact methods. Immersion biometry results—particularly with contact techniques—are highly operator-dependent. For this reason, contact biometry is best performed by senior staff and gradually delegated to junior personnel under supervision [2].

Additional examinations commonly performed include keratometry, biometry, specular microscopy, and retinometry. Among these, biometry requires particular attention. In certain cases, optical biometry cannot be performed due to inherent device limitations, necessitating a follow-up with immersion biometry. Since immersion biometry involves direct contact with the patient's globe, topical anesthesia is required. This examination demands specific expertise to ensure both accuracy and result validity; therefore, it is recommended that immersion biometry be performed as the final step in the diagnostic workflow [3, 4].

Additional diagnostic evaluations for advanced cataract cases may include macular evaluations by optical coherence tomography (OCT), corneal topography, OCT evaluations for glaucoma and retinal nerve fiber layer (RNFL), visual field testing, fundus photography, or ultrasonography (USG) [1–4].

Patients scheduled for multifocal IOL implantation require fundus photography, macular OCT, corneal topography, and glaucoma OCT. All of these ancillary tests are noncontact, with the exception that fundus photography typically requires pharmacologic dilation, unless the center is equipped with ultra-widefield retinal imaging (Optos camera (Optos, Dunfermline, UK), or Clarus 700 (Carl Zeiss Meditec, Dublin, CA)). Therefore, dilated examinations can be performed after corneal topography or visual field testing, with no specific sequence required for these ancillary assessments.

12.4 Special Populations in Public Eye Hospitals

High-volume public hospitals manage complex cataract cases: mature cataracts, subluxated lenses, traumatic cataracts, postvitrectomy, uveitic, and pediatric eyes. Each requires adapted biometry strategies. These complexities highlight the importance of flexible protocols, experienced supervision, and outcome tracking [8–11].

Postvitrectomy eyes may have deeper ACDs; Haigis or Barrett is preferred. Uveitic eyes demand careful IOL positioning and inflammation control. Pediatric cases require undercorrection and exam under anesthesia. Subluxated and traumatic eyes often necessitate intraoperative IOL decision-making [10, 11].

For patients with coexisting glaucoma, an initial assessment of disease severity (mild to advanced) is essential. These investigations can be integrated into the cataract surgery work-up, but must account for whether pharmacologic dilation is necessary or not. This evaluation is critical due to the risk of postoperative "wipe-out" vision in severe glaucoma [9, 12, 13].

Cataract patients with retinal pathology also require tailored examinations to determine disease severity. In diabetic patients, it is crucial to assess for macular edema or diabetic retinopathy prior to cataract surgery. Certain cases may require preoperative argon laser photocoagulation or intravitreal antivascular endothelial growth factor (anti-VEGF) injection. For dense cataracts with limited retinal visualization, cataract extraction may be performed first, followed by close postoperative monitoring by the retina team [6, 7, 14].

USG of the globe is particularly important as a primary tool in dense bilateral or unilateral cataracts or when posterior segment visualization is absent, to rule out vitreous hemorrhage or retinal detachment prior to surgery. If the vitreous is clear and the retina attached, further evaluations can proceed. However, if retinal pathology is detected, consultation with a retina specialist is warranted before proceeding with cataract surgery [8, 13].

12.5 Electronic Medical Record (EMR) Integration

Transcription errors and manual data entry can undermine high-volume workflows, potentially leading to costly mistakes in IOL selection. Manual processes such as printing medical records require paper, ink, storage space, and staff time for manual data transfer—all of which increase the risk of data errors. Such mistakes may result in financial losses for physicians and clinics, patient dissatisfaction, or even legal claims due to unsatisfactory surgical outcomes. In some cases, errors can be corrected by procedures such as toric IOL rotation for axis misalignment, IOL exchange, or postcataract surgery laser refractive surgery (LVC) [1, 2, 6, 15].

The use of EMR also presents challenges. For certain ancillary tests, results often need to be printed and scanned into the EMR system, creating workflow bottlenecks in the print–scan–upload process. By contrast, most modern diagnostic devices are equipped with direct data transfer capabilities, eliminating the need for intermediate printing [2, 6].

Reliable internet or intranet connectivity is therefore a fundamental requirement in centers with EMR-integrated systems, particularly those with multiple branches. A strong network backbone, complemented by redundant backup systems, ensures uninterrupted functionality even during network failures. Such robust EMR networking is especially valuable in ophthalmology centers with high patient volumes, enabling faster and more efficient service delivery [2, 5].

An EMR system can also serve as a valuable tool for evaluating patient flow efficiency, from initial registration through to the cashier. In the context of preoperative cataract evaluation, EMR enables the detection and assessment of whether additional diagnostic equipment is required. A well-designed EMR queue management system can identify which diagnostic devices represent workflow bottlenecks within a clinic or hospital. This is particularly relevant for ancillary testing stations where rapid print–scan integration is needed, or where newer devices are available that can transmit data directly into the EMR without intermediate steps [4, 6].

For example, the IOLMaster can be integrated directly with EMR systems. Furthermore, the Zeiss Forum platform allows surgeons to perform IOL calculations directly in the clinic room without relying on printed biometry reports. Zeiss also provides integration with surgical microscopes through the Callisto system (Carl Zeiss Meditec, Dublin, CA), which enables markerless toric IOL alignment. This markerless technology significantly improves the efficiency of the preoperative workflow and enhances accuracy in toric IOL implantation [4, 5].

12.6 Quality Control Measure

Quality control measures are essential to improving the standard of care. Biometry outcomes can be evaluated by sampling regular cases to assess the accuracy of biometry predictions in routine patients. Ultrasound contact biometry, in particular, is highly operator-dependent. To enhance accuracy, contact biometry should be restricted to designated staff, which also facilitates quality evaluation of results [2].

Immersion ultrasound biometry is less operator-dependent and generally easier to perform. This task can be delegated to staff who have received appropriate immersion biometry training. Evaluation can be conducted by comparing postoperative refractive outcomes against preoperative refractive targets [2, 6, 15].

Optical biometry requires minimal specialized training. Its advantage lies in higher accuracy of keratometry and axial length measurements, as well as simplified workflow without the need for extensive operator expertise [2, 4].

Quality control in biometry is critical because it directly affects surgical outcomes. Consistency must be maintained not only in measurement technique—particularly in contact and immersion methods—but also in relation to the IOL used, since A-constants vary among lens types [1, 3, 6].

Outcome evaluation should also account for workflow efficiency in high-volume settings, such as when the clinic is overcrowded and long waiting times occur. This includes monitoring for erroneous biometry measurements or refractive surprises postoperatively. Special or atypical cases—such as irregular astigmatism, postpterygium surgery, keratoconus, silicone-filled eyes, post-LVC eyes, or patients scheduled for IOL exchange—should be clearly flagged in the workflow. Nurses should communicate these cases to supervising staff or surgeons to avoid redundant examinations and delays. In such scenarios, communication between nursing staff and surgeons regarding the IOL type is essential to ensure accurate integration of biometry results into the EMR [1, 3, 7, 15].

In high-volume clinics, quality monitoring also requires robust data speed and storage capacity. As patient data accumulate, server upgrades and higher internet/

intranet capacity may eventually be required. Data transfer processes (exporting/importing) carry risks of data loss, underscoring the importance of a capable IT team within the hospital or clinic. Safeguarding patient data must remain a top priority, as both personal and medical information are strictly confidential [1, 5, 6].

References

1. Norrby S. Sources of error in intraocular lens power calculation. J Cataract Refract Surg. 2008;34(3):368–76. https://doi.org/10.1016/j.jcrs.2007.10.031.
2. Karimi S, Arabi A, Shahraki T, Javadi MA, Safi S. Resident-performed phacoemulsification cataract surgery: impact of resident-level characteristics. J Curr Ophthalmol. 2023;35(1):29–35. Published 2023 Aug 11. https://doi.org/10.4103/joco.joco_58_21.
3. Rossi T, Romano MR, Iannetta D, et al. Cataract surgery practice patterns worldwide: a survey. BMJ Open Ophthalmol. 2021;6(1):e000464. Published 2021 Jan 13. https://doi.org/10.1136/bmjophth-2020-000464.
4. Darcy K, Gunn D, Tavassoli S, Sparrow J, Kane JX. Assessment of the accuracy of new and updated intraocular lens power calculation formulas in 10 930 eyes from the UK National Health Service. J Cataract Refract Surg. 2020;46(1):2–7. https://doi.org/10.1016/j.jcrs.2019.08.014.
5. Eckert KA, Carter MJ, Das AV, Lansingh VC. The prediction capability of a cataract surgery risk stratification model based on a large electronic medical record dataset. Indian J Ophthalmol. 2022;70(11):3948–53. https://doi.org/10.4103/ijo.IJO_1489_22.
6. Srinivas SP, Young AL, Behndig A, et al. Controversies, consensuses and guidelines on modern cataract surgery by the academy of Asia-Pacific professors of ophthalmology (AAPPO). Asia Pac J Ophthalmol (Phila). 2025;14(4):100224. https://doi.org/10.1016/j.apjo.2025.100224.
7. Ryu S, Jun I, Kim TI, Kim EK, Seo KY. Accuracy of the Kane formula for intraocular lens power calculation in comparison with existing formulas: a retrospective review. Yonsei Med J. 2021;62(12):1117–24. https://doi.org/10.3349/ymj.2021.62.12.1117.
8. Roessler GF, Huth JK, Dietlein TS, et al. Accuracy and reproducibility of axial length measurement in eyes with silicone oil endotamponade. Br J Ophthalmol. 2009;93(11):1492–4. https://doi.org/10.1136/bjo.2008.152637.
9. Ozates S, Berker N, Cakar Ozdal P, Ozdamar Erol Y. Phacoemulsification in patients with uveitis: long-term outcomes. BMC Ophthalmol. 2020;20(1):109. Published 2020 Mar 17. https://doi.org/10.1186/s12886-020-01373-5.
10. Nihalani BR, VanderVeen DK. Benchmarks for outcome indicators in pediatric cataract surgery. Eye (Lond). 2017;31(3):417–21. https://doi.org/10.1038/eye.2016.240.
11. Wójcik-Niklewska B, Nocoń-Bratek M, Szala K. Intraocular lens power calculation in pediatric cataract surgery: a narrative review. Medicine (Baltimore). 2025;104(14):e42072. https://doi.org/10.1097/MD.0000000000042072.
12. Vanags J, Laganovska G. Long-term outcome of cataract surgery in eyes with pseudoexfoliation syndrome associated with weak Zonules: a case report. Case Rep Ophthalmol. 2020;11(1):54–9. Published 2020 Jan 29. https://doi.org/10.1159/000505720.
13. Foster GJL, Allen QB, Ayres BD, et al. Phacoemulsification of the rock-hard dense nuclear cataract: Options and recommendations. J Cataract Refract Surg. 2018;44(7):905–16. https://doi.org/10.1016/j.jcrs.2018.03.038.
14. Yang Y, Chen H, An J, Fan W. Long-term effects of phacoemulsification and intraocular lens implantation in a patient with pathologic myopia and extremely long axial length: A case report. Medicine (Baltimore). 2020;99(37):e22081. https://doi.org/10.1097/MD.0000000000022081.
15. Jain P, Nema N. Incidence of refractive surprise after phacoemulsification in patients of cataract with primary pterygium. Saudi J Ophthalmol. 2023;37(2):79–82. Published 2023 Feb 27. https://doi.org/10.4103/sjopt.sjopt_211_21.

Chapter 13
Optimized Calculation Methods for Mass, Charitable, and Rural Cataract Surgery Programs: Phacoemulsification

Darmawan M. Sophian, Vidyapati Widiarto Mangunkusumo, and Faraby Martha

13.1 Introduction

Cataracts remain the leading cause of avoidable blindness worldwide, affecting approximately 94 million people, and account for a significant proportion of visual impairment, particularly in low- and middle-income countries [1, 2]. The prevalence of cataract-induced visual impairment is significantly higher in rural areas compared to urban centers, primarily due to disparities in healthcare access, availability of skilled ophthalmologists, and socioeconomic challenges that delay diagnosis and treatment [3]. The cataract surgery rate (CSR), the number of cataract surgeries performed per million population per year, is the key indicator used to benchmark a country's capacity to address cataract-induced blindness, and global CSRs range from as low as 36 to as high as 12,800 per million population [1, 2].

This variability is not simply a matter of resource availability; it is fundamentally a planning and calculation problem. Mass, charitable, and rural cataract programs such as Aravind Eye Care System and Tilganga Eye Centre achieve CSRs many multiples higher than the regional average not because they have more surgeons per

---

All authors declare no financial interest.

Vidyapati Widiarto Mangunkusumo has died before the publication of this book.

D. M. Sophian (✉)
Saruni Eye Clinic, Pandeglang, Banten, Indonesia

V. W. Mangunkusumo
JEC Eye Hospitals & Clinics, Jakarta, Indonesia

F. Martha
Cipto Mangunkusumo Hospital, Jakarta, Indonesia

Universitas Indonesia, Jakarta, Indonesia

G. Pardianto (ed.), *Intraocular Lens (IOL) Power Calculation*,
https://doi.org/10.1007/978-981-92-1223-1_13

capita, but because they have engineered every stage of the program, patient flow, IOL power selection, supply consumption, and unit cost, around explicit, reproducible calculations. In India, mass campaigns increased the number of cataract surgeries performed annually from 1.2 million in 1992 to 3.86 million in 2003, a scale-up that was only possible because patient throughput, consumable use, and surgical capacity were modeled quantitatively rather than managed ad hoc [4].

This chapter departs from a purely descriptive treatment of mass cataract programs. Its purpose is to make explicit the arithmetic that underlies four decisions every program director or operating surgeon must make repeatedly: (1) which intraocular lens (IOL) power formula to apply and how to compute the implanted power from biometric inputs; (2) how to size daily surgical capaacity and screening throughput from a target backlog-clearance time; (3) how to model the true unit cost of a case and locate the program's break-even volume; and (4) how to interpret population-level outcome data to decide where calculation-method choices most affect a program's results. Each of these is presented with the governing equation, the input parameters, and a fully worked numerical example so that the method can be applied directly to a program's own data rather than merely recognized by name.

13.2 Challenges in Mass Cataract Surgery Programs

High-volume cataract surgery programs face five recurring constraints that any calculation framework must take as inputs rather than ignore. Resource scarcity limits the number of surgical instrument sets, intraocular lenses, and trained personnel available at a rural site, which caps daily throughput regardless of patient demand [2]. Patient mobilization requires outreach and education capacity that determines how many of the eligible candidates identified by screening actually present on surgical day [5]. Quality assurance becomes harder to sustain as volume rises, since low complication rates depend on supervision and training that do not scale linearly with case count [1]. Cost management requires balancing free or subsidized surgery against the program's financial sustainability [4]. Follow-up care is often the most difficult constraint to satisfy in remote settings, where return visits are limited by distance and transport cost [6]. Each of these constraints reappears as a parameter in following sections: resource scarcity bounds the daily case capacity used in the patient-flow model; mobilization yield determines the screening-to-surgery conversion ratio; and cost management is the direct subject of the cost model in Section 13.6.

13.3 Key Parameters for Optimization

Five categories of parameters must be quantified, not merely named, before a mass cataract program can be optimized: patient flow, surgical capacity, cost structure, logistics, and quality control. The remainder of this chapter develops the calculation method for each. Patient flow parameters are generated by the screening funnel: individuals screened, then candidates confirmed eligible for surgery, then patients who present on surgical day. The conversion ratios between these stages, the eligibility yield and the attendance yield, must be measured locally and updated after each campaign, because the calculations in Section 13.5 (daily quota, screening targets) are directly proportional to these ratios. Surgical capacity parameters are bounded by the number of operating tables or microscopes, the effective operating time per session, and the mean procedure time per case, including turnover time between cases; these combine in Section 13.5 into a single daily-throughput equation. Cost structure parameters separate into a fixed component, independent of case volume over the planning horizon (equipment depreciation, venue, core staff salaries), and a variable component per case (IOL, viscoelastic, sutures, disposables, and consumable medication); total program cost at volume Q is the fixed cost plus the variable cost per case multiplied by Q, the formula developed fully in Section 13.6. Logistics parameters require consumable inventory, such as IOLs and viscoelastics, to be matched to expected case volume with a safety buffer, since understocking halts surgery mid-campaign while over-stocking ties up scarce charitable funding in unused supplies; Section 13.5 develops the reorder-point calculation used to size this buffer. Quality control parameters are tracked through intraoperative complication rate and the proportion of eyes achieving postoperative best-corrected visual acuity of 6/18 or better, both of which should be measured per surgeon, per session, and per IOL formula in use.

13.4 Optimized Calculation Methods

To obtain the desired targeted postoperative refractive outcome and minimize the PE, clinical measurements and IOL calculation have to be accurate. Most of the error source is inaccuracy in the IOL formula's predictions of the postoperative IOL position (35.5%), postoperative refraction determination (27%), inaccuracies in AL (17%), and keratometry measurements (10.1%) [7].

Accurate IOL power calculation is essential for optimal visual outcomes post-cataract surgery. In urban settings, advanced diagnostic tools and technologies facilitate precise measurements of ocular parameters, leading to better refractive outcomes. Conversely, rural areas may lack access to such sophisticated equipment, potentially compromising the accuracy of IOL power calculations [2, 7, 8].

In large-scale cataract surgery programs, especially those conducted in resource-limited settings, adopting efficient and reliable methods for IOL power calculation is crucial. However, the accuracy of IOL power calculation remains a challenge [7]. Various formulas have been developed to enhance the accuracy of these calculations (Table 13.1). Among the numerous available formulas, studies indicate that third-generation formulas, particularly Sanders-Retzlaff-Kraff/Theoretical (SRK/T) and Holladay 1, provide highly accurate outcomes for eyes with medium-long AL (24.50–25.99 mm), and Hoffer Q is suitable for short eyes [9]. These formulas

Table 13.1 Common IOL power calculation formulas and their applications [7, 9]

Formula	Best for axial length	Key features
SRK/T	Medium-long	Widely available, robust
Holladay 1	Medium-long	Integrates ACD, surgeon factor
Hoffer Q	Short	Optimal for small eyes
Barrett Universal II (BUII)	All ranges	Requires advanced biometry

remain widely utilized in clinical practice and continue to be effective for IOL power calculations in a broad range of patient cases. The SRK/T formula is widely accessible due to its incorporation in numerous biometric measuring devices, making it a prevalent tool for calculating intraocular lens power. In clinical practice, the SRK/T formula serves as a readily available resource, enabling clinicians to achieve relatively accurate calculation outcomes even in constrained hardware environments. Its accessibility and practicality underscore its significant clinical application value in the field of ophthalmology [7, 9].

Beyond formula selection, the underlying calculation itself should be made explicit. The original SRK formula, still embedded as a fallback in many low-cost biometers used in outreach settings, is a linear regression on two variables: $P = A - 2.5L - 0.9K$, where P is the implant power in diopters, A is a lens-specific constant supplied by the manufacturer, L is the axial length in millimeters, and K is the mean corneal power in diopters. The SRK II formula extends this with an axial-length-dependent correction term C: $P = A - 2.5L - 0.9K + C$, with $C = +3.0$ for $AL < 20.0$ mm, +2.0 for 20.0-20.99mm, +1.0 for 21.0-21.99mm, 0 for 22.0-24.49 mm, and -0.5 for $AL \geq 24.5$ mm. Consider a patient screened during a rural outreach camp with optical biometry measurements of axial length $L = 23.50$ mm and mean keratometry $K = 44.00$ D, targeting emmetropia, with an IOL whose manufacturer-supllied A-constant is 118.0. Applying the SRK formula: $P = 118.0 - (2.5 \times 23.50) - (0.9 \times 44.00) = 118.0 - 58.75 - 39.60 = 19.65$ D. Available IOL powers are typically stocked in 0.5 D steps; the program would implant the 19.5 D or 20.0 D lens depending on whether slight myopic or hyperopic target is preferred. Manufacturer A-constants are population averages and rarely match a program's own combination of biometer, technique, and IOL stock exactly. The constant can be back-calculated from accumulated postoperative refraction data: $A = P(\text{implanted}) + 2.5L + 0.9K$, where the ideal power is $P(\text{ideal}) = P(\text{implanted}) + (RE \times RF)$, RE being the achieved postoperative refractive error and RF a refractive factor (commonly 1.5). For example, a patient implanted with 20.0 D and a stable postoperative refraction of +1.0 D would have an ideal power of $20.0 + (1.0 \times 1.5) = 21.5$ D. Averaging this back-calculation across 50–100 recent cases per IOL model, repeated annually, yields the program's own optimized constant for prospective use.

13.5 Calculation Methods for Patient Flow and Surgical Capacity

Effective management of large patient volumes in mass cataract surgical operations involves integration of structured operational protocols, strategic workforce arrangement, and real-time technological solutions.

Preoperative efficiency can be significantly enhanced through the arrangement of community health workers equipped with mobile screening applications, which allow for accurate identification, triage, and prioritization of surgical candidates prior to the event, thereby reducing congestion and improving patient preparedness.

On the surgical day, principles of queuing theory can be systematically applied to regulate patient movement through preoperative evaluation, anesthesia administration, surgical intervention, and postoperative recovery, ensuring optimal use of surgical team capacities. Comprehensive patient education, initiated during prescreening and reinforced upon arrival at the surgical site, mitigates confusion and anxiety, contributing to smoother patient flow and better compliance with procedural instructions.

Furthermore, the implementation of real-time data-tracking systems through smartphone applications empowers program managers to monitor patient progress dynamically and reallocate human resources swiftly to critical points along the workflow, thereby preserving operational fluidity despite the inherent unpredictability of high-volume environments [11]. Collectively, these integrated strategies form a scalable, adaptive model capable of sustaining high-quality surgical outcomes in mass cataract surgery initiatives. Managing large patient volumes is, at its core, a capacity-planning problem. The maximum number of cases a program can complete per day is bounded by the number of operating stations (m), the effective operating time per session in minutes (T), the mean procedure time per case (tp), and the turnover time between cases (to): $Q(max) = m \times [T / (tp + to)]$. For example, a camp running $m = 4$ operating stations for $T = 480$ minutes (an 8-hour session), with mean procedure time $tp = 12$ minutes and turnover time $to = 3$ minutes, gives $Q(max) = 4 \times [480 / (12 + 3)] = 4 \times 32 = 128$ cases per day. Programs typically plan to 80–85% of this ceiling to absorb variability in individual case time without cascading delay through the schedule. If a campaign's surgical-day target is N(surg) cases, and the program's historical eligibility yield (the fraction of screened individuals confirmed as candidates) is Ye and attendance yield (the fraction of eligible candidates who present on surgical day) is Ya, then the number of individuals who must be screened is: $N(screen) = N(surg) / (Ye \times Ya)$. Using representative yields of $Ye = 0.35$ and $Ya = 0.70$, reaching a surgical-day target of 100 cases requires screening $N(screen) = 100 / (0.35 \times 0.70) = 100 / 0.245 \approx 408$ individuals. A program that screens only 200 individuals against the same yields should expect roughly 49 surgical cases, not 100, a shortfall that calculation in advance allows the program to correct before the campaign, rather than discover on surgical day. Consumable inventory should be governed by a defined reorder point (ROP) rather than depleted to zero before reordering: ROP = (d × LT) + SS, where SS = z × σd × $\sqrt{LT}$, d is the expected daily consumption rate, LT is the supplier lead time in days, σd is the day-to-day standard deviation in consumption, and z is a service-level factor (commonly 1.65 for approximately 95% service level). For a program consuming a mean of d = 25 IOLs per day with σd = 5 and a supplier lead time of LT = 6 days: SS = 1.65 × 5 × $\sqrt{6}$ ≈ 20 units, and ROP = (25 × 6) + 20 = 170 units, a reorder should be triggered when stock falls to 170 units, not when it is exhausted.

13.6 Cost Calculation Methods for Mass and Charitable Programs

Total program cost at case volume Q can be modeled as C(Q) = F + (V × Q), where F is the fixed cost over the planning period (equipment depreciation, facility rent, core salaried staff) and V is the variable cost per case (IOL, viscoelastic, sutures, disposables). If the program receives an average blended revenue R per case (subsidy plus paying-patient cross-subsidy), the break-even volume is Q* = F / (R – V), for R > V. A program with annual fixed costs F = USD 80,000, variable cost V = USD 25 per case, and blended revenue R = USD 45 per case reaches break-even at Q* = 80,000 / (45 – 25) = 4,000 cases per year. Below this volume the program operates at a deficit covered by donor funding; above it, additional volume contributes margin that can cross-subsidize free cases for the poorest patients. A published micro-costing study from the Aravind Eye Hospital in southern India itemized cost per procedure across three surgical techniques: phacoemulsification averaged USD 25.55 in provider direct cost and USD 12.37 in patient direct and indirect cost; manual small-incision surgery (MSICS) averaged USD 17.03 provider cost and USD 12.37 patient cost; and extracapsular extraction with IOL averaged USD 16.25 provider cost and USD 19.85 patient cost [10]. MSICS combines the lowest total societal cost with outcomes reported as broadly comparable to phacoemulsification, which is why it remains the dominant technique in high-volume, low-resource mass programs. A separately published cost-utility analysis of the Aravind Eye Care System found a total cost per operation of USD 120 and a cost-utility ratio of USD 195 per quality-adjusted life-year (QALY) gained. Applied at population scale, the same analysis estimated that eliminating cataract-related blindness and low vision in India would cost USD 2.6 billion while yielding a net societal benefit of USD 13.5 billion.

13.7 Recommendations for Future Programs

Building directly on the calculation methods developed above, programs seeking to close the urban-rural outcome gap should adopt an explicit, axial-length-stratified IOL formula protocol as a written standard operating procedure for every biometer in use, and should re-optimize the lens constant for each IOL model at least annually using the program's own accumulated postoperative refraction data. To further enhance the effectiveness of mass cataract surgery programs, it is recommended to standardize prescreening protocols across different regions to ensure uniform patient selection criteria, and to calculate and publish the program's own daily capacity ceiling, screening targets, and reorder points before each campaign, comparing achieved volumes against calculated targets afterward to refine local yield estimates. A universal costing framework that can be adapted to local economic contexts should be developed and maintained as a running fixed and variable cost model, rather than reconciled only retrospectively, so that subsidy requirements are known before a funding shortfall occurs. Artificial intelligence tools could be employed to better predict patient turnout and surgical supply needs [3]. Implementing real-time data tracking systems during surgical camps would facilitate more dynamic management and prompt adjustments. Additionally, building strong partnerships with local communities is vital for sustainable follow-up care [11].

13.8 Conclusion

Mass, charitable, and rural cataract surgery programs are, at their operational core, calculation problems: which IOL power formula to apply and how to derive implant power from biometric inputs; how many patients a fixed surgical capacity can absorb and how large a screening campaign must be to fill that capacity; and what a case truly costs once fixed and variable inputs are itemized, and at what volume a program becomes self-sustaining. By incorporating explicit, auditable calculations rather than inherited rules of thumb, programs can significantly enhance surgical outputs while maintaining high standards of care. The success of existing models such as Aravind and Tilganga highlights the transformative potential of optimized planning, available to every program regardless of resource setting, in the fight against avoidable blindness.

References

1. Huang W, Huang G, Wang D, Yin Q, Foster PJ, He M. Outcomes of cataract surgery in urban southern China: the Liwan Eye Study. Invest Ophthalmol Vis Sci. 2011;52(1):16–20. Published 2011 Jan 5. https://doi.org/10.1167/iovs.10-5382.

2. Cicinelli MV, Buchan JC, Nicholson M, Varadaraj V, Khanna RC. Cataracts. Lancet. 2023;401(10374):377–89. https://doi.org/10.1016/S0140-6736(22)01839-6.
3. Mohammed J, Assegid S, Fekadu L, Kabeta T. Cataract surgery visual outcome and associated factors among adults attended Jimma University Medical Center, Jimma, Southwest Ethiopia. Clin Ophthalmol. 2023;17:3341–51. Published 2023 Nov 3. https://doi.org/10.2147/OPTH.S434453.
4. Hashemi H, Fayaz F, Hashemi A, Khabazkhoob M. Global prevalence of cataract surgery. Curr Opin Ophthalmol. 2025;36(1):10–7. https://doi.org/10.1097/ICU.0000000000001092.
5. Truong PN, Merlinsky EA, Maamari NC, Weng CY, Lee AG. Tools and methods for cataract recognition in low-resource settings: A narrative review. PLOS Glob Public Health. 2025;5(5):e0004619. Published 2025 May 16. https://doi.org/10.1371/journal.pgph.0004619.
6. Khanna RC, Pallerla SR, Eeda SS, Gudapati BK, Mettla AL, Cicinelli MV, et al. Barriers to cataract surgery and strategies to overcome them in rural India: a qualitative study. Clin Ophthalmol. 2020;14:3269–78.
7. Gupta A, Singh P. Intraocular Lens Power Calculation. [Updated 2022 Dec 8]. In: StatPearls [Internet]. Treasure Island: StatPearls Publishing; 2025 Jan-. Available from: https://www.ncbi.nlm.nih.gov/books/NBK589643/
8. Vijaya L, George R, Rashima A, et al. Outcomes of cataract surgery in a rural and urban south Indian population. Indian J Ophthalmol. 2010;58(3):223–8. https://doi.org/10.4103/0301-4738.62648.
9. Stopyra W, Voytsekhivskyy O, Grzybowski A. Accuracy of 20 intraocular lens power calculation formulas in medium-long eyes. Ophthalmol Ther. 2024;13(7):1893–907. https://doi.org/10.1007/s40123-024-00954-7.
10. Ginel J, Burguera N, Piñero D, Sáez-Martín A, Haro De Rosario A, Fernández J. Economic evaluations in cataract surgery: a narrative review. Eye (Lond). 2024;38(8):1418–24. https://doi.org/10.1038/s41433-024-02965-x.
11. Bastawrous A, Rono HK, Livingstone IA, Weiss HA, Jordan S, Kuper H, et al. Development and validation of a smartphone-based visual acuity test (Peek Acuity) for clinical practice and community-based fieldwork. JAMA Ophthalmol. 2019;137(8):930–7. https://doi.org/10.1001/jamaophthalmol.2015.1468.

Chapter 14
Biometry for Outreach Microsurgical Clinic (OMEC): Combined Mass Surgeries of Manual Small Incision Cataract Surgery (MSICS) and Phacoemulsification

Sanduk Ruit, Sagar Ruit, Anil Boyaju, Swechha Sharma, and Satenla Ruit

14.1 Introduction

Cataract is the leading cause of blindness worldwide. Nearly 20 million people are blinded by it [1]. Cataracts directly impact a person's quality of life when the blindness limits them from living a normal life. Blindness from cataract not only becomes a barrier for the patient but extends to their family, community, and even the country. The effect of visual impairment from cataract can grossly affect the patient's quality of life and impose financial burden on their family and community.

Nepal is a beautiful yet topographically challenged country with mountains and hills running through the majority of its land. This becomes a major concern for patients blinded by cataracts, limiting them from mobility and navigation through the difficult terrains. Another important factor we cannot ignore is the economical constraints of the patient that prevent them from reaching out for eye care.

To solve this, Tilganga Institute of Ophthalmology (TIO), Nepal, has pioneered and has been working on the concept of high-quality, sustainable community cataract surgery for the last three decades. TIO has expertise in the different areas of community cataract surgery, focusing on a fine-tuned system to provide a successful, high-quality outcome [1].

All authors declare no financial interest.
Authors declare that all figures and tables belong to them.

S. Ruit (✉) · S. Ruit · A. Boyaju · S. Sharma · S. Ruit
Tilganga Institute of Ophthalmology, Kathmandu, Nepal

G. Pardianto (ed.), *Intraocular Lens (IOL) Power Calculation*,
https://doi.org/10.1007/978-981-92-1223-1_14

Outreach Microsurgical Clinic (OMEC) is a temporary surgical setup for providing surgical facilities in communities that would otherwise face difficulty in accessing a surgical eye care provider due to difficult geography and/or financial constraints (Fig. 14.1). The overall objective of OMEC is to eliminate avoidable blindness and visual impairment by delivering high-quality eye care services to those in need at their doorstep [1].

The surgical results are significant in addressing the massive problem of cataract blindness in the third world [2]. For a successful OMEC with good postoperative results, an accurate and efficient biometry is important.

Biometry is the measurement of the eye that takes into account dimensions of the corneal curvature, axial length (AL), lens thickness, and anterior chamber depth (ACD). This helps in the calculation of the power of intraocular lens to be implanted during cataract surgery [3].

The importance of biometry lies in the visual outcome of the patients in the postoperative stage. For a good visual outcome following cataract surgery, good biometry is mandatory.

Biometry includes the measurement of two ocular parameters:

(i) Keratometry:

- The determination of the curvature of the anterior corneal surface
- Includes the flattest meridian (K1) and steepest meridian (K2)
- Commonly done

(ii) Axial length (AL)

- Distance from anterior surface of the cornea to the retinal pigment epithelium
- 1 mm error in axial length measurement will lead to refractive error of 3 D postoperatively

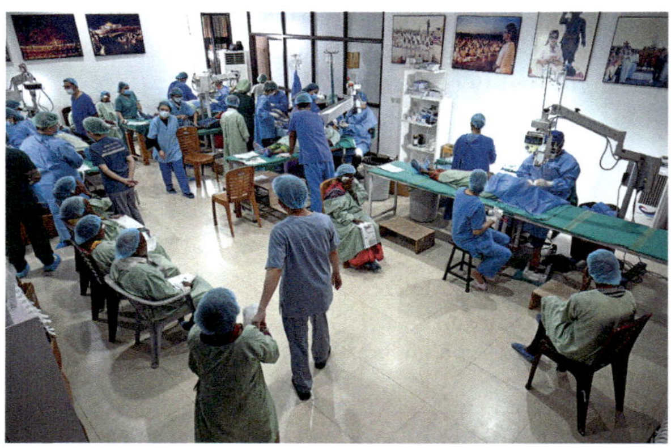

Fig. 14.1 Operation theatre setup in a high-volume OMEC

- It should be more accurate in shorter eyes than longer eyes (refractive error of 3.75 D/mm in 20 mm eye, while only 1.75 D/mm in 30 mm long eye postoperatively

Techniques for Biometry

(i) Keratometry:

  (a) Manual keratometry

    - Bausch and Lomb type: Fixed object size
    - Javal-Schiotz type: Fixed image size

  (b) Automated keratometry: Can be either

    - Standalone automated keratometers
    - Autorefractor-keratometer (ARK) combos
    - Optical biometers with integrated keratometry
    - Corneal topographers with keratometry
    - Handheld or portable keratometers (best for OMEC setup)

(ii) Axial length measurement technique:

  (c) A-scan ultrasonography:

    - Contact method (best for OMEC setup)
    - Immersion method

  (d) Optical biometry

Biometry in OMEC for High-Volume Patients

Room setup (Fig. 14.2):

- Standard room illumination.
- Adequate room temperature to avoid overheating of machine.
- Check with voltmeter and adequate voltage supply of electricity (around 220 Volts). Low voltage can make the machine nonfunctional, and high voltage can lead to system failure of the machine (Fig. 14.3).

Instruments Required:

- Portable handheld automated keratometer (Fig. 14.4)
- A-scan machine (manual) (Fig. 14.5)

Calibration of Machines

- Critical quality control step to ensure accuracy and reliability in IOL power calculation
- Must be done every day before starting mass calculation
- Usually done with model eye with known dimensions provided with the machine or can be done with the auto calibration depending on the machine (Fig. 14.6)

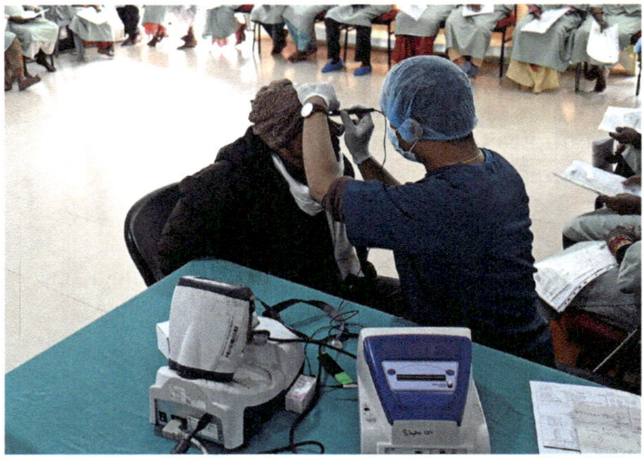

Fig. 14.2 Biometry setup in OMEC

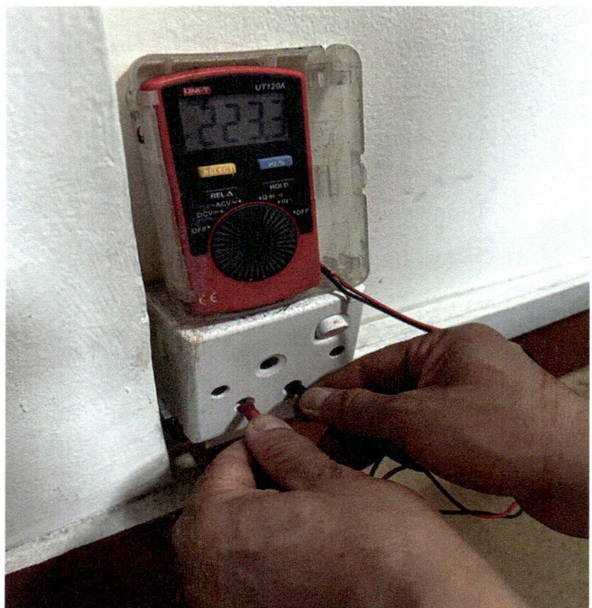

Fig. 14.3 Examination of the voltage supply while setting up the room for biometry

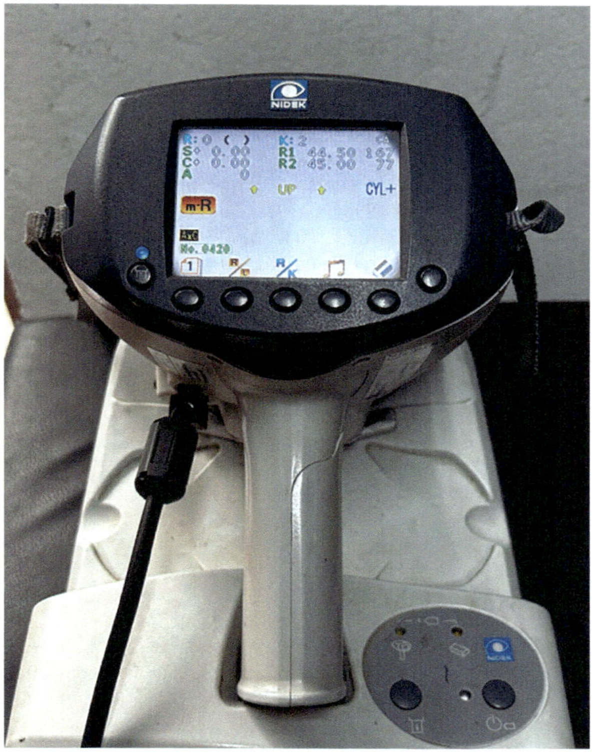

Fig. 14.4 Portable handheld automated keratometer

Sterilization

- Ensuring proper sterilization and disinfection of the contact probe and patient interface components is critical to prevent cross-contamination and maintain patient safety during high-volume OMEC setting
- Done by wiping the probe with alcohol swab (70% isopropyl alcohol) after every patient (Fig. 14.7)

Steps for General Health Status

- Registration: Maintain record of patient undergoing cataract surgery in a register book.
- Check BP/blood test: Blood pressure should be examined. Blood test such as sugar and serology examined by glucometer and rapid antigen kits, respectively.
- Check drug allergy history.

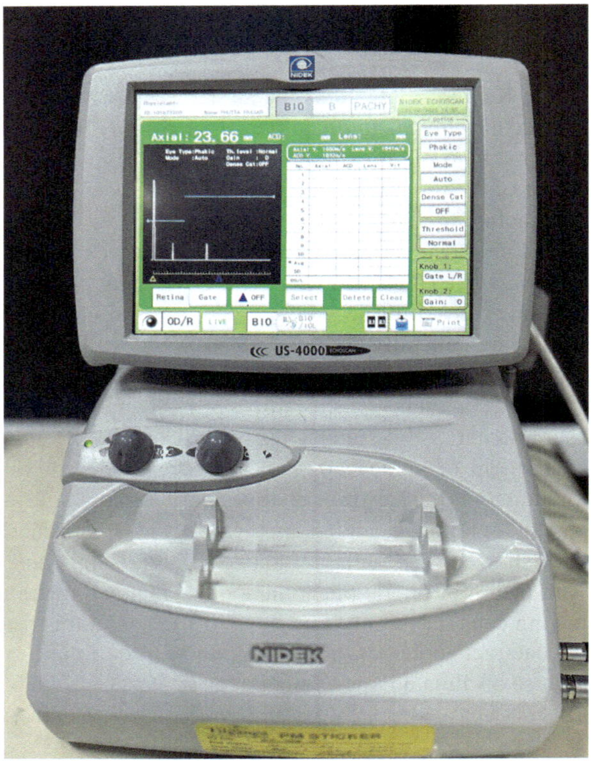

Fig. 14.5 A-scan machine

Steps for Keratometry

- Ask patient to look at a fixation target (can be a green/red light or an image of a hot air balloon) in machine.
- Machine will detect K reading value automatically.
- Focus light at the center of cornea.
- Ensure adequate tear film at the ocular surface, which can be confirmed by the proper Mires formation.
- If Mires are distorted, instill low-viscosity lubricating eye drops.
- If Mires are eccentric, centralize the mires at the center of cornea.
- Take average of three readings of each eye.
- Note down the values in the patient document (Figs. 14.8, 14.9, and 14.10).

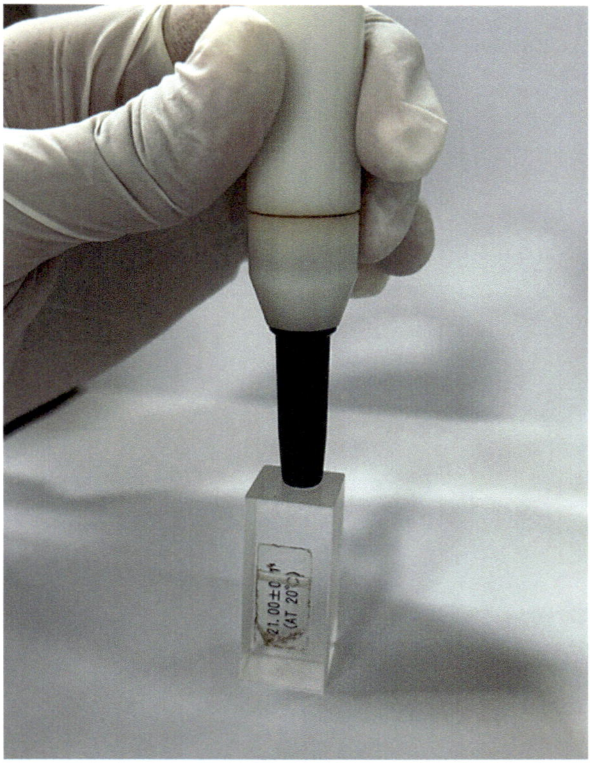

Fig. 14.6 Calibration of A-scan machine

A-Scan Biometry (Figs. 14.11 and 14.12)

Contact Method

- Document patient details.
- Ask the patient to sit comfortably in a sitting position.
- Anesthetize patient's cornea with the topical drop proparacaine (0.5%) or lignocaine (4%) in both eyes.
- Ask the patient to look straight at the fixation target at a distance.
- Retract eyelids without applying pressure on the globe to avoid change in the corneal curvature and artificially shorten axial length calculation, resulting in a false reading.
- Select the lowest gain at which the best spikes are obtained (usually 70 decibels (dB) but differs according to different machines).

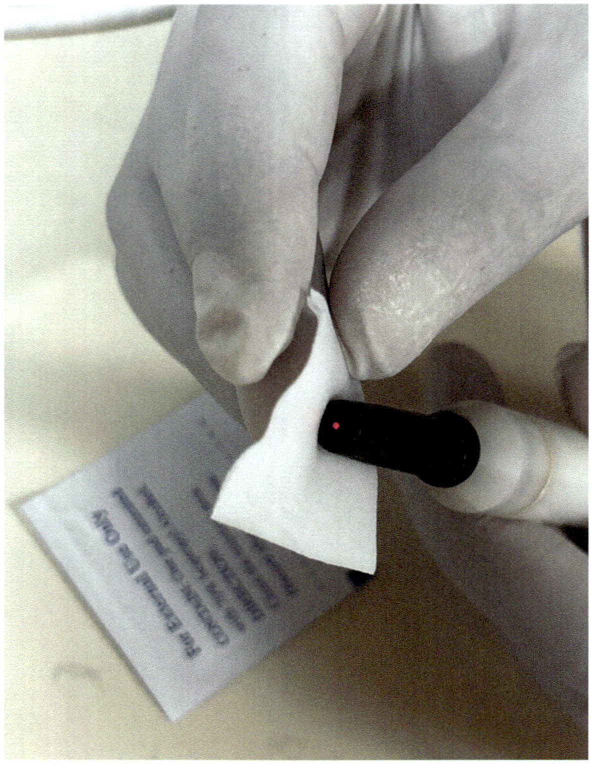

Fig. 14.7 Sterilization of A-scan probe

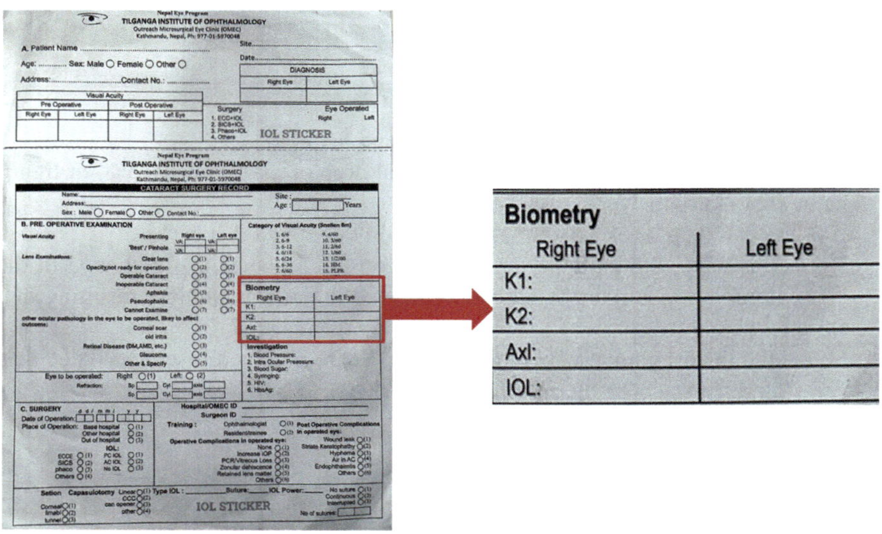

Fig. 14.8 Patient document during OMEC with the parameters of biometry, which must be filled

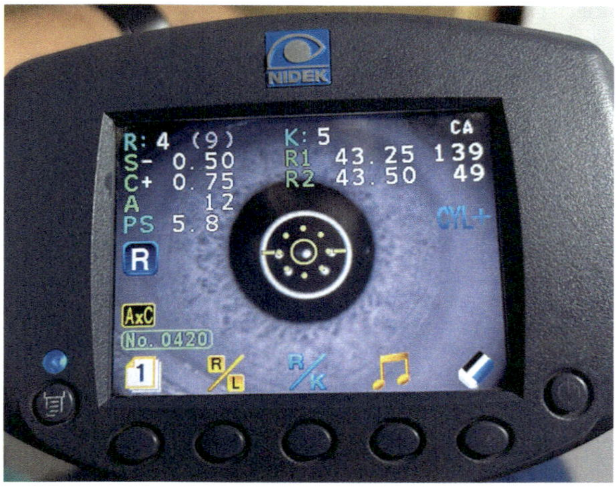

Fig. 14.9 Good keratometry reading with well-formed Mires

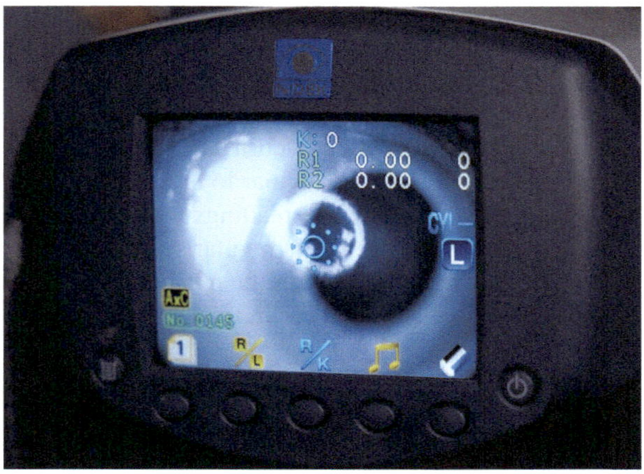

Fig. 14.10 Bad keratometry reading with eccentric and distorted mires

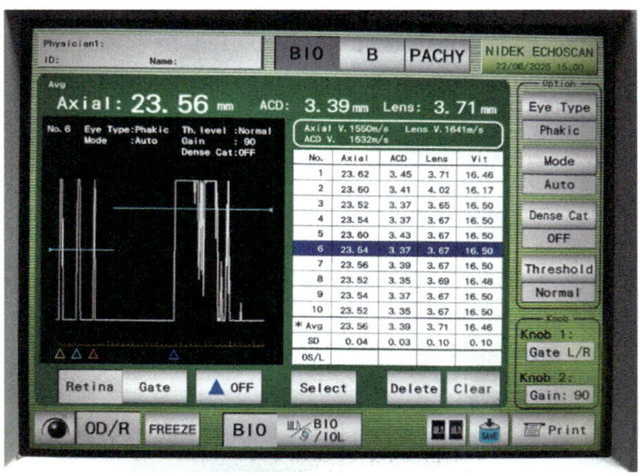

Fig. 14.11 A-scan reading with good spikes

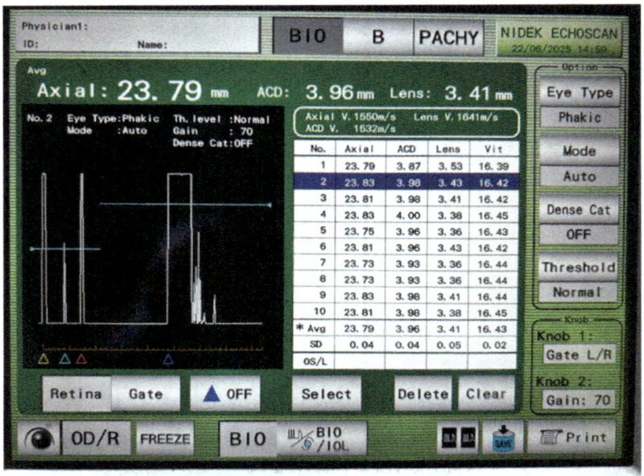

Fig. 14.12 A-scan reading with false spikes

- Select A constant value. This differs from the IOL being used in the OMEC (For Tilganga IOL Flex / Tetra, A-constant =118; for Tilganga PMMA, A-constant = 118.3 for Sanders-Retzlaff-Kraff (SRK)-II formula).
- Select a formula for IOL calculation (usually SRK II) but differs in different eyes.
- Gently touch the patient's cornea, avoiding excess corneal compression, while the probe is held perpendicular to the corneal apex.
- Acquire 8–10 consecutive readings with standard deviation less than 0.05.
- Each reading should have a regular spike of good amplitude.
- Enter the K reading value in the machine, then calculate the power of IOL.
- Record the final IOL power in the patient's document and encircle the eye to be operated.

Immersion Technique

- Instill topical anesthetic drops.
- Position the patient comfortably in a semireclined chair or in a bed of appropriate height.
- Explain the procedure to the patient and ask them to fixate on the probe.
- Place the immersion shell on the eye, and fill it with sterile normal saline.
- Insert the A-scan probe into the shell, keeping it centered and perpendicular to the corneal apex.
- Acquire at least five consistent AL readings with clear and tall spikes.
- Record and save the best readings, and calculate the IOL power using the appropriate formula.
- Remove shell and rinse it thoroughly.
- Repeat for the other eye.
- Disinfect the shell after use.

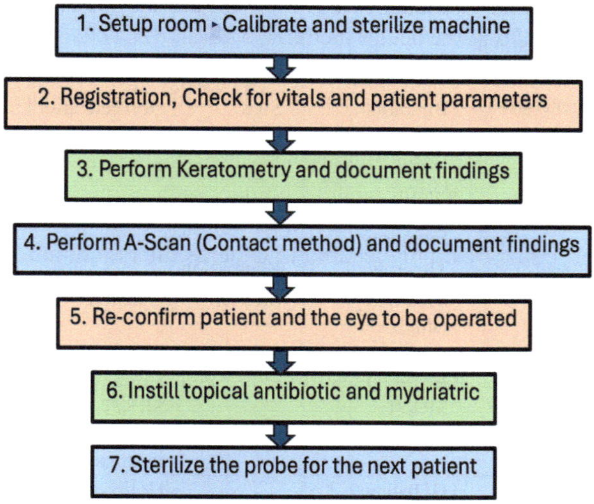

Fig. 14.13 Flowchart showing the steps of biometry in an OMEC

After Biometry

- Reconfirm the patient and the eye to be operated on.
- Sterilize the probe before using it on the next patient (Fig. 14.13).
- Instill an antibiotic drop (ciprofloxacin 0.3% or ofloxacin 0.3%).
- Instill pupil dilating drops (tropicamide 1%).
- Form completion: Fill up all data and take consent before investigation and surgery.
- Recheck: Confirm patient details and the eye to be operated on.

14.2 Classification of IOL Power Calculation Formula

Although IOL power calculation began as an optical approach using theoretical formulas, the majority of methods used in clinical practice over the past 25 years have been based on empirical methods that have used "fudged" formulas to compensate for the unknowns in the system. However, the advent of better diagnostic equipment and ever-improving surgical techniques has decreased the number of unknowns, and optical methods now hold sway in IOL power calculation (Table 14.1) [4].

Table 14.1 Classification of IOL power calculation formula

Generations			
1st generation	Theoretical	Regression	
	Binkhorst Colenbrander-Hoffer Gills Clayman Fyodorov	SRK	Obsolete aren't used nowadays
2nd generation	Theoretical	Regression	
	Modified Binkhorst	SRK-II	Obsolete
3rd generation	Holladay 1 Hoffer Q SRK/T		Holladay 1:24.6 mm–26.0 mm Hoffer Q: < 22 mm SRK/T: 22–27 mm, extreme axial lengths (>27 mm) require Wang-Koch adjustment for increased accuracy
4th generation	Holladay 2 Haigis Olsen		Holladay 2: short–long[a] eyes Haigis (a0, a1, a2 optimized): short– long[a] eyes Olsen: Short to long
Newer generation	Barrett-Universal II Kane Hill-RBF OKULIX		Barrett-Universal II: Long to short, recommended as more accurate in axial length >25 mm Kane: Long to short, recommended in case of keratoconus

[a]Haigis formula where a0 = offset constant, a1 = anterior chamber depth, and a2 = axial length

14.3 Commonly Used IOL Power Calculation Formula in OMEC

1. *SRK Formula*: [5]

$$P = A - 2.5L - 0.9K$$

A = A constant
P = IOL power
L = Axial length
K = *Average K reading*

2. *Hoffer Q*: [6]

$$P = 1336 / A - C - 0.05 - 1.336 / \{(1.336 / K + R) - (C + 0.05 / 1000)\}$$

A = Axial length
C = Anterior chamber depth

K = Average corneal diopter
R = Refractive error

3. *Haigis Formula*: [7]

$$D = a0 + \left(a1^{*}\,\mathrm{ACD}\right)\left(a2^{*}\,AL\right)$$

ACD: *Preoperative* ACD
AL: Axial length
$a0$, $a1$, & $a2$: Constants
$a0$: Shifts the entire power prediction curve up or down
$a1$: Linked to the measured anterior chamber depth
$a2$: Linked to the measured axial length

14.4 Challenging Situations During Biometry in High-Volume OMEC Setup

Environment condition:

- Crowd management in high-volume setup: Use the help of volunteers for line management and counselling.
- Have to work at extremes of climate. Ensure patient comfort before anything else.
- Chances of power cut. Requires backup electrical supply.

Patient's General Condition

- Uncooperative or mentally impaired patients: Good and clear counselling is key, and refer to hospital setup if required
- Medical emergencies such as hypoglycemia/hyperglycemia, heat stroke, anxiety, hypotension, hypertension, and seizure: Call for help, monitor vitals, treat and delay surgery if needed
- Blind patients: Ensure safe mobilization by providing verbal and physical support during positioning and testing
- Head nodding (Parkinson's disease): Stabilize head with head rests or manual support, and proceed carefully to avoid probe misalignment and corneal trauma
- Pediatric patients: Selection of cooperative children who can undergo surgery under local anesthesia. Lens calculation varies according to age group
- Language barriers: Use translators or local volunteers. Use visual cues to direct patients
- Hearing impairment: Highlight the case to alert other team members, and use visual cues to direct patients for the steps

Patient Ocular Condition

- Eyelids and adnexa:
  - Lid masses such as stye or hordeolum, chalazion, and lid tumors can induce mechanical astigmatism and lead to false reading of the corneal curvature. Treat the lid mass and delay surgery.
- Ocular surface and cornea:
  - Pterygium: If large enough to cover the visual axis, take eccentric reading or advise for excision first.
  - Corneal scar: May lead to false reading. If the scar is central, then eccentric reading can be taken. If the scar is dense, use the reading from the fellow eye.
  - Astigmatism: Highlight the case and inform the operating doctor.
  - Keratoconus and high astigmatism: Can lead to false reading. Refer for surgery after corneal topography.
  - Contact lens wear: Discontinue lens before biometry (rigid gas permeable lens and scleral lens: 2 weeks and soft lens: 48 h).
- Anterior chamber (AC):
  - Shallow AC can risk corneal compression, giving false readings; repeat to confirm IOL power.
  - Glaucoma: Cornea may be hazy; reduce high intraocular pressure (IOP) before the reading, and increase gain until spike is seen (study).
- Lens and zonules:
  - Mature/hypermature cataracts: Increase A-scan gain. Do B-scan to confirm if the retina is intact.
  - Aphakia: Use the aphakic mode (sound velocity around 1532 m/s). Plan for secondary IOL.
  - Pseudophakia in the fellow eye: Use the pseudophakic mode for that eye as the sound velocity mode is changed (differs according to material of IOL).
  - Traumatic cataract: Check for subluxation/dislocation and highlight the case.
  - Subluxation/weak zonules: Highlight the case for possible use of a capsular tension ring (CTR) or an AC IOL power (subtract 3 D), or use the rule of 9 table for sulcus placement.
- Vitreous:
  - Vitreous hemorrhage: Determined by the poor spikes on the A-scan.
  - Silicon oil: Refer for optical biometry.

- Retina:
  - Retinal detachment: Causes false posterior spike and underestimation of axial length. Confirm with B-scan and refer. Fellow eye reading can be taken for approximation.
- High refractive error:
  - High myope: Use Holladay 2 or Barrett formula. Highlight the case for retrobulbar/peribulbar anesthesia to prevent globe rupture. If a calculated lens is not available, refer the case or plan for secondary implantation.
  - High hyperope: Use Hoffer Q formula for accurate IOL power calculation.
- Strabismus:
  - Nonparalytic: Occlude the fixating eye and maintain fixation in the nonfixating eye to take the reading.
  - Paralytic: Adjust the head position for better exposure, and refer if fixation cannot be maintained.
- Posterior staphyloma: Leads to false reading due to focal increase in the axial length. Use the immersion technique for more accurate technique.
- Nystagmus: May require biometry under local anesthesia or in the operating theatre (OT) table for better control.
- Proptosis: Check for exposure keratopathy.

  Any false spike or abnormality faced during the biometry must be informed to the operating surgeon before posting the case for surgery and referred or managed accordingly.

User Challenges
- Limited resources, extreme geographical location
- Human error
- Wrong documentation
- Exhaustion
- Experience and user variability

Complications of Biometry
- Corneal abrasion: Avoid by a gentle approach, and counsel patients to avoid abrupt movement.
- Epithelial defect: Treat the defect first and delay surgery.
- Infection: Proper sterilization is required to avoid cross-contamination.
- Wrong IOL: Plan for IOL exchange.
- Post-operative refractive surprise: Counsel patients regarding the need of glasses and keep in close follow-up.

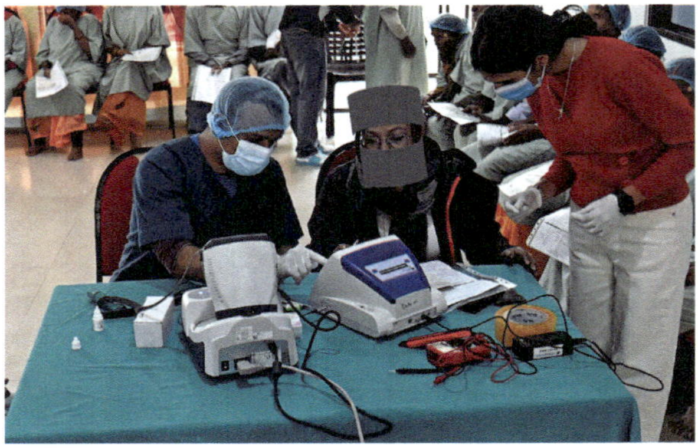

Fig. 14.14 Biometry training by Tilganga outreach team

Training Staff for High-Quality Biometry During OMECs (Fig. 14.14)

- Make a designated team with good mentors and enthusiastic trainees.
- Conduct routine training prior to the OMEC.
- Familiarize them with the machine and the lenses available at the OMEC.
- Educate them regarding special conditions and how to manage them accordingly.

Future Direction

- Routine B-scan in all cases
- Managing patients who have undergone refractive surgery
- Portable optical biometry
- Electronic medical record (EMR) for better documentation
- Use of artificial intelligence (AI)
- Better counselling

14.5 Difference Between Hospital-Based Biometry and OMEC-Based Biometry

Cataract surgery at a hospital, even though with similar volume, is different from cataract surgery at OMEC (Table 14.2).

Table 14.2 Difference between hospital-based biometry and OMEC-based biometry

Parameters	Hospital-based biometry	OMEC-based biometry
Patient volume	Moderate volume	High-volume, rapid screening
IOL choice	Wide choice including toric, multifocal, extended-depth-of-focus (EDOF)	Limited stock, mostly monofocal, minimal astigmatic correction
Condition-specific calculations	Available for postrefractive, keratoconus, etc.	Not feasible; default formulas used
Biometry machine type	IOLMaster (Carl Zeiss Meditec, Dublin, CA), Lenstar (Haag-Streit, Köniz, Switzerland), advanced optical biometers	Mostly A-scan, manual keratometry
Positioning for measurement	Sitting position for IOLMaster	Sitting or supine position
Invasiveness	Noninvasive optical biometry	Invasive contact A-scan
Sterilization required	No (noncontact)	Yes (probe disinfection essential)
Instrumentation	Full access to topographers, optical biometers, and immersion setups	Limited to basic A-scan and handheld keratometers
Counseling	Detailed counseling with diagnostic backup	Limited time for counseling, mostly generic
IOL formulas available	Full access to multiple formulas (Holladay 2, Barrett, Haigis)	Basic formulas (SRK II, SRK/T) due to limited digital access
Accuracy	High-accuracy, multiple parameters (AL, K, ACD, central corneal thickness (CCT)) measured	Moderately accurate; less precise readings
User-friendliness	Software guided; technician friendly	Requires manual skill and experience
Portability	Low-hospital-bound machines	High-compact and transportable equipment
Cost per patient	Higher due to setup and equipment	Lower, optimized for mass screening
Postop refractive surprise	Minimal with full workup	Higher due to limited customization
Mature/ hypermature cataracts	Optical biometry fails; use B-scan + immersion A-scan	Direct use of A-scan; B-scan may be available selectively

References

1. Pardianto G, Tassignon MJ, editors. Innovation in cataract surgery. Singapore: Springer; 2024. https://doi.org/10.1007/978-981-97-5192-1.
2. Ruit S, Tabin GC, Nissman SA, Paudyal G, Gurung R. Low-cost high-volume extracapsular cataract extraction with posterior chamber intraocular lens implantation in Nepal. Ophthalmology. 1999;106(10):1887–92. https://doi.org/10.1016/S0161-6420(99)90397-4.
3. Sahin A, Hamrah P. Clinically relevant biometry. Curr Opin Ophthalmol. 2012;23(1):47–53. https://doi.org/10.1097/ICU.0b013e32834cd63e.

4. Olsen T. Calculation of intraocular lens power: a review. Acta Ophthalmol Scand. 2007;85(5):472–85. https://doi.org/10.1111/j.1600-0420.2007.00879.x.
5. Sanders DR, Retzlaff J, Kraff MC. Comparison of the SRK II formula and other second-generation formulas. J Cataract Refract Surg. 1988;14(2):136–41. https://doi.org/10.1016/s0886-3350(88)80087-7.
6. Hoffer KJ. The Hoffer Q formula: a comparison of theoretic and regression formulas. J Cataract Refract Surg. 1993;19(6):700–12. https://doi.org/10.1016/s0886-3350(13)80338-0.
7. Haigis W, Hoffer KJ. The Haigis Formula. In: Aramberri J, Hoffer KJ, Olsen T, Savini G, Shammas HJ, editors. Intraocular lens calculations. Essentials in ophthalmology. Cham: Springer; 2024. p. 625–36. https://doi.org/10.1007/978-3-031-50666-6_41.

Chapter 15
Optimizing Intraocular Lens Calculation in Emergency Intraoperative Complications: A Surgical Challenge

Budiman and Novita Sitompul

15.1 Introduction

Cataract surgery is one of the most frequently performed surgical procedures worldwide, with over 28 million cases annually, and its success hinges on precise intraocular lens (IOL) power calculation to achieve optimal refractive outcomes [1]. Advances in biometry and IOL formulas (e.g., Barrett Universal II (BUII), Holladay 2) have reduced postoperative refractive surprises. Still, emergency intraoperative complications—such as posterior capsule rupture, zonular dehiscence, or vitreous loss—dramatically alter the surgical landscape. These events disrupt preoperative assumptions about effective lens position (ELP), anterior chamber depth (ACD), and IOL fixation, demanding rapid recalibration of calculations to avoid hyperopic or myopic surprises that compromise patient satisfaction and surgical success [2].

IOL power formulas rely heavily on accurate predictions of ELP and the postoperative position of the lens relative to the cornea and retina. ELP is estimated using preoperative axial length (AL), keratometry (K), and ACD in uncomplicated cases. However, intraoperative complications often force surgeons to abandon in-the-bag IOL placement instead of sulcus fixation, scleral fixation, or anterior chamber IOLs.

All author declare no financial interest

Budiman (✉)
Universitas Padjadjaran, Bandung, Indonesia

Cicendo National Eye Hospital, Bandung, Indonesia

Bandung Eye Center, Bandung, Indonesia

Dago Vision Care, Bandung, Indonesia

N. Sitompul
Priangan Medical and Eye Center, Bandung, Indonesia

G. Pardianto (ed.), *Intraocular Lens (IOL) Power Calculation*,
https://doi.org/10.1007/978-981-92-1223-1_15

Each alternative placement shifts the ELP anteriorly or posteriorly, altering the adequate power of the lens. For example, a sulcus-fixated IOL typically requires a 0.5–1.0 diopter (D) reduction compared to in-the-bag placement due to its anterior shift [3]. Similarly, scleral-fixated IOLs may necessitate adjustments for AL elongation caused by suture-induced pseudophakic accommodation [4].

Emergencies introduce time-sensitive dilemmas: surgeons must balance immediate anatomical stabilization (e.g., managing vitreous loss) with refractive accuracy. Traditional formulas assume ideal conditions, but complications like capsular rupture or zonular weakness invalidate these assumptions. Patients risk suboptimal visual outcomes without real-time adjustments, necessitating secondary procedures such as IOL exchange or laser correction. Furthermore, tools such as intraoperative aberrometry (e.g., Optiwave Refractive Analysis (ORA) System (WaveTec Vision, Aliso Viejo, CA) may be unavailable or unreliable in unstable eyes, emphasizing the need for surgeon-driven strategies [5–7].

15.2 Common Intraoperative Complications Affecting IOL Calculation

Intraoperative complications during cataract surgery can disrupt preoperative biometry assumptions, necessitating rapid adjustments to IOL power calculations. Below is an in-depth analysis of key complications, their impact on IOL optimization, and evidence-based management strategies.

15.2.1 Posterior Capsule Rupture (PCR)

During phacoemulsification or irrigation/aspiration, the posterior capsule's tear occurs in 0.5–2% of cases [8]. Impact on IOL calculation is ELP shift: prevents in-the-bag IOL placement, forcing sulcus fixation or anterior chamber IOLs. Sulcus placement shifts the ELP anteriorly, reducing adequate IOL power by 0.5–1.0 D [9]. There, for adjustments needed, subtract 0.5–1.0 D from the in-the-bag power for sulcus-fixated IOLs and use three-piece IOLs (e.g., Tecnis ZA9003 (Abbott Medical Optics, Abbott Park, IL)) for sulcus stability; avoid one-piece lenses due to iris chafing risk [10].

15.2.2 Zonular Dehiscence

The weakness or rupture of zonular fibers is often due to trauma, pseudoexfoliation, or intraoperative stress. The impact on IOL Calculation will be capsular Instability, which may require capsular tension rings (CTRs) or segments (e.g.,

Cionni ring) to stabilize the bag. CTRs preserve ELP but may slightly interiorize the IOL [11]. If zonular support is <50%, consider scleral-fixated or iris-claw IOLs, adjusting for ELP changes. For CTR-stabilized bags: Use standard formulas, but reduce target refraction by 0.25–0.5 D to account for subtle ELP shifts [12]. Apply Wang-Koch adjustment (+1.0–2.0 D) for scleral fixation to counteract AL elongation [4].

15.2.3 Vitreous Loss

Prolapse of vitreous into the anterior chamber during capsular rupture or nucleus drop has an impact on IOL Calculation caused by (1) AL shortening: vitreous loss reduces intraocular volume, shortening the AL by 0.2–0.5 mm, (2) anterior chamber instability: post-vitrectomy fluid/gas use alters ACD, and (3) invalidating preoperative keratometry. Formula adjustments for these events will increase IOL power by 0.5–1.5 D if AL is not remeasured intraoperatively, and intraoperative ultrasound biometry will be used to reassess AL [13, 14].

15.2.4 Dropped Nucleus/IOL

Dislocation of lens fragments or IOL into the vitreous cavity has an impact on IOL calculation due to secondary IOL strategies: (1) requires pars plana vitrectomy followed by scleral-fixated or anterior chamber IOL implantation, and (2) ELP variability: Scleral-fixated IOLs sit posteriorly, mimicking natural ELP, but may induce pseudo-accommodation [15]. For scleral-fixated IOLs, the Wang-Koch formula (+1.0–2.0 D) or Sanders-Retzlaff-Kraff/Theoretical (SRK/T) with A-constant reduced by 0.5–1.0 is applicable. For anterior chamber IOLs, apply vertex distance correction (e.g., Hoffer Q with ACD set to 3.0 mm) [4, 16].

15.2.5 Expulsive Hemorrhage

This rare, sight-threatening bleeding from choroidal vessels occurs in 0.03–0.06% of cases. Expulsive hemorrhage can result in delayed IOL implantation, requiring secondary IOL implantation several weeks to months after the initial surgery. Posthemorrhage scarring or hypotony may alter corneal curvature and AL. Repeated biometrics will be needed once the eye stabilizes (4–6 weeks post event), prioritizing the anterior chamber or iris-claw IOLs if capsular support is lost [17].

15.3 Challenges in IOL Optimization During Emergencies

Intraoperative complications in cataract surgery introduce unique obstacles to achieving optimal refractive outcomes. These challenges arise from sudden anatomic disruptions, time-sensitive decision-making, and limitations in available tools. Below is an expanded analysis of key challenges supported by clinical evidence and practical insights.

15.3.1 *Altered ELP*

IOL power formulas (e.g., BUII, Holladay 2) rely on accurate prediction of the postoperative ELP—the distance between the IOL and the cornea. Intraoperative emergencies often force deviations from planned in-the-bag placement, leading to anterior or posterior shifts in ELP. For example, sulcus fixation: Anterior displacement reduces the IOL's adequate power by 0.5–1.0 D compared to in-the-bag placement, as the lens sits closer to the cornea. Scleral-fixated IOLs: Posterior placement near the retina mimics the natural lens position but may induce AL elongation due to suture tension, necessitating a +1.0–2.0 D adjustment. Anterior chamber IOLs: Positioned far anteriorly, these lenses increase adequate power, requiring vertex distance corrections (e.g., adjusting Hoffer Q formulas for shallow anterior chambers) [2–4, 16, 18].

15.3.2 *Time Constraints and Decision-Making Under Pressure*

Emergencies demand rapid eye stabilization (e.g., managing vitreous loss, controlling hemorrhage), leaving little time for meticulous IOL recalculation. Surgeons must balance immediate anatomical repair and refractive accuracy to avoid postoperative dissatisfaction. Studies show that time pressure increases the risk of cognitive errors, such as overlooking ELP adjustments or miscalculating A-constants. For example, failing to subtract 0.75 D for a sulcus IOL in a rushed setting can result in hyperopic surprise.

15.3.3 *Limited Access to Intraoperative Tools*

Intraoperative aberrometry (e.g., ORA System) and advanced biometry devices are often unavailable or unreliable in unstable eyes. For instance, vitreous loss: ORA measurements may be skewed by fluidics imbalance or corneal edema. Many hospitals lack intraoperative optical coherence tomography (OCT) or real-time biometry, which makes surgeons revert to manual calculations, increasing reliance on preoperative data that may no longer reflect the eye's altered state (e.g., shortened AL after vitrectomy) [19].

Portable A-scan devices can remeasure AL intraoperatively but require technical skill [20]. Seasoned surgeons often use heuristic adjustments (e.g., "+1.0 D if vitreous lost") based on prior outcomes.

15.3.4 IOL Model Swaps and A-Constant Variability

Emergencies may necessitate switching IOL models (e.g., from one-piece acrylic to three-piece Polymethyl methacrylate (PMMA)). Each IOL has a unique A-constant, which influences ELP predictions. A-constants for sulcus-fixated three-piece IOLs (e.g., Tecnis ZA9003) are typically 0.5–1.0 lower than in-the-bag one-piece IOLs. Using the wrong A-constant can lead to ±1.5 D errors. For instance, implanting a scleral-fixated IOL without adjusting the A-constant may result in myopic surprise [21]. Preloaded A-constants are recommended, and ensure operating room staff have A-constants for backup IOL models readily available, and also use the SRK/T formula with manufacturer-specific A-constants for scleral-fixated IOLs.

15.4 Strategies for Intraoperative Optimization of IOL Calculations

Intraoperative complications in cataract surgery demand rapid, evidence-based strategies to optimize IOL power calculations. This section outlines practical approaches to mitigate refractive surprises, combining preoperative preparation, intraoperative tools, formula adjustments, and clinical judgment.

15.4.1 Preoperative Preparation

Anticipate complications in high-risk eyes to streamline intraoperative decision-making.

(a) *High-risk patients*: Identify eyes with pseudoexfoliation, shallow anterior chambers, or dense cataracts. Use multiple IOL formulas (e.g., BUII, Holladay 2, and Hill-Radial Basis Function (RBF)) to calculate a range of potential powers [22].
(b) *Backup IOLs*: Ensure availability of three-piece, scleral-fixated, or anterior chamber IOLs in the operating room.

(c) *Document biometry*: Verify AL, K, and ACD preoperatively. Repeat biometry to minimize errors in eyes with borderline AL measurements (e.g., nanophthalmos or high myopia).

15.4.2 Intraoperative Tools

15.4.2.1 Intraoperative Aberrometry (e.g., ORA System)

Intraoperative aberrometry provides real-time aphakic refraction in stable eyes. Studies show it reduces refractive errors by 0.3 D compared to preoperative formulas [19]. Limitations are unreliable in eyes with vitreous loss, corneal edema, or unstable capsules due to fluid imbalances [23].

15.4.2.2 Ultrasound Biometry

Remeasure AL intraoperatively if posterior segment changes (e.g., vitreous loss) are suspected. A 10 MHz A-scan probe with an immersion technique can improve accuracy [22]. In cases requiring vitrectomy, AL may shorten by 0.2–0.5 mm, requiring a +0.5–1.5 D IOL power adjustment [24].

15.4.3 Formula Adjustments for Alternative IOL Placements

15.4.3.1 Sulcus-Fixated IOLs

For intraocular lenses (IOLs) implanted in the ciliary sulcus, an overall length of 13.0–13.5 mm is recommended to ensure stability and prevent lateral subluxation. Due to their inadequate fixation, single-piece IOLs with plate-shaped haptics are contraindicated in sulcus placement. Additionally, single-piece IOLs made of hydrophilic acrylic material have large, thick haptics, making them unsuitable for ciliary sulcus implantation. The C-Flex 570C and Superflex 620H (Rayner Intraocular Lenses Limited, East Sussex, United Kingdom) are hydrophilic foldable acrylic IOLs with closed planar haptics. While the manufacturer indicates that these lenses can be placed in the ciliary sulcus, there is a risk of iris chafing and pigment dispersion. According to Chang et al., the square-edge design and shorter overall length of these IOLs—12.0 mm for the 570C and 12.5 mm for the 620H—pose the same risks as other hydrophobic single-piece acrylic lenses when implanted in the sulcus. Use three-piece lenses (e.g., Alcon MA60AC (Alcon Laboratories Inc., Fort Worth, TX)) to avoid iris chafing. Avoid one-piece acrylic IOLs in the sulcus [10, 25, 26].

Given these factors, cataract surgeons recommend using a three-piece posterior chamber IOL with a larger 6 mm optic diameter. The haptics should be made of PMMA, as its stiffness provides better stability and facilitates proper placement in the ciliary sulcus. The IOL calculation recommended is to subtract 0.5–1.0 D from in-the-bag power to account for anterior ELP shifts [26].

The required IOL power adjustment depends on the planned initial dioptric power for in-the-bag implantation. The general principle is that higher-power posterior chamber IOLs require a greater dioptric reduction when implanted in the sulcus, whereas very low-power IOLs may not require any adjustment [26]. To estimate the necessary IOL power adjustment. For example, if the calculated IOL power for capsular bag implantation is +17.50 D, a reduction of 1.00 D would be applied for sulcus placement, resulting in an adjusted IOL power of +16.00 D [26].

15.4.3.2 Scleral-Fixated IOLs

Wang-Koch adjustment is added +1.0–2.0 D to the in-the-bag power to compensate for suture-induced AL elongation. A-constant modification reduces the A-constant by 0.5–1.0 (e.g., from 119.0 to 118.5) for sutured lenses [4].

15.4.3.3 Anterior Chamber IOLs

For anterior chamber IOL placement, vertex distance correction is needed by adjusting the Hoffer Q formula by setting ACD to 3.0 mm (shallow chamber assumption). For a target refraction of −0.5 D, use +1.0 D more than the in-the-bag calculation [27].

15.4.4 Clinical Judgment and Heuristics

15.4.4.1 Surgeon Experience

For every 1.0 mm decrease in AL due to vitreous loss, increase IOL power by +2.0–3.0 D [28]. In eyes with zonular weakness, target −0.25 D to offset CTR-induced ELP shifts [29].

15.4.4.2 Quick-Reference

A quick reference for complication and its adjustment can be learned as follows: If a posterior capsule rupture complication occurs, the IOL power needs to be adjusted by −0.75 D for the IOL sulcus. If vitreous loss occurs, it needs to be adjusted by +1.0 D if AL is not remeasured. And if a scleral fixation procedure is required, an adjustment of +1.5 D is required (Wang-Koch method) [28, 29]:

15.4.5 Postoperative Salvage Techniques

Piggyback IOLs implant a supplementary lens in the ciliary sulcus and can be used to correct residual refractive errors. For laser vision correction, surgeons can use laser in-situ keratomileusis (LASIK) or photorefractive keratectomy (PRK) for stable eyes with >1.0 D surprises [30, 31].

15.5 Postoperative Management: Navigating Refractive Surprises and Complications

Intraoperative complications, including refractive errors, inflammation, and IOL instability, often lead to postoperative challenges. This section provides a structured approach to managing these issues.

15.5.1 Managing Refractive Surprises

15.5.1.1 Causes and Magnitude

Refractive errors exceeding ±1.0 D are common after emergency complications due to ELP shifts (e.g., sulcus vs. bag fixation), AL changes from vitreous loss or hemorrhage, and inaccurate formula adjustments under time pressure [32].

15.5.1.2 Corrective Strategies

Piggyback IOLs

Implant a supplementary IOL in the ciliary sulcus (e.g., +3.0 D lens for −3.0 D hyperopia). The advantages of this procedure are minimally invasive and preserves corneal integrity [31].

IOL Exchange

Replace the IOL, which is suggested to be performed within 6–8 weeks if capsular support allows. Preoperative biometry adjusted for postoperative ELP measurements [33].

Laser Vision Correction

LASIK/PRK is used for stable corneas (>3 months postop) and contraindicated for patients with corneal edema and unstable IOL [30].

15.5.2 Monitoring for Inflammation and IOL Stability

15.5.2.1 Early Postoperative Phase (1–7 Days)

For inflammation control, intensive topical steroids (e.g., prednisolone acetate 1% hourly) and nonsteroidal anti-inflammatory drug (NSAID) (e.g., bromfenac BID (bis in die, or twice a day)) are needed to prevent cystoid macular edema (CME). Oral steroids (e.g., prednisone 40 mg/day) are required for severe uveitis [34]. IOL stability checks for IOL tilt, decentralization, or iris chafing (common with sulcus-fixated IOLs) are mandatory. Ultrasound biomicroscopy (UBM) can assess the haptic position in scleral-fixated IOLs [35].

15.5.2.2 Intermediate Phase (1–3 Months)

Refractive stabilization was assessed 8–12 weeks before planning enhancements; corneal edema and IOL position may shift. OCT macula for subclinical edema, especially in eyes with vitreous loss [36].

15.6 Future Directions: Innovations in IOL Calculation and Complication Management

The field of cataract surgery is rapidly evolving, driven by technological advancements, artificial intelligence (AI), and collaborative research. This chapter explores emerging trends poised to revolutionize IOL optimization in complex cases, addressing current limitations and enhancing surgical outcomes.

15.6.1 Real-Time Intraoperative Biometry and Imaging

15.6.1.1 Intraoperative OCT

High-resolution, real-time OCT integrated into surgical microscopes (e.g., Opmi Lumera RESCAN 700 (Carl Zeiss Meditec, Inc., Dublin, CA)) enables visualization of capsule integrity, zonular status, and IOL position during surgery. This allows immediate ELP adjustments if complications arise (e.g., detecting posterior capsule rupture early). In fact, two large prospective clinical trials, PIONEER (Prospective Intraoperative and Perioperative Ophthalmic Imaging with Optical Coherence Tomography) and DISCOVER (Determination of Feasibility of Intraoperative Spectral-Domain Microscope Combined/Integrated OCT Visualization during En Face Retinal and Ophthalmic Surgery) studies, demonstrated that (microscope integrated) intraoperative optical coherence tomography (iOCT) may alter intraoperative decision-making in a significant percentage of anterior-segment and posterior-segment surgeries [37, 38].

15.6.1.2 AI-Driven IOL Formulas

Machine learning algorithms (e.g., Hill-RBF 4.0) analyze thousands of surgical outcomes to predict optimal IOL power, even in eyes with irregular anatomy. AI models trained on complication-specific datasets (e.g., postvitrectomy eyes) could automate intraoperative adjustments [39].

15.6.2 Advanced IOL Designs and Materials

15.6.2.1 Adjustable-Power IOLs

Light-adjustable (LAL) IOLs (RxSight, Inc., Aliso Viejo, CA) enable postoperative refractive tweaks via ultraviolet (UV) light, which is ideal for eyes with unpredictable ELP. This lens can correct residual errors (±2.0 D) after scleral-fixated or sulcus IOL placement [40, 41].

15.6.2.2 Modular IOL Systems

"Lens-in-a-lens" designs (e.g., HARMONI Modular IOL System (ClarVista Medical, Aliso Viejo, CA) allow surgeons to add toric or multifocal components postoperatively, reducing reliance on perfect intraoperative calculations [42].

15.6.3 Collaborative Research and Standardization

Global Consensus Guidelines by multisociety efforts (American Society of Cataract and Refractive Surgery (ASCRS), American Academy of Ophthalmology (AAO), and European Society of Cataract and Refractive Surgeons (ESCRS)) are needed to standardize complication IOL adjustment protocols (e.g., unified Wang-Koch formula for scleral fixation). Patient-reported outcome measures (PROMs) using validated questionnaires (e.g., Catquest-9SF) integrated into electronic health records can prioritize patient satisfaction in IOL studies [43].

15.7 Conclusion

The optimization of IOL power calculations in the face of emergency intraoperative complications demands a synthesis of meticulous preparation, real-time adaptability, and evidence-based innovation. As cataract surgery evolves into a refractive discipline, surgeons must balance cutting-edge tools—such as intraoperative aberrometry and AI-driven formulas—with time-tested clinical judgment to navigate anatomic disruptions such as posterior capsule rupture or zonular dehiscence. Postoperative strategies, including piggyback IOLs or laser enhancements, offer salvage pathways for refractive surprises. In contrast, emerging technologies such as adjustable-power IOLs and gene therapy promise to redefine precision in complex cases. Ultimately, success hinges on a proactive, systematic approach: leveraging preoperative planning, intraoperative recalibration, and collaborative research to mitigate uncertainties and elevate patient outcomes. By embracing both technological advancements and the art of surgical improvisation, ophthalmologists can transform intraoperative crises into opportunities for refractive excellence, ensuring that even the most challenging surgeries culminate in visual clarity and patient satisfaction.

References

1. World Health Organization. Blindness and vision impairment: cataract surgical coverage. Geneva: World Health Organization; 2021.
2. Hoffer KJ, Savini G. IOL power calculation in short and long eyes. Asia-Pac J Ophthalmol (Philadelphia, PA). 2017;6:330–1. https://doi.org/10.22608/APO.2017338.
3. Wang L, Koch DD, Hill W, Abulafia A. Pursuing perfection in intraocular lens calculations: III. Criteria for analyzing outcomes. J Cataract Refract Surg. 2017;43(8):999–1002. https://doi.org/10.1016/j.jcrs.2017.08.003. PMID: 28917430
4. Wang L, Koch DD. Modified axial length adjustment formulas in long eyes. J Cataract Refract Surg. 2018;44(11):1396–7. https://doi.org/10.1016/j.jcrs.2018.07.049, indexed in Pubmed: 30274847.
5. Ianchulev T, Hoffer KJ, Yoo SH, Chang DF, Breen M, Padrick T, Tran DB. Intraoperative refractive biometry for predicting intraocular lens power calculation after prior myopic refractive surgery. Ophthalmology. 2014;121(1):56–60. https://doi.org/10.1016/j.ophtha.2013.08.041. Epub 2013 Oct 30. PMID: 24183339.
6. ASCRS Cataract Clinical Committee. Calculating IOL power in eyes with prior refractive surgery. American Society of Cataract and Refractive Surgery; 2022. https://ascrs.org/tools/clinical-resources. Accessed 15 Aug 2023.
7. Chang DF. Managing intraoperative complications in cataract surgery. In: Focal points: clinical modules for ophthalmologists. San Francisco: American Academy of Ophthalmology; 2018: Module 12.
8. Gimbel HV, Sun R. Management of posterior capsule tears. Surv Ophthalmol. 2001;45(1):3–26. https://doi.org/10.1016/S0039-6257(00)00145-3.
9. Abdelghany AA, Alio JL. Surgical options for correction of refractive error following cataract surgery. Eye Vis (Lond). 2014;1:2. https://doi.org/10.1186/s40662-014-0002-2.
10. Chang DF, Masket S, Miller KM, et al. Complications of sulcus placement of single-piece acrylic intraocular lenses: recommendations for backup IOL implanta-

tion following posterior capsule rupture. J Cataract Refract Surg. 2009;35(8):1445–58. https://doi.org/10.1016/j.jcrs.2009.04.027.
11. Cionni RJ, Osher RH. Endocapsular ring approach to the subluxed cataractous lens. J Cataract Refract Surg. 1995;21(3):245–9. https://doi.org/10.1016/s0886-3350(13)80126-5.
12. Cionni RJ, Osher RH. Management of profound zonular dialysis or weakness with a new endocapsular ring designed for scleral fixation. J Cataract Refract Surg. 1998;24:1299–306. https://doi.org/10.1016/s0886-3350(98)80218-6.
13. Aramberri J. IOL calculation in vitreoretinal pathology and surgery. In: Aramberri J, Hoffer KJ, Olsen T, Savini G, Shammas HJ, editors. Intraocular lens calculations. Essentials in ophthalmology. Cham: Springer; 2024. p. 945–61. https://doi.org/10.1007/978-3-031-50666-6_68.
14. Arbisser LB. Comprehensive strategies for unplanned vitrectomy for the anterior segment surgeon. Cataract Refract Surg Today. 2012;1(Suppl):3–20. Accessed 22 Mar 2021.
15. Melamud A, Topilow JS, Cai L, He X. Pars Plana vitrectomy combined with either secondary scleral-fixated or anterior chamber intraocular lens implantation. Am J Ophthalmol. 2016;168:177–82. https://doi.org/10.1016/j.ajo.2016.05.006. Epub 2016 May 14. PMID: 27189930.
16. Hoffer KJ. The Hoffer Q formula: a comparison of theoretic and regression formulas. J Cataract Refract Surg. 1993;19(6):700–12. https://doi.org/10.1016/s0886-3350(13)80338-0. PMID: 8271165
17. Davison JA. Acute intraoperative suprachoroidal hemorrhage in extracapsular cataract surgery. J Cataract Refract Surg. 1986;12(6):606–22. https://doi.org/10.1016/s0886-3350(86)80075-x. PMID: 3491206
18. Xia T, Martinez CE, Tsai LM. Update on intraocular lens formulas and calculations. Asia Pac J Ophthalmol (Phila). 2020;9(3):186–93. https://doi.org/10.1097/APO.0000000000000293. PMID: 32501896; PMCID: PMC7299214.
19. Ianchulev T, Salz J, Hoffer K, Albini T, Hsu H, Labree L. Intraoperative optical refractive biometry for intraocular lens power estimation without axial length and keratometry measurements. J Cataract Refract Surg. 2005;31(8):1530–6. https://doi.org/10.1016/j.jcrs.2005.01.035. PMID: 16129287.
20. Chan NSW, Lim JS, Mohanram LS, Chee SP. Ultrasound biomicroscopy in the management of complex cataract and intraocular lens: a review. Clin Experiment Ophthalmol. 2024;52(2):186–206. https://doi.org/10.1111/ceo.14321. Epub 2024 Jan 12. PMID: 38214059.
21. Aristodemou P. IOL constant optimization. In: Aramberri J, Hoffer KJ, Olsen T, Savini G, Shammas HJ, editors. Intraocular lens calculations. Essentials in ophthalmology. Cham: Springer; 2024. p. 551–76. https://doi.org/10.1007/978-3-031-50666-6_36.
22. Wang Q, Jiang W, Lin T, Zhu Y, Chen C, Lin H, Chen W. Accuracy of intraocular lens power calculation formulas in long eyes: a systematic review and meta-analysis. Clin Experiment Ophthalmol. 2018;46(7):738–49. https://doi.org/10.1111/ceo.13184. Epub 2018 Mar 24. PMID: 29498180.
23. Pantanelli SM, Hatch K, Lin CC, Steigleman WA, Al-Mohtaseb Z, Rose-Nussbaumer JR, Santhiago MR, Keenan TDL, Kim SJ, Jacobs DS, Schallhorn JM. Intraoperative Aberrometry versus preoperative biometry for intraocular lens power calculations: a report by the American Academy of ophthalmology. Ophthalmology. 2025;132(2):238–52. https://doi.org/10.1016/j.ophtha.2024.08.007.
24. Markatia Z, Hudson J, Leung EH, Sajjad A, Gibbons A. The post-vitrectomy cataract. Int Ophthalmol Clin. 2022;62(3):79–91. https://doi.org/10.1097/IIO.0000000000000440. Epub 2022 Jun 22. PMID: 35752887; PMCID: PMC10187786
25. Oh J, Shin HH, Kim JH, Kim HM, Song JS. Direct measurement of the ciliary sulcus diameter by 35-megahertz ultrasound biomicroscopy. Ophthalmology. 2007;114(9):1685–8. https://doi.org/10.1016/j.ophtha.2006.12.018.
26. Fang JP, Hill W, Wang L, Chan V, Koch DD. Advanced intraocular lens power calculations. In: Kohnen T, Koch DD, editors. Cataract and refractive surgery. Essentials in ophthalmology. Berlin/Heidelberg: Springer; 2006. p. 31–46. https://doi.org/10.1007/3-540-30796-6_4.

27. Findl O, Hirnschall N, Kronschläger M. Anterior chamber depth and IOL calculations. In: Aramberri J, Hoffer KJ, Olsen T, Savini G, Shammas HJ, editors. Intraocular lens calculations. Essentials in ophthalmology. Cham: Springer; 2024. p. 537–50. https://doi.org/10.1007/978-3-031-50666-6_35.
28. Retzlaff J. Posterior chamber implant power calculation regression formulas. Am Intra-Ocular Implant Soc J. 1980;6:268–70. https://doi.org/10.1016/s0146-2776(80)80076-0.
29. Sanders DR, Retzlaff J, Kraff MC. Comparison of empirically derived and theoretical aphakic refraction formulas. Arch Ophthalmol. 1983;101(6):965–7. https://doi.org/10.1001/archopht.1983.01040010965024.
30. Gayton JL, Sanders V, Van Der Karr M, et al. Piggybacking intraocular implants to correct pseudophakic refractive error. Ophthalmology. 1999;106:56–9. https://doi.org/10.1016/S0161-6420(99)90005-2.
31. Alio JL, Abdelghany AA, Fernández-Buenaga R. Management of residual refractive error after cataract surgery. Curr Opin Ophthalmol. 2014;25(4):291–7. https://doi.org/10.1097/ICU.0000000000000067. PMID: 24865171.
32. Gale RP, Saldana M, Johnston RL, Zuberbuhler B, McKibbin M. Benchmark standards for refractive outcomes after NHS cataract surgery. Eye (Lond). 2009;23(1):149–52. https://doi.org/10.1038/sj.eye.6702954.
33. Alsetri H, Masket S, Fram N, Sandoval H, Cabang J, McLachlan J. Clinical outcomes and complications following intraocular lens exchange in the setting of an open or intact posterior capsule. J Cataract Refract Surg. 2023;49(5):499–503. https://doi.org/10.1097/j.jcrs.0000000000001138.
34. Wielders LHP, ESCRS PREMED Study Group, et al. European multicenter trial of the prevention of cystoid macular edema after cataract surgery in nondiabetics: ESCRS PREMED study report 1. J Cataract Refract Surg. 2018;44(4):429–39. https://doi.org/10.1016/j.jcrs.2018.01.029.
35. Yamane S, Sato S, Maruyama-Inoue M, Kadonosono K. Flanged intrascleral intraocular lens fixation with double-needle technique. Ophthalmology. 2017;124(8):1136–42. https://doi.org/10.1016/j.ophtha.2017.03.036.
36. Gulkilik G, Kocabora S, Taskapili M, Engin G. Cystoid macular edema after phacoemulsification: risk factors and effect on visual acuity. Can J Ophthalmol. 2006;41(6):699–703. https://doi.org/10.3129/i06-062. PMID: 17224950
37. Ehlers JP, Modi YS, Pecen PE, et al. The DISCOVER study 3-year results: feasibility and usefulness of microscope-integrated intraoperative OCT during ophthalmic surgery. Ophthalmology. 2018;125(7):1014–27. https://doi.org/10.1016/J.OPHTHA.2017.12.037.
38. Ehlers JP, Dupps WJ, Kaiser PK, et al. The prospective intraoperative and perioperative ophthalmic ImagiNg with optical CoherEncE TomogRaphy (PIONEER) study: 2-year results. Am J Ophthalmol. 2014;158(5):999–1007. https://doi.org/10.1016/j.ajo.2014.07.034.
39. Nuliqiman M, Xu M, Sun Y, Cao J, Chen P, Gao Q, Xu P, Ye J. Artificial intelligence in ophthalmic surgery: current applications and expectations. Clin Ophthalmol. 2023;17:3499–511. https://doi.org/10.2147/OPTH.S438127. PMID: 38026589; PMCID: PMC10674717.
40. Hengerer FH, Dick HB, Conrad-Hengerer I. Clinical evaluation of an ultraviolet light adjustable intraocular lens implanted after cataract removal: eighteen months follow-up. Ophthalmology. 2011;118(12):2382–8. https://doi.org/10.1016/j.ophtha.2011.05.030. Epub 2011 Aug 27. PMID: 21872939.
41. Chayet A, Sandstedt C, Chang S, Rhee P, Tsuchiyama B, Grubbs R, Schwartz D. Use of the light-adjustable lens to correct astigmatism after cataract surgery. Br J Ophthalmol. 2010;94(6):690–2. https://doi.org/10.1136/bjo.2009.164616. PMID: 20508043
42. MacLean KD, Werner L, Kramer GD, et al. Evaluation of stability and capsular bag opacification of a new foldable adjustable intraocular lens. Clin Experiment Ophthalmol. 2015;43(7):648–54. https://doi.org/10.1111/ceo.12526.
43. Sparrow JM, Grzeda MT, Frost NA, et al. Cataract surgery patient-reported outcome measures: a head-to-head comparison of the psychometric performance and patient acceptability of the Cat-PROM5 and Catquest-9SF self-report questionnaires. Eye (Lond). 2018;32(4):788–95. https://doi.org/10.1038/eye.2017.297.

Chapter 16
Calculation for Miscellaneous Cases

Vidyapati Widiarto Mangunkusumo, Rio Rhendy, and Andrew Maximillian Herman Knoch

16.1 Introduction

Biometry in ophthalmology refers to the measurement and analysis of the eye's physical characteristics, such as its shape, size, and curvature. This technology has revolutionized the field of eye care, enabling accurate diagnoses, personalized treatment plans, and improved surgical outcomes. By leveraging advanced diagnostic tools and techniques, biometry helps ophthalmologists to better understand the unique anatomy of each patient's eye, ultimately leading to more effective and precise care [1].

All authors declare no financial interest.

Vidyapati Widiarto Mangunkusumo has died before the publication of this book.

V. W. Mangunkusumo (✉)
JEC Eye Hospitals & Clinics, Jakarta, Indonesia

R. Rhendy
Cipto Mangunkusumo Hospital, Jakarta, Indonesia

Universitas Indonesia, Jakarta, Indonesia

A. M. H. Knoch
Universitas Padjadjaran, Bandung, Indonesia

Cicendo National Eye Hospital, Bandung, Indonesia

Bandung Eye Center, Bandung, Indonesia

G. Pardianto (ed.), *Intraocular Lens (IOL) Power Calculation*,
https://doi.org/10.1007/978-981-92-1223-1_16

16.2 Biometry Measurements in Eyes with Long Axial Length (AL)

Eyes with long ALs pose unique challenges for biometry measurements. Several factors can contribute to inaccuracies, including:

1. Optical coherence tomography (OCT) limitations: OCT imaging may struggle to accurately capture the entire AL of highly myopic eyes, leading to measurement errors.
2. Ultrasound biometry limitations: Ultrasound waves can be affected by the altered anatomy of long eyes and the density of the vitreous body, potentially causing inaccuracies in AL measurements.
3. Formula selection: Standard formulas for intraocular lens (IOL) power calculation may not be optimized for eyes with extreme ALs, leading to errors in IOL power selection.
4. Retinal shape and curvature: Irregularities in retinal shape and curvature can affect biometry measurements, particularly in eyes with posterior staphyloma.
5. Instrument calibration and quality control: Ensuring proper calibration and quality control of biometry instruments is crucial to minimize measurement errors.
6. Operator experience and technique: The skill and experience of the operator performing biometry measurements can significantly impact accuracy [2, 3].

To mitigate these challenges, it is essential to:

1. Use advanced biometry instruments: Utilize modern biometry devices that incorporate advanced technologies, such as swept-source OCT (SS-OCT) or partial coherence interferometry. SS-OCT is a laser beam with a rapidly changing wavelength that scans the eye and creates reflected light from the eye that interferes with the reference beam. The interference forms patterns that are used to create high-resolution images of the ocular structures, including the retina and choroid. Advanced algorithms reconstruct detailed images of the eye. The advantage of SS-OCT allows deeper penetration into ocular structures, high-resolution images, and enables rapid image acquisition.
2. Select appropriate formulas: Choose formulas specifically designed for eyes with long ALs or consider using newer, more advanced formulas.
3. Consider multiple measurements: Take multiple measurements and verify their consistency to ensure accuracy.
4. Account for individual variations: Be aware of individual variations in eye anatomy and adjust measurements accordingly [4].

16.3 Three Best Formulas for IOL Calculation in Long Eyes

- Barrett Universal II (BUII): This formula is accurate in long eyes and has performed well in various studies. It is also easily accessible online and preinstalled on several biometers, including Aladdin (Topcon, Tokyo, Japan), ANTERION

(Heidelberg Engineering, Heidelberg, Germany), and IOLMaster 700 (Carl Zeiss Meditec, Dublin, CA). However, it may be less accurate in short eyes or with high-power lenses.
- Kane: This blended formula, combining vergence, regression, and artificial intelligence, has shown high accuracy in long eyes (AL $\geq$26 mm). It is also accurate in short eyes and extreme anterior chamber depths.
- Emmetropia Verifying Optical (EVO) 2.0: This vergence formula has demonstrated accuracy in long eyes (26 mm $\leq$ AL $<$ 28 mm) and accounts for optical dimensions and different IOL geometries. Although it is not pre-installed on many biometers, it is easily accessible online [5].

Additionally, other formulas, such as Hoffer QST (Kenneth J. Hoffer Q/Giacomo Savini/Leonardo Taroni), Olsen-C, and PEARL-DGS (postoperative spherical Equivalent prediction using ARtificial intelligence and Linear algorithms by Guillaume Debellemanière, Damien Gatinel, and Alain Saad), may also be suitable for long eyes, but more evidence is needed to confirm their correlation to consider individual patient characteristics, and optimize biometry measurements for the best outcome [6].

16.4 Biomechanical Properties of Eyes That Can Influence Biometry Measurements

1. Corneal properties: Corneal thickness (CT), curvature, and stiffness can affect biometry measurements, particularly when using optical or ultrasound-based methods.
2. Scleral rigidity: Variations in scleral rigidity can impact the accuracy of AL measurements, especially in eyes with extreme ALs elasticity of the zonules, are correlated to different measurement outcomes.
3. Intraocular pressure (IOP): IOP fluctuations can influence corneal shape and thickness, potentially affecting biometry measurements.
4. Retinal shape and curvature: Irregularities in retinal shape and curvature, such as posterior staphyloma, can impact difficulty in finding the exact location of the macula during biometry measurements [7–9].

16.5 Ultrasound (A-Scan or Amplitude Mode Scan/Display) Biometry for IOL Calculation

When using A-scan ultrasound biometry for IOL calculation, some modifications to the formulas may be necessary, due to potential differences in measurement accuracy compared to optical biometry. These are some considerations:

- Velocity adjustment: A-scan ultrasound biometry assumes a fixed velocity of sound in the ocular media. However, this velocity can vary slightly between individuals and ocular structures. Some formulas allow for adjustments in velocity or use different velocities for different densities and segments of the eye.
- Measurement technique: A-scan biometry requires careful technique to ensure accurate measurements. The formulas might need to account for potential variations in measurement technique, such as immersion vs. contact A-scan.
- Correction for corneal indentation: Contact A-scan can cause corneal indentation, potentially leading to underestimation of anterior chamber depth.
- Using specific A-scan-based formulas: Certain formulas, such as the Holladay 1 or Hoffer Q, can be optimized for use with A-scan biometry. These formulas might incorporate specific constants or adjustments to account for the characteristics of A-scan measurements [9–11].

16.6 Significant Role of Scleral Rigidity in the Accuracy of Ocular Biometry in Eyes with Long ALs

1. Underestimation of AL: Eyes with long ALs often have thinner sclerae, which can lead to increased ocular wall compliance. This might cause the ultrasound signal in biometry measurements to be affected, potentially leading to inaccuracies in AL measurements.
2. Impact on IOL power calculation: Inaccurate AL measurements can significantly affect IOL power calculations. Underestimation or overestimation of AL can lead to errors in IOL power selection, potentially resulting in postoperative refractive surprises.
3. Consideration for formulas: Some biometry formulas might not accurately account for variations in scleral rigidity. This could further contribute to errors in IOL power calculation, especially in eyes with extreme ALs [4, 12].

16.7 Significant Role of Scleral Rigidity in the Accuracy of Ocular Biometry in Eyes with Short ALs

Scleral rigidity in eyes with short ALs can also impact biometry measurements:

- Overestimation or underestimation: Eyes with short ALs often have stiffer, more rigid sclerae. This increased rigidity might affect the accuracy of ultrasound signal penetration and reflection, potentially leading to overestimation or underestimation of AL.
- IOL power calculation challenges: Inaccurate AL measurements in eyes with short ALs can significantly impact IOL power calculations. Errors in AL measurement can lead to incorrect IOL power selection, potentially resulting in postoperative refractive errors.

- Formula limitations: Standard biometry formulas might not perfectly account for the unique characteristics of eyes with short ALs and increased scleral rigidity. This could further contribute to errors in IOL power calculation [13].

16.8 Challenges in Short Eyes

1. Increased curvature: Short eyes often have steeper corneal curvatures, which can affect biometry measurements.
2. Higher IOL power requirements: Short eyes typically require higher IOL powers, making accurate biometry crucial.
3. Formula selection: Standard formulas may not be optimized for short eyes, potentially leading to errors in IOL power calculation.

16.9 Strategies for Accurate Biometry

1. Use advanced biometry instruments: Utilize modern biometry devices that incorporate advanced technologies, such as SS-OCT or partial coherence interferometry (PCI).
2. Select appropriate formulas: Choose formulas specifically designed for short eyes or consider using newer, more advanced formulas.
3. Take multiple measurements: Verify the consistency of measurements to ensure accuracy.
4. The User Group for Laser Interference Biometry (ULIB) provides optimized A-constants for various IOL models, which can be useful for accurate calculations in eyes with short ALs [13, 14].

Using optimized A-constants from ULIB can help improve the accuracy of IOL power calculations by accounting for the specific characteristics of the IOL model being used. By incorporating ULIB's optimized A-constants, clinicians can refine their calculations and provide more precise IOL power predictions for patients with short ALs [14].

16.10 Biometry Roles in Diagnosing and Treating Astigmatism

To correct astigmatism with toric intraocular lenses (tIOLs), clinicians need accurate measurements of corneal astigmatism. Several methods are used, including:

- Keratometry: Measures the curvature of the corneal front surface using manual or automated keratometers, such as the IOLMaster 700 [15, 16].
- Corneal tomography: Measures the curvature of both corneal surfaces using devices like the Galilei G4 or the newer version G6 (Ziemer, Biel, Switzerland), providing a more comprehensive understanding of corneal astigmatism [16].

16.11 Challenges in Measuring Corneal Astigmatism

Different measurement modalities may yield inconsistent results. The study highlights the importance of considering the corneal back surface measurement, as it can add against-the-rule astigmatism. Moreover, the disparity between refractive cylinder and keratometric astigmatism may include noncorneal components such as lens tilt or decentration [15, 16].

16.12 Prediction Models

To improve accuracy, prediction models can be used to map measured corneal astigmatism to reconstructed corneal power (recCP). Two approaches are:

- Feedforward neural networks (NET): Can perform well but may over-fit data.
- Linear regression (REG): Offers similar performance to NET with easier implementation [15].

16.13 Calculating IOL Power for Eyes Undergoing Limbal Relaxing Incisions (LRIs) to Correct Astigmatism

16.13.1 Astigmatism Correction

LRIs can reduce corneal astigmatism, affecting IOL power calculation. Clinicians should:

- Measure preoperative astigmatism: Accurately assess corneal astigmatism using keratometry or corneal tomography.
- Plan LRI: Determine the location, length, and depth of LRIs based on the amount and axis of astigmatism. [17]

16.13.2 IOL Calculation

When calculating IOL power, consider the expected change in corneal astigmatism after LRI:

- Adjust keratometry values: Account for the anticipated reduction in corneal astigmatism.
- Use toric IOL calculators: Some calculators can account for the effect of LRIs on corneal astigmatism [15–17].

16.13.3 Nomograms and Guidelines

Several nomograms and guidelines are available to help plan LRIs, including:

- LRI nomograms: Provide guidance on incision length and location based on astigmatism magnitude and axis.
- Toric IOL calculators: Can account for LRI-induced changes in corneal astigmatism [15, 16].

When combining IOL implantation with LRIs, consider:

- Variability in response: Individual responses to LRIs can vary, affecting astigmatism correction.
- Coupling effects: LRIs can induce changes in corneal curvature, potentially affecting the spherical power of the IOL, which has to be compensated by increasing the spherical power by ½ x astigmatism [17].

16.14 Biometry in Congenital Lens Dislocation Is Crucial for Planning Surgical Interventions

Congenital lens dislocation often occurs in Marfan syndrome, homocystinuria, or other conditions affecting ocular structures. Accurate biometry is essential but can be challenging due to ocular dimensions, which include:

- Lens subluxation or dislocation: Affects the accuracy of keratometry and AL measurements and asymmetric zonular dimensions, which affect IOL centration.
- Retinal abnormalities: May impact the exact macular location during biometric measurements.

To overcome these challenges, clinicians use advanced biometric techniques:

- PCI: Provides accurate AL measurements, even in eyes with lens subluxation.
- Scheimpflug imaging or OCT: Helps align the central cornea to lens anatomy.

Accurate biometry enables precise IOL power calculation, which is critical in congenital lens dislocation cases. Clinicians may use intraoperative aberrometry, which helps fine-tune IOL power selection on the line of sight.

Biometry informs surgical decisions, such as:

- IOL placement: Choosing the optimal IOL type (ULIB) and placement location.
- Scleral fixation: Planning suture placement for IOL fixation [14, 18, 19].

By combining advanced biometric techniques with clinical expertise, surgeons can achieve better outcomes in congenital lens dislocation cases.

16.15 Biometry Plays a Crucial Role in Calculating Piggyback IOL Power

When implanting a piggyback IOL, accurate calculation of the additional IOL power is essential. Biometry helps determine:

- Residual refractive error: Measuring the remaining refractive error after primary IOL implantation [6].
- Additional IOL power: Calculating the power of the piggyback IOL needed to achieve the desired refractive outcome [20].

To calculate piggyback IOL power, clinicians use:

- Subjective refraction: Measuring the residual refractive error.
- Keratometry: Assessing corneal power and astigmatism.
- AL measurement.

Several methods are used to calculate piggyback IOL power, including:

- Empirical formulas: Based on clinical experience and regression analysis.
- Theoretical formulas: Using optical principles to calculate IOL power.
- Online calculators: Utilizing specialized software to determine piggyback IOL power [20].

When calculating piggyback IOL power, clinicians must consider:

- IOL type and material: Different IOLs may interact differently with the primary IOL.
- Haptic design and placement: Ensuring proper positioning and stability of both IOLs [6, 20].

16.16 Postmyopic Laser Correction

Postmyopic laser in-situ keratomileusis (LASIK)/photorefractive keratectomy (PRK) correction, also known as post-LASIK/PRK hyperopia or hyperopic shift, can be challenging. After myopic LASIK/PRK, the cornea may become too flat, leading to:

- Hyperopic shift: Difficulty achieving accurate IOL power calculation due to altered corneal shape.
- Inaccurate keratometry: Traditional keratometry may not accurately reflect corneal power in flat corneas. [21]

Several methods can help calculate IOL power:

- History-based methods: Utilize preoperative refraction and keratometry values [4, 5].
- No-history methods: Rely on postoperative keratometry and tomography measurements [4–6].
- Advanced calculation methods: Incorporate corneal tomography and ray-tracing analysis [21–23].

When calculating IOL power for postmyopic LASIK/PRK eyes, consider:

- Corneal irregularity: Altered corneal shape can affect IOL power calculation.
- Previous ablation profile: Understanding the previous laser treatment can help inform IOL power calculation [21].

To achieve optimal results, clinicians should:

- Use advanced diagnostic tools: Utilize corneal tomography and wavefront analysis.
- For eyes that have undergone myopic laser vision correction (LVC), calculating IOL power can be challenging due to altered corneal shape and power.

Corneal tomography and wavefront analysis can be valuable tools in this context [4–6, 16].

16.17 Corneal Tomography

1. Accurate corneal mapping: Provides detailed information about the corneal shape, curvature, and power.
2. Improved IOL power calculation: Helps clinicians account for the altered corneal shape and power after LVC.

16.18 Wavefront Analysis

1. Total corneal power calculation: Wavefront analysis can provide information about the total corneal power, including the posterior corneal surface.
2. Customized IOL power calculation: Allows clinicians to consider the unique optical characteristics of each eye [4–6, 16].

By combining corneal tomography and wavefront analysis, clinicians can develop more accurate IOL power calculations for patients who have undergone myopic LVC, ultimately leading to better outcomes.

Keratometry accuracy can be challenging in flat corneas. Flat corneas can lead to:

- Measurement errors: Keratometry may struggle to accurately measure corneal curvature.
- Inaccurate IOL power calculation: Errors in keratometry can affect IOL power calculation.

Several factors contribute to keratometry inaccuracies in flat corneas:

- Instrument limitations: Keratometers may have limited measurement ranges or accuracy in very flat or steep corneas.
- Corneal irregularity: Aspheric or irregular corneal shapes can affect keratometry measurements [16, 21].

To improve keratometry accuracy in flat corneas:

- Use advanced diagnostic tools: Utilize corneal tomography, such as Scheimpflug imaging or optical coherence tomography [4–6, 16].
- Multiple measurement methods: Combine keratometry with other measurement methods, like corneal topography or ray-tracing analysis. Ray tracing analysis in ophthalmology is a computational method that simulates the path of light through the eye's optical system. [22, 23]

16.19 Ray-Tracing Analysis

1. Models corneal and lenticular surfaces: Accurately represents the shape and refractive properties.
2. Tracks light rays: Simulates how light interacts with the eye's optics.
3. Calculates optical properties: Provides detailed information about the eye's optical performance.

Ray tracing analysis is useful for:

1. IOL power calculation: Improves accuracy, especially in complex cases.
2. Corneal analysis: Helps understand corneal shape and power.
3. Optical performance evaluation: Assesses the eye's optical quality [22, 23].

16.20 Conclusion

Accurate AL is essential in IOL calculation in any kind of eye. For myopic eyes, ALs between 26.0 mm and 28.0 mm, optical and A-scan resolve in similar accuracy. For AL more than 28.0 mm, optical biometry with SS-OCT is superior due to pathologic changes in the posterior pole.

In short eyes, choosing the correct IOL lens depends on a precise A-constant selection. This can be achieved by ULIB confirmation.

In flat corneas (post LVC) and dislocated crystalline lens, AL measurement should be combined with ray tracing for simulating the exact center of the cornea or the lens.

References

1. Pathak M, Sahu V, Kumar A, Kaur K, Gurnani B. Current concepts and recent updates of optical biometry: a comprehensive review. Clin Ophthalmol. 2024;18:1191–206. https://doi.org/10.2147/OPTH.S464538.
2. Abulafia A, Barrett GD, Rotenberg M, et al. Intraocular lens power calculation for eyes with an axial length greater than 26.0 mm: comparison of formulas and methods. J Cataract Refract Surg. 2015;41(3):548–56. https://doi.org/10.1016/j.jcrs.2014.06.033.
3. Stopyra W, Voytsekhivskyy O, Grzybowski A. Comparison of the accuracy of twenty intraocular lens power calculation formulas in long eyes. Asia Pac J Ophthalmol (Phila). 2025;14(3):100198. https://doi.org/10.1016/j.apjo.2025.100198.
4. Chen C, Xu X, Miao Y, Zheng G, Sun Y, Xu X. Accuracy of intraocular lens power formulas involving 148 eyes with long axial lengths: a retrospective chart-review study. J Ophthalmol. 2015;2015:976847. https://doi.org/10.1155/2015/976847.
5. Kane JX, Van Heerden A, Atik A, Petsoglou C. Intraocular lens power formula accuracy: comparison of 7 formulas. J Cataract Refract Surg. 2016;42(10):1490–500. https://doi.org/10.1016/j.jcrs.2016.07.021.
6. Melles RB, Holladay JT, Chang WJ. Accuracy of intraocular lens calculation formulas. Ophthalmology. 2018;125(2):169–78. https://doi.org/10.1016/j.ophtha.2017.08.027.
7. Esporcatte LPG, Salomão MQ, Lopes BT, et al. Biomechanical diagnostics of the cornea. Eye Vis (Lond). 2020;7:9. https://doi.org/10.1186/s40662-020-0174-x. Published 2020 Feb 5.
8. Wilson A, Marshall J. A review of corneal biomechanics: mechanisms for measurement and the implications for refractive surgery. Indian J Ophthalmol. 2020;68(12):2679–90. https://doi.org/10.4103/ijo.IJO_2146_20.
9. Kojima T, Tamaoki A, Ichikawa K, et al. Effect of intraocular lens power calculation formula optimization in the sum-of-segments optical biometer. Clin Ophthalmol. 2024;18:2545–53. https://doi.org/10.2147/OPTH.S477006. Published 2024 Sep 6.
10. Tehrani M, Krummenauer F, Blom E, Dick HB. Practicality of optical biometry and applanation ultrasound in 253 eyes. J Cataract Refract Surg. 2003;29(4):741–6. https://doi.org/10.1016/s0886-3350(02)01740-6.
11. Rose LT, Moshegov CN. Comparison of the Zeiss IOLMaster and applanation A-scan ultrasound for IOL calculation. Clin Experiment Ophthalmol. 2003;31(2):121–4. https://doi.org/10.1046/j.1442-9071.2003.00617.x.
12. Wang L, Shirayama M, Ma XJ, Kohnen T, Koch DD. Optimizing intraocular lens power calculations in eyes with axial lengths above 25.0 mm. J Cataract Refract Surg. 2011;37(11):2018–27. https://doi.org/10.1016/j.jcrs.2011.05.042.

13. Shrivastava AK, Nayak S, Mahobia A, Anto M, Pandey P. Accuracy of intraocular lens power calculation formulae in short eyes: a systematic review and meta-analysis. Indian J Ophthalmol. 2022;70(3):740–8. https://doi.org/10.4103/ijo.IJO_934_21.
14. Wang Y, Liu Y, Li J, et al. Lens biometry in congenital lens deformities: a swept-source anterior segment optical coherence tomography study. Front Med (Lausanne). 2021;8:774640. https://doi.org/10.3389/fmed.2021.774640.
15. Abulafia A, Barrett GD, Kleinmann G, Ofir S, Levy A, Marcovich AL, et al. Prediction of refractive outcomes with toric intraocular lens implantation. J Cataract Refract Surg. 2015;41(5):936–44. https://doi.org/10.1016/j.jcrs.2014.08.036.
16. Savini G, Taroni L, Jeon S, et al. Comparison of keratometry and total corneal power, as measured by an SS-OCT-based optical biometer, for intraocular lens power calculation in Asian eyes. J Cataract Refract Surg. 2024;50(11):1117–22. https://doi.org/10.1097/j.jcrs.0000000000001515.
17. Müller-Jensen K, Fischer P, Siepe U. Limbal relaxing incisions to correct astigmatism in clear corneal cataract surgery. J Refract Surg. 1999;15(5):586–9. https://doi.org/10.3928/1081-597X-19990901-12.
18. Chen X, Song Q, Yan W, et al. Evaluation of multimodal biometric parameters for diagnosing acute angle closure secondary to lens subluxation. Ophthalmol Ther. 2023;12(2):839–51. https://doi.org/10.1007/s40123-022-00638-0.
19. Kristianslund O, Østern AE, Drolsum L. Astigmatism and refractive outcome after late in-the-bag intraocular lens dislocation surgery: a randomized clinical trial. Invest Ophthalmol Vis Sci. 2017;58(11):4747–53. https://doi.org/10.1167/iovs.17-22723.
20. Norrby S. Sources of error in intraocular lens power calculation. J Cataract Refract Surg. 2008;34(3):368–76. https://doi.org/10.1016/j.jcrs.2007.10.031.
21. Coulibaly R. Underestimation of intraocular lens power for cataract surgery after myopic PRK. Ophthalmology. 2000;107(2):222–3. https://doi.org/10.1016/s0161-6420(99)00103-7.
22. Pérez-Merino P, Aramberri J, Quintero AV, Rozema JJ. Ray tracing optimization: a new method for intraocular lens power calculation in regular and irregular corneas. Sci Rep. 2023;13(1):4555. Published 2023 Mar 20. https://doi.org/10.1038/s41598-023-31525-8.
23. Ghaffari R, Abdi P, Moghaddasi A, Heidarzadeh S, Ghahvhechian H, Kasiri M. Ray tracing versus thin-lens formulas for IOL power calculation using swept-source optical coherence tomography biometry. J Ophthalmic Vis Res. 2022;17(2):176–85. Published 2022 Apr 29. https://doi.org/10.18502/jovr.v17i2.10788.

Chapter 17
IOL Calculation in Phakic Eye (Phakic IOL Calculation)

Hadi Prakoso Wreksoatmodjo and Sharita Rosalyne Siregar

17.1 Introduction

As we all know, phakic intraocular lens (pIOL) is an intraocular lens that is implanted surgically into the eye to correct refractive errors without removing the natural crystalline lens (also known as "phakos," hence the term). Phakic intraocular lens is indicated for patients with high refractive errors when the usual laser vision corrections (LVC) (such as photorefractive keratectomy (PRK), Lasik, or laser lenticule extraction) are not suitable or contraindicated due to some reasons (myopia over −12 Diopters (D)) or corneal thickness less than 500 microns, or corneal thickness not sufficient for patient's refractive error correction). Phakic IOL also gives a clear postoperative vision without inducing any high-order aberration (spherical aberration) to the patient.

Over more than three decades, phakic intraocular lenses (pIOLs) have become an important component of refractive surgery. Currently, three main categories of pIOLs are available: angle-supported pIOLs, including the AcrySof Cachet (Alcon Surgical, Fort Worth, Texas, USA) and Baikoff ZB5M (Domilens, Lyon, France); iris-fixated (iris-claw) pIOLs, including the Artisan (Ophtec BV, Groningen, the Netherlands) and Verisyse (Johnson & Johnson Vision, Irvine, California, USA); and sulcus-supported pIOLs, including the Visian Implantable Collamer Lens (ICL) (STAAR Surgical, Monrovia, California, USA), Eyecryl Phakic (Biotech Healthcare,

All authors declare no financial interest.

H. P. Wreksoatmodjo (✉)
IEC Eye Care, Jakarta, Indonesia

S. R. Siregar
JEC Eye Hospitals & Clinics, Jakarta, Indonesia

G. Pardianto (ed.), *Intraocular Lens (IOL) Power Calculation*,
https://doi.org/10.1007/978-981-92-1223-1_17

Luzern, Switzerland), and AddOn Implantable Phakic Intraocular Lens (IPCL) (1stQ, Mannheim, Germany).

Since angle support was reported widely with associated long-term complications such as corneal decompensation due to excessive endothelial cells loss, chronic uveitis, and glaucoma, this kind of lens was gradually abandoned by surgeons around the world.

The aim of calculating the IOL power is to get optimum vision after surgery, which may happen if the postoperative refraction were as close to the wishes of the patient (and the surgeon) and to the possibilities of the eye under consideration. Since it is different to correction with spectacles or contact lens, which can easily be replaced when it does not perfectly overcome the refractive error, the IOL power should be calculated carefully before surgery. Because when the surgeon fails to achieve optimum postoperative refractive error correction, it will be more complicated or almost impossible to replace the lens.

Determination of the intraocular lens power in a phakic eye is totally different from a cataract eye, where the power of the cataractous lens could be ignored. In cataract patients, the IOL power was predicted by calculating several parameters, such as corneal refractive power, axial length, and effective lens position of the IOL inside the globe. In a phakic eye, the clear crystalline lens, which still exists, plays an important role in focusing the image at the macula. Thus, an inaccuracy of the focus on the retina may also, in some parts, be a "mistake" of the crystalline lens. So, in contrast to IOL in cataract surgery, where the IOL is replacing the power of the cataractous lens, in the phakic eye, the IOL power that will be implanted will replace the power of the spectacle that corrected the refractive error of the patient.

In a virgin eye with myopia refractive error, the incoming beam will be refracted by the cornea and also the crystalline lens and focused in front of the macula. A spectacle with a specific power (minus lens) will diverge the incoming beam before it is translated into the eye through the cornea and the crystalline lens and falls on a focal point at the macula. It means that the spectacle power is decreasing the combined vergence power of the cornea and the human crystalline lens. The closer we put the spectacles to the cornea (the lesser the vertex distance), the smaller the power of the spectacles needed to correct the refractive error. In a similar situation applied to the determination of contact lens power to overcome myopia, the power of the contact lens is almost always less than the power of the spectacles. If the correction of myopia is replaced with an IOL that is placed behind the cornea, the rays emanating from an object are first refracted by the cornea, then by the IOL, and next by the crystalline lens. In contrast to the myopia case, in hyperopia, the closer the spectacles correction to the cornea (and nearer to the retina as well), the higher the power of the lens.

In such a condition where the IOL is addressed to replace the power of the spectacles, in myopia or hyperopia, the IOL power calculation should be done rigorously. Basically, if a phakic IOL is implanted inside the phakic eye, the two most important refractive surfaces (the cornea and the crystalline lens) remain unaltered. Thus, a direct calculation of the power needed can be done based on preoperative refraction, corneal power, and vertex distance [1]. Calculating the thickness and refractive index of the crystalline lens or even measuring the axial length of the eye is unnecessary. The other factor to consider is the desired postoperative refraction. It must be considered also that inaccurate corneal curvature measurement due to long-term contact lens wear and previous keratorefractive surgery may lead to error in power calculation [1–3].

Some authors had proposed mathematical calculations, such as van der Heijde, Holladay, and Olsen. But the most established and most commonly used for anterior chamber phakic IOL is the formula of van der Heijde [1, 2].

17.2 IOL Power Calculation of Anterior Chamber Iris Claw pIOL (Artisan/Verisyse)

The important parameters for phakic intraocular lens (pIOL) calculation are the best spectacle correction (subjective refraction), corneal power (K), and the pIOL position. The pIOL position is defined by the distance between the pIOL and the posterior surface of the cornea (*d*), also referred to as the back vertex distance, which will be discussed later.

According to van der Heijde, first of all we need to determine the power of the spectacles (at the vertex distance) if we move to the corneal plane [3]. If we denote ***S*** as the power of the spectacles at vertex distance (***t***), then the effective power of the spectacles at the corneal plane (***S′***) is:

$$S' = \frac{S}{1 - t.S}$$

The second step is calculating ***K′*** or the sum of the power of the spectacles at the corneal plane (***S′***) and the power of the cornea (*K*):

$$K' = K + S' = K + \frac{S}{1 - t.S}$$

The position of the IOL toward the back vertex of the cornea (***d***), or usually named as ELP (Effective Lens Position), may be measured as follows:

- The distance between the back vertex and the crystalline lens is ACD (anterior chamber depth).
- It should be known that ACD results on biometric readings are mostly a distance between the anterior surface of the cornea (epithelium). And to get the “pure” ACD from the back vertex (endothelium), we need to subtract it from the central corneal thickness (measured with pachymetry).
- The distance between the IOL and the crystalline lens for Artisan/Verisyse, as factors advised by Ophtec BV (manufacturer of Artisan):
  - Artisan/Verisyse hyperopia lens: 0.6 mm.
  - Artisan/Verisyse myopia lens: 0.8 mm.

- The ELP (***d***) of Artisan/Verisyse IOL = ACD (endothelium)—0.6 mm or 0.8 mm.

Finally, the spherical power of the pIOL (Artisan/Verisyse) turns out as:

$$\text{Piol} = \frac{n}{\frac{n}{K'(\text{preop})} - d} - \frac{n}{\frac{n}{K'(\text{postop})} - d}$$

P = power of pIOL
N = refractive index of aqueous (1.336)
K = corneal power in Diopters = K' (post op)
K' = sum of corneal power and spectacle power at the corneal plane
D = effective lens position (in meter)

If we put the d in mm, the n should be multiplied by 1000, and the equation become:

$$\text{Piol} = \frac{1336}{\frac{1336}{K'(\text{preop})} - d} - \frac{1336}{\frac{1336}{K'(\text{postop})} - d}$$

To facilitate the power calculation for surgeons all over the world who want to implant Artisan/Verisyse pIOL, the company that produces those IOLs (Ophtec BV, Groningen, the Netherlands) provides an online IOL calculator:

ArtiCalc (https://calculator.ophtec.com)

17.3 IOL Power Calculation of Sulcus Supported pIOL/Posterior Chamber pIOL (Visian ICL, Eyecryl Phakic IOL, etc.)

The posterior chamber phakic IOL calculation may also be done using the van der Heijde method. However, there is another alternative formula by Olsen for posterior chamber phakic IOL, which is as follows:

$$\text{Piol} = \frac{1336}{\frac{1336}{K + \text{ECL} - T - \text{ACD} - 0.1}} - \frac{1336}{\frac{1336}{K - T - \text{ACD} - 0.1}}$$

1336 = aqueous refractive index multiplied by 1000 (because all distances in this formula are in mm)
K = corneal power in D
ECL = equivalent of contact lens power at the corneal level

T = corneal thickness in mm
ACD = anterior chamber depth in mm

Calculating posterior chamber phakic IOL using van der Heijde or Olsen formulae provides excellent postoperative results, assuming the initial measurements of all parameters were done accurately [3]. However, another important factor that must be taken into account in selecting posterior chamber phakic IOL is sizing.

Choosing the right size of the lens involves the measurement of the WTW (white-to-white) horizontal corneal diameter. By this measurement we can determine the lens size, assuming that the horizontal sulcus diameter is equivalent to WTW + 0.5 mm [2, 4]. According to a report, for an average European with a WTW distance of 11.7 mm, the ATA (angle to angle) distance is 11.9 mm and the sulcus-to sulcus (STS) measurement is 11.7 mm. Measuring the STS more accurately is reported using more complicated equipment, such as AS-OCT or Anterior Segment Optical Coherence Tomography (Visante (Carl Zeiss Meditec, Dublin, CA) and UBM or Ultrasound Biomicroscopy (Artemis-2 VHFUS (Scott Philips Engineering, Victoria, BC, Canada)).

Accurate sizing is particularly important for posterior chamber phakic IOLs because if the STS diameter is overestimated and a larger-sized IOL is implanted, vaulting of the lens can occur, resulting in angle narrowing and pigment dispersion. Conversely, if the IOL size is too small, due to underestimated STS diameter measurement, the phakic IOL may move freely, inducing an anterior subcapsular cataract [2, 4].

For easier and simpler calculation of posterior chamber phakic IOL, the companies that produce the IOL provide an online power calculator:

- STAAR Surgical/Online Calculation & Ordering System (OCOS) for EVO ICL: https://evo-ocos.staarag.ch/live/ [6].
- For Eyecryl phakic IOL: http://biotechcalculators.com

17.4 IOL Calculation of Toric Phakic IOL (TPIOL)

The calculation of the astigmatic power of TPIOL is more complicated than calculating the spherical power of phakic IOL. In hyperopia, the power of spherical correction at the spectacle plane is increasing at the corneal plane, meaning that the power of spherical correction in the IOL plane is even higher according to the equations of van Heijde and Olsen. This means that the power of plus cylindrical correction at the IOL plane will also be higher when compared to the power of plus cylindrical correction at the spectacle plane.

Sarver and Sanders proposed a method that combines Holladay's step-along method with the astigmatic decomposition technique described by Bennett and Rabbett to yield equations to calculate the ideal toric power of a TPIOL to predict the postoperative refraction for selected TPIOL, and then calculate a simple optimization parameter to remove bias in the predicted postoperative refraction error of spherical equivalent for a given data set [5]. After a series of complicated equations, the Sarver method gives a calculation of the ideal TPIOL for a given eye and desired post-operative spectacle power. It also gives prediction postoperative spectacle power for a selected TPIOL other than the ideal power (the TPIOL power provided by the manufacturer is in a series of powers with an increment of 0.50 D, or 1.0 D in certain series of powers). That means that, for example, the ideal TPIOL power is S-12.35 C-3.63 with 47° axis; you can select TPIOL with power as S-12.50 C-3.50 with 45° axis.

To facilitate surgeons who intend to implant a TPIOL, all TPIOL manufacturers, such as Ophtec BV (Artisan), Johnson & Johnson Vision (Verisyse), STAAR Surgical (Visian ICL), and Biotech Healthcare (Eyecryl Phakic), provide toric power calculation that is incorporated in their online IOL calculator. Once the surgeon enters all parameter data required for the calculation, the online calculator will provide a series of selected powers with their predicted postoperative refraction of each selected power. Then the surgeon may be able to choose a certain selected power that is closest to the desired postoperative refraction.

17.5 IOL Calculation After pIOL Explantation

As patients with pIOLs age, the need for cataract surgery after pIOL explantation becomes increasingly common. However, accurate IOL power prediction post explantation remains challenging due to changes in corneal structure and the anterior segment after pIOL implantation.

17.6 Clinical Considerations

1. *Explanted IOL data*: The model, power, vault, and orientation (for TPIOL) should all be documented prior to explantation to guide refractive targeting.
2. *Surgical approach*: Whether the explantation and cataract extraction are performed simultaneously or staged will affect the timing and accuracy of biometry measurements.
3. *Corneal alterations*: pIOL implantation may induce subtle changes in corneal topography and biomechanics, which can affect the accuracy of postoperative refractive targeting [7].

17.7 Biometry and Formula Selection

For postexplantation IOL calculations, standard parameters such as AL, K, and ACD should be measured accurately. Modern IOL power calculation formulas such as Barrett Universal II (BUII), Emmetropia Verifying Optical (EVO) 2.0, and Olsen are recommended, as they account for changes in corneal and anterior segment anatomy that may occur after pIOL implantation. The use of ray-tracing techniques and Swept-Source Optical Coherence Tomography (SS-OCT) biometry (e.g., IOLMaster 700 (Carl Zeiss Meditec, Dublin, CA), ARGOS (Movu, Aichi, Japan)) can also enhance accuracy.

17.8 Use of Historical and Empirical Data

In cases where corneal data is altered by the presence of a pIOL, the surgeon may need to rely on historical data, such as the previous manifest refraction, pIOL vault, or toric axis, to guide refractive targeting. In cases where these data are unavailable, intraoperative aberrometry or aphakic refraction methods may be employed to refine the IOL power calculation during surgery.

17.9 Conclusion

IOL power calculation in phakic and postphakic eyes requires careful consideration of the unique anatomical and optical characteristics of the eye. For phakic IOL implantation, using appropriate formulas such as Van der Heijde or Olsen can provide accurate results when the correct input parameters are used. In postexplantation cataract surgery, precise biometry, the correct choice of formula, and modern imaging technologies are crucial for ensuring optimal postoperative outcomes.

References

1. Holladay JT. Refractive power calculations for intraocular lenses in the phakic eye. Am J Ophthalmol. 1993;116:63–6. https://doi.org/10.1016/s0002-9394(14)71745-3.
2. Lovisolo CF, Reinstein DZ. Phakic intraocular lenses. Surv Ophthalmol. 2005;50:549–87. https://doi.org/10.1016/j.survophthal.2005.08.011.
3. Van der Heijde GL. Some optical aspects of implantation of an IOL in a myopic eye. Doc Ophthalmol. 1987;65(3):301–10.
4. Zhang GM, Zhao LJ, Xie HT, Wu MF. Anterior segment biometry during accommodation after posterior chamber phakic implantable collamer lens implantation. J Refract Surg. 2024;40(3):e164–72. https://doi.org/10.3928/1081597X-20240212-01.

5. Cano-Ortiz A, et al. Astigmatism correction with toric implantable collamer lens in low and high astigmatism groups. Eur J Ophthalmol. 2022;32(1):183–92. https://doi.org/10.1177/1120672121999991.
6. STAAR Surgical. EVO/EVO+ Visian ICL product information and sizing guidelines. Monrovia: STAAR Surgical; 2023. Available at: STAAR Surgical/Online Calculation & Ordering System (OCOS) for EVO ICL: https://evo-ocos.staarag.ch/live/ (login required).
7. Yang W, Zhao J, Sun L, et al. Four-year observation of the changes in corneal endothelium cell density and correlated factors after Implantable Collamer Lens V4c implantation. Br J Ophthalmol. 2021;105(5):625–30. https://doi.org/10.1136/bjophthalmol-2020-316144.

Chapter 18
Femtosecond Laser-Assisted Cataract Surgery (FLACS): Is There Any Adjustment Needed for IOL Calculations?

Steve A. Arshinoff and Chinmayi H. Vyas

18.1 Introduction

Modern cataract surgery has progressed from basic displacement of an opacified lens, initially by couching, first reported by Sushruta in 600 BCE (before the common era), followed 2200 years later by the dramatic improvement of extracapsular cataract surgery by Jacques Daviel in 1747, to which Sir Nicholas Harold Lloyd Ridley contributed monumentally 200 years later with intraocular lenses in 1949, completing the groundwork to set the stage for modern enhancements. Charles David Kelman introduced phacoemulsification in 1967, which led to smaller incisions and foldable intraocular lens (IOL). Cataract surgery is now progressing, in the 2000s, to include astigmatic and presbyopia correcting IOLs, laser-based corneal refractive correction techniques, and now femtosecond laser-assisted cataract surgery (FLACS). Cataract surgery has become a highly refined, individualized refractive procedure aimed at optimizing postoperative visual outcomes for every eye. This evolution has also depended upon the development of increasingly sophisticated IOL power calculation formulas and progressively accurate preoperative measurement techniques. As always happens with progress, patient expectations jump ahead of realistic expectations and now extend to spectacle independence and

All authors declare no financial interest.

S. A. Arshinoff (✉)
Department of Ophthalmology and Vision Sciences, University of Toronto, Toronto, ON, Canada

C. H. Vyas
Department of Surgery, Vitreoretinal Surgery Service, McMaster University, Hamilton, ON, Canada

G. Pardianto (ed.), *Intraocular Lens (IOL) Power Calculation*,
https://doi.org/10.1007/978-981-92-1223-1_18

excellent visual quality, irrespective of the starting point, often exceeding anything the patients have ever experienced before in their lives [1].

As standard cataract surgery and refractive lens exchange have merged in their goals, the emphasis has moved from preventing complications, the incidence of which has progressively declined, to enhancing surgical precision, predictability, and customization to manage whatever problems the patient presented with. Building on the established success of laser technology in refractive surgery, the introduction of femtosecond laser technology into cataract procedures represents a natural evolutionary step toward greater surgical accuracy and predictability, but like everything new, the initial price tag is always shocking, and that led to skepticism. Since its approval in 2010, FLACS has emerged as a powerful tool to meet increasing patient expectations. By automating some critical surgical steps of conventional phacoemulsification cataract surgery (CPCS) that were most subject to individual variability (capsulorhexis, nucleus fragmentation, astigmatic keratotomies, and incision creation), FLACS enhances reproducibility and precision and assures more consistent effective lens position of the IOL. Through this integration, FLACS has demonstrated the potential to improve safety, minimize intraocular energy use (thereby decreasing surgical-induced corneal endothelial damage), and deliver superior refractive outcomes.

This chapter explores the role of FLACS as a tool in optimizing IOL power calculation outcomes, with a focus on how greater surgical precision contributes to improved lens positioning and visual performance.

18.2 Overview of Femtosecond Cataract Laser Types

Femtosecond (fs) lasers emit at 1053 nm (YAG (Yttrium Aluminum Garnet) lasers emit at 1064 nm). The pulses emitted are extremely short with durations of about 400 femtoseconds (fs = 10^{-15} s, YAG pulses are about 10 picoseconds (ps = 10^{-12} s), so a femtosecond laser pulse is about 1/25th the duration of a YAG laser picosecond pulse). Both fs and YAG lasers work by photodisruption, creating tiny plasmas that enable tissue destruction, but fs laser photodisruption volumes per pulse are much smaller and cause much less collateral damage.

The most widely used femtosecond laser platforms, such as LenSx® (Alcon Laboratories, Inc., Fort Worth, TX), VICTUS® (Bausch & Lomb, Bridgewater, NJ), Catalys® (Johnson & Johnson Vision, Jacksonville, FL), and LENSAR® (LENSAR, Inc., Orlando, FL), are higher energy, lower frequency systems that emit pulses in the microjoule (μJ) range at repetition rates of kilohertz (kHz) frequencies. In contrast, the Femto LDV Z8® (Ziemer Ophthalmic Systems AG, Port, Switzerland) utilizes a compact handpiece with closer proximity to the eye, allowing for lower energy delivery in nanoJoules (nJ), a smaller spot size, and megahertz (MHz) repetition rates, maintaining high precision, and resulting in less gas bubble formation during photodisruption, thereby decreasing possible collateral damage.

Docking of the laser to the eye is critical for femtosecond lasers. Some lasers use a rigid curved contact lens to applanate the cornea, such as LenSx® and VICTUS®. The applanation can produce corneal folds, which may compromise imaging quality and result in more frequent anterior capsular tags or tears, and reduced incision precision. Others, such as Catalys®, LensAR®, and Femto LDV Z8®, use nonapplanating interfaces employing a fluid immersion system combined with a scleral suction ring, creating a vacuum seal without directly flattening the cornea.

All femtosecond lasers must image the interior of the eye to function. The majority use integrated anterior segment optical coherence tomography, whereas LensAR® uses a Scheimpflug 3D ray-tracing system. Each has its own proprietary imaging software and claimed benefits over competitors.

18.3 What Does FLACS Address?

We are always content with the procedures we perform that become familiar and reliably reproducible for cataract surgery, accepting their limitations, until something better comes along and proves its unquestionable superiority. In the "good old days," when extracapsular cataract extraction (ECCE) with 10 mm sutured incisions was the norm, we simply accepted that just about every patient would develop 1–2 diopters of against-the-rule astigmatism (plus cylinder of glasses oriented at 180°) over the first year or two, as surgical incisions were always made at 90° at that time. When phacoemulsification appeared and incisions shrank from 10 mm to 6 mm, postoperative astigmatism shrank dramatically, and then foldable IOLs and clear corneal incisions permitted surgically induced astigmatism to approach zero, dramatically improving vision. However, as each progressive step appeared, numerous surgeons claimed that the innovative procedural addition was only being done to make more money, but it eventually proved to be a significant quality enhancement.

FLACS is a similar iterative improvement. Without FLACS, capsulorhexes are unavoidably variable in size and centration, due to the fact that cataracts come in endless gradations of density in eyes of widely varying axial lengths and anterior chamber depth, and patients vary widely in degrees of cooperation during surgery. Some stay completely calm and still, while others squirm and squeeze. Cataracts come in widely different degrees of density; some patients have small pupils, pseudoexfoliation, or other issues, so manual phacoemulsification is by necessity prolonged for some cases, and increased surgical duration carries a higher degree of risk for almost all possible complications. These factors result in suboptimal IOL positioning in many patients. Astigmatism correction is fraught with its own limitations. We measure every patient with at least two different machines (currently immersion ultrasound, IOLMaster (Carl Zeiss Meditec, Dublin, CA), ANTERION (Heidelberg Engineering, Heidelberg, Germany), and Zeiss corneal tomography. In the majority of cases, the steep astigmatic axis differs slightly with different machines, perhaps because the patient inserts his/her head slightly differently into each machine, varying tilt. And then if a toric IOL is used, careful postop assessment will show that they are rarely exactly on the chosen axis, which itself may have been off due to measurement error. Radial alignment is generally close, but rarely perfect. The only way to measure astigmatism perfectly is to perform a manifest refraction 2 or more weeks postoperatively, treating the postop eye as a physical black box, and simply measuring the manifest optical error. This is one reason why the light-adjustable IOL has achieved such rave reviews, despite its high cost. FLACS addresses the capsulorhexis by making them all precisely the same. It also can soften dense nuclei, rendering all nuclear removal aspects of the surgery very much the same from case to case, dramatically decreasing variability. FLACS can also make all incisions precisely the same, an advantage for less experienced surgeons, whereas very experienced surgeons may choose to make manual incisions, as they can be adjusted slightly to tweak astigmatic management, especially when the corneal topographic axes are not orthogonal. FLACS can correct corneal astigmatism with precise corneal relaxing incisions in the vast majority of cases. There are a number of nomograms available, and some surgeons, such as the senior author, choose to create their own. An advantage of corneal relaxing incisions is that they can be placed anywhere on the cornea and can be left imperforate on the anterior surface, so suboptimal results can be enhanced by simply opening the incisions at the slit lamp (another example of a desirable postop black box refraction and then correction method). Considering all of the above, even a brief experience with FLACS makes the surgeon aware that some cases benefit from FLACS greatly, whereas in other "more routine" cases, the benefit may be only marginal.

18.4 Which Cases Definitely Benefit Greatly from FLACS?

Our group produced a very interesting paper on FLACS in 2019. What we demonstrated is that the more difficult a cataract procedure is assessed to be, preoperatively, the greater the benefit of performing FLACS [2]. I have compiled a list of cataract types, which, when I encounter, I strongly advise patients to undergo FLACS because it is safer and the results are considerably better in my hands.

1. Dense cataracts. There is simply no question that dense cataracts become much easier with FLACS. We have two special settings in our CATALYS™ laser: one for dense and one for very dense cataracts. For both the laser divides the nucleus into octants and delivers double or triple the number of pulses to the nucleus to soften it. This has made a huge difference for these cases.
2. Fuchs endothelial dystrophy and other cases of low endothelial cell loss (ECL) counts. The laser results in much less required phaco time and, along with ophthalmic viscosurgical devices (OVD) soft shell techniques, greatly assists in the preservation of ECLs [3].
3. Shallow anterior chambers. Performing the capsulotomy and breaking up the lens prior to entering with the phaco makes these more difficult cases much easier and safer.

4. Pseudoexfoliation (PXF). PXF cases are known to frequently suffer dislocation of the IOL bag complex up to two decades, or more, postoperatively. FLACS greatly diminishes the intraoperative stress on the zonules and is expected to decrease the frequency of PXF IOL-bag dislocations as time goes on and we collect data.
5. Posterior polar cataracts. True posterior polar cataracts are more difficult in the performance of cataract surgery and in-the-bag placement and centration of the IOL, and many have devised techniques to gently remove the interior of the nucleus before slowly peeling off the peripheral cortex afterwards. FLACS does that by simply preserving a relatively thick cortical layer posteriorly as it softens the central nucleus. After performing many of these surgeries, I now advise all posterior polar cataract patients that FLACS will greatly reduce their cataract surgical risk.
6. Fibrotic anterior capsules. Fibrotic capsules make the capsulorhexis difficult, resulting in higher complication rates. With FLACS and the dimple-down and FLACS OVD Press techniques, these cases are no longer a problem [4, 5].
7. Hypermature cataracts. FLACS creates the capsulotomy and softens the nucleus before the anterior chamber is entered. Therefore, since there is no pressure gradient in any part of the eye prior to entering the eye, the capsulotomies are always perfect, and the procedure is much easier and safer.
8. Myotonic dystrophy. These patients have very elastic capsules, making a manual capsulorhexis much more difficult. FLACS makes it easy.
9. Postvitrectomy cataracts. These patients have unsupported posterior capsules. FLACS simply removes most of the risk associated with these patients' surgeries.
10. Patients on tamsulosin and similar drugs often exhibit intraoperative floppy iris syndrome (IFIS). By creating the capsulotomy, dividing the lens into sextants, and softening the nucleus, most of the risky work is done before the eye is opened. Simply dilating the pupil at surgery with intracameral phenylephrine and xylocaine, then expanding the pupil with a highly viscous cohesive OVD, such as Healon5 (Johnson & Johnson Vision, Jacksonville, FL), and performing the surgery with low-flow techniques (aspiration 15–20 cc./min.) make these cases easy.

18.5 Relative Contraindications to FLACS

There are a few contraindications to FLACS, and those tend to decrease with surgeon experience and familiarity with the fs laser system being employed. Relative contraindications include:

1. Significant corneal scarring precluding good imaging of the anterior segment by the optical coherence tomography (OCT) and obstructing the laser's performance. If the scar is mild and only results in a small gap in the complete capsu-

lorhexis, the dimple-down and FLACS OVD Press techniques can overcome the obstacle.
2. Poor dilation (usually with posterior synechiae or tamsulosin use). A pupil size of 4.5–5 mm is generally needed for performance of FLACS.
3. Very deep-set eyes, unless the patient can compensate with head positioning.
4. Inadequate patient cooperation due to a physical restriction in positioning, extreme anxiety, etc.

18.6 Biometry and Outcomes

Performing all of the above, we make no changes to our routine biometric program. We perform immersion ultrasound (Sanders-Retzlaff-Kraff/Theoretical (SRK/T) equation), IOLMaster (Haigis, Hoffer Q, Olsen, and Kane formulas), Anterion (Barret Universal II (BUII) and Kane equations), and Zeiss OCT corneal tomography on every patient. In postrefractive patients, we perform the Barrett True-K equation as well, whether the patient is undergoing phaco or FLACS. The only difference we notice is that the accuracy is slightly better for FLACS patients, and slightly worse in phaco patients, especially if that patient had dense cataracts or one of the other FLACS-preferred issues above and refused FLACS.

18.7 Summary

We are convinced that FLACS is simply a significant enhancement compared to manual phacoemulsification or CPCS. It does not require any significant changes to the methods of biometry and IOL power calculation used but yields greater accuracy. Femtosecond lasers are complex devices, and it is recommended that every surgeon read the engineering manual of their chosen laser and then review the laser with the company educator, before embarking on FLACS. Even then, FLACS has a fairly long learning curve similar to manual phacoemulsification. It is a better, but different operation. It is expected that, like with the history of the evolution of phacoemulsification, we are still in the infancy of FLACS, and it will likely improve dramatically over the next 10–15 years.

References

1. Arshinoff SA, editor. Immediately Sequential Bilateral Cataract Surgery (ISBCS). 1st ed. Academic; 2023.
2. Nithianandan H, Jegatheeswaran V, Dalal V, et al. Refractive laser-assisted cataract surgery versus conventional manual surgery: comparing efficacy and safety in 3144 eyes. Am J Ophthalmol. 2019;206:32–9. https://doi.org/10.1016/j.ajo.2019.04.010.

3. Arshinoff SA, Norman R. Tri-soft shell technique. J Cataract Refract Surg. 2013;39(8):1196–203. https://doi.org/10.1016/j.jcrs.2013.06.011.
4. Arbisser LB, Schultz T, Dick HB. Central dimple-down maneuver for consistent continuous femtosecond laser capsulotomy. J Cataract Refract Surg. 2013;39(12):1796–7. https://doi.org/10.1016/j.jcrs.2013.09.009.
5. Arshinoff SA. FLACS OVD Press to prevent radial anterior capsular tears. Can J Ophthalmol. 2020;55:461–3. https://doi.org/10.1016/j.jcjo.2020.05.016.

Chapter 19
A Focus on IOL Master Optical Biometry, A-Scan Biometry and Intraoperative Aberrometry: A Practical Guide

John Steven Jarstad

19.1 Introduction

Intraocular lens (IOL) power calculation is a critical component of cataract surgery, directly influencing visual outcomes postoperatively. Accurate measurements of the eye's dimensions and characteristics are essential for selecting the appropriate IOL power. This chapter will discuss the primary methods for measuring intraocular lens power, with particular emphasis on the IOL Master and A-scan biometry.

19.2 Understanding IOL Power Calculation

The goal of IOL power calculation is to determine the correct lens strength needed to achieve optimal postoperative vision. Several factors influence this calculation, including the axial length of the eye, the curvature of the cornea, and the depth of the anterior chamber. The two most common methods for obtaining these measurements are the IOL Master and A-scan biometry.

Author declares no financial interest.
Author declares that figure is under permission from its manufacturer.

J. S. Jarstad (✉)
Morsani School of Medicine, University of South Florida, Tampa, FL, USA

G. Pardianto (ed.), *Intraocular Lens (IOL) Power Calculation*,
https://doi.org/10.1007/978-981-92-1223-1_19

19.3 IOLMaster Biometry

The IOLMaster (Carl Zeiss Meditec, Dublin, CA) is a noncontact optical device that utilizes laser technology to measure key ocular parameters. It has gained widespread acceptance and is considered the gold standard in modern ophthalmic practice due to its precision and ease of use. Carl Zeiss offers two versions of the IOLMaster. The IOL Master 500 employs partial coherence interferometry (PCI) to measure axial length, which is crucial for accurate IOL power calculation. Meanwhile, the IOLMaster700 employs a Swept Source Optical Coherence Tomography (SS-OCT) with its three OCT images to measure Axial Length (AL) and Anteriopr Chamber Depth (ACD) for every single calculation. This device uses a tunable swept laser, which eliminates the deployment of a spectrometer, providing faster scan speeds and potentially greater and better sensitivity at deeper scanning depths [1].

Advantages:

1. Accuracy: The IOL Master provides highly repeatable measurements with minimal variability, reducing the risk of measurement errors that can occur with other methods.
2. Comprehensive measurements: In addition to axial length, the IOL Master measures keratometry (corneal curvature) and anterior chamber depth, allowing for more comprehensive assessments in a single session.
3. User-friendly interface: The device is designed for ease of use, requiring minimal patient cooperation and reducing the time needed for measurement acquisition. It is "user-friendly" in that a relatively inexperienced ophthalmic technician is able to master taking measurements in a short time with a fairly easy learning curve.
4. Efficiency of measurement time: "With the Zeiss IOLMaster 700 you can measure both eyes in less than 45 seconds" (Zeiss.com), adding high efficiency to a busy, high-volume cataract and refractive surgery practice.
5. Additional measurements: With the Zeiss IOLMaster 700, corneal topography can also be measured, and penetration through dense cataracts is successful in approximately 99% [1].

Disadvantages:

1. Cost: The IOLMaster is relatively expensive, which might limit its availability in certain healthcare settings, although the cost has decreased to between 7000 and 10,000 USD at the time of this publication.
2. Limited accessibility: As a sophisticated device, it may not be available in all clinics, particularly in rural or underserved areas, and is not particularly portable for use in developing countries or on eye mission work.

19.4 A-Scan Biometry

Amplitude mode scan/display (A-scan biometry) is the traditional method for measuring ocular dimensions that uses ultrasound to obtain data. This technique involves placing a probe on the eye's surface to emit sound waves, which reflect off the internal structures of the eye. The time taken for the sound waves to return is used to calculate distances, including axial length.

Advantages:

1. Cost-effectiveness: A-scan devices are generally more affordable than advanced optical biometry systems, making them accessible for many practices.
2. Portability: A-scan equipment is often more portable, allowing for use in various clinical settings, including those that may not have the infrastructure for more advanced technology. In fact, a portable device can be purchased for between 1500 and 4000 USD and is even available in a hand-held Palm Pilot version (Fig. 19.1) of Micro Medical Device (MMD) PalmScan AP2000 (MicroMedical Devices, Inc., Calabasas, CA).
3. Compact features:

   - This A-scan device includes immersion A-scan capability, as well as corneal compression detection for contact biometry, which helps ensure more precise measurements.
   - It is capable of measuring anterior chamber depth, lens thickness, and axial length, and includes Holladay, Hoffer Q, SRK/T (Sanders-Retzlaff-Kraff/Theoretical), and Haigis IOL calculation formulas.
   - Corneal curvature measurements are available via a dedicated keratometry probe attachment, designed with 16-point lens keratometry to ensure accurate corneal power and astigmatism measurements.
   - Additionally, MMD PalmScan AP2000 offers a pachymetry probe attachment for central and peripheral corneal thickness measurements.
   - The device also features a limbal relaxing incision (LRI) module that allows users to create a customized LRI surgical plan to alleviate astigmatism.

4. Proven reliability: A-scan biometry has a long history of use in ophthalmology, and many practitioners are familiar with its operation and interpretation.

Disadvantages:

1. Operator dependency: The accuracy of A-scan measurements can be significantly affected by the operator's skill. Inexperienced technicians may produce inconsistent results. One of my nurse/technicians was noted to be "heavy-handed" and always pressed too firmly with the probe, making her scan results of the AL too short, resulting in postop overcorrection and leaving the patient with a myopic rather than an emmetropic refractive outcome.
2. Limited data: A-scan primarily focuses on axial length and may not provide comprehensive data on other ocular parameters, such as corneal curvature, anterior chamber depth, or concerning topographical changes without additional measurements [2].

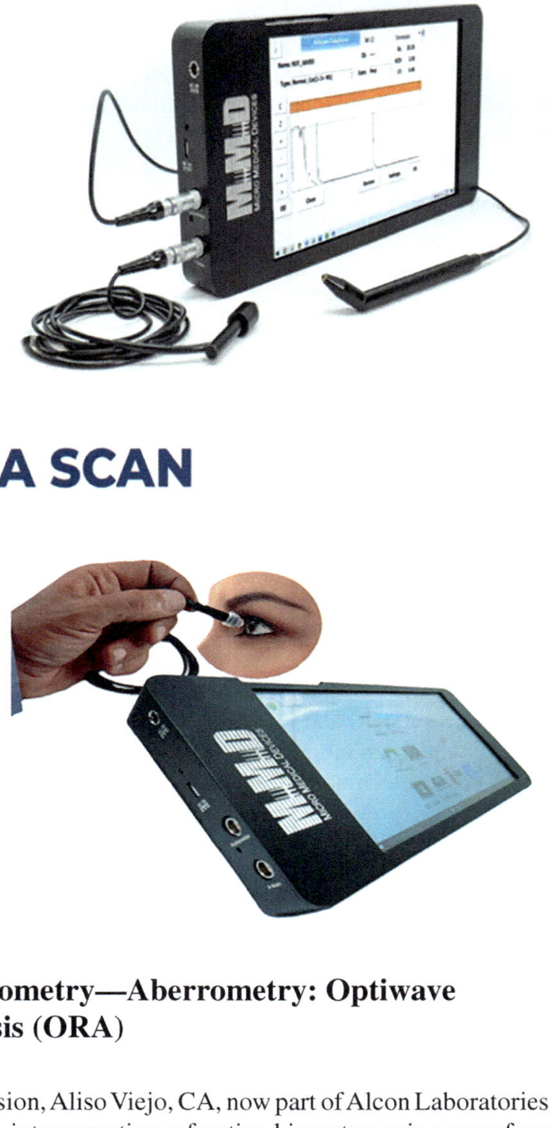

Fig. 19.1 A-scan biometry MMD PalmScan AP2000 [2]

19.5 Intraoperative Biometry—Aberrometry: Optiwave Refractive Analysis (ORA)

The ORA System (WaveTec Vision, Aliso Viejo, CA, now part of Alcon Laboratories, Inc., Fort Worth, TX) employs intraoperative refractive biometry, using wavefront aberrometry data to measure and analyze the refractive power of the eye during cataract surgery, both in the aphakic state immediately after cataract removal and following implantation of the artificial lens implant. This is particularly helpful in axis alignment in the use of toric and multifocal lens implants [3].

Advantages:

1. High accuracy in alignment of toric IOLs. When alignment of the toric IOL is correct, the ORA-VerifEye+ will show "No Rotation Recommended" or NRR to confirm alignment [4].
2. Confirmation of IOL power in premium IOLs, where small errors often lead to a 5% need for photorefractive keratectomy (PRK) or laser in-situ keratomileusis (LASIK) 'touch ups."

Disadvantages:

1. Cost: Current cost is around 55,000 USD for the initial purchase, with an additional monthly fee of 3000 USD for unlimited use.
2. Added time during surgery: Taking accurate measurements repeatedly following IOL placement of toric IOLs can sometimes take an additional 5 minutes to a case [3].

19.6 My "Guestimate" Approach

In cases where it is impossible to obtain measurements with a sophisticated device such as the ORA or a nonportable A-scan, I have found success in patients who were wheelchair- or stretcher-bound or in uncooperative patients with disabilities such as Down's Syndrome and those with white mature or hypermature cataracts in our university referral tertiary practice to use one of two methods [3–6]:

1. Use the SRK/T formula ($P = A - 2.5\ L - 0.9 \times \text{Kavg}$), where P is the calculated IOL power to be used, A is the A-constant for a given IOL, and L is axial length (AL) from portable A-scan (MMD PalmScan AP2000), while patient is sedated in the operating theatre, and K is the average keratometry (K) readings). For example, for a patient using a manufacturer's A constant of 119.3, an axial length of 22.5 mm, and an average K reading of 44.50 Diopter (D), we calculate using the SRK-T formula $P = 119.3 - (2.5 \times 22.5) - 44.5 = 18.55$ or 18.50 D IOL [2].
2. On a visit to North Korea, where we were not certain whether a keratometry would be available, I took an average of the K readings from 30 of my Korean American patients and found it to be 44.50 D. This was inserted into the SRK-T formula along with the measured axial length result from a pocket MMD PalmScan AP2000 IOL biometer, with surprisingly good results [2, 4].

When all else fails, I have requested the patient's family to provide the last known eyeglass prescription and added or subtracted algebraically 50% of that eyeglass prescription from 19.00 D. (In many settings in developing countries where donated IOLs are the norm, all patients receive a 19.00 D donated lens implant and correction with eyeglasses is done postoperatively) [4]. For the patient with hand movement (HM) dense cataract or light perception (LP) mature cataracts, this has been a happy outcome, and, often, we have had surprising 20/25 uncorrected vision using this approach [6].

19.7 Comparative Analysis

When comparing the IOLMaster and A-scan biometry, several factors come into play. The IOL Master is often favored for its superior accuracy and comprehensive measurements, leading to better surgical outcomes [1]. However, A-scan biometry remains a valuable tool, particularly in settings where cost, accessibility, and portability are significant concerns [2].

Recent studies suggest that while both methods can yield satisfactory results, the IOL Master tends to produce fewer refractive surprises postoperatively, making it the preferred choice in many modern practices. However, it is essential for surgeons to consider the specific context of their practice, including patient population, available resources, and individual expertise.

In any case, when I started my career in the 1990s, with the advent of small incision phacoemulsification surgery rather than extracapsular procedures using multiple astigmatism-causing sutures, it was considered acceptable and met the minimal standard of care for patient postoperative results within +/− 1 D to meet the standard of care and resulted in higher patient satisfaction [4]. Today, with the newer IOL Master technology, we have 99% of our patients passing driving license vision requirements without spectacles and about 50% of our patients reaching 20/20 (1.0 or 6/6) vision without spectacles [1].

19.8 Conclusion

IOL calculation is a fundamental aspect of cataract surgery that directly affects patient outcomes and patient satisfaction. The choice of measurement technique, whether the advanced IOL Master or the traditional A-scan biometry, along with newer and future advancements, depends on various factors, including accuracy requirements, cost considerations, and clinical setting. As technology continues to evolve, ongoing research and development in biometry will likely yield even more precise and efficient methods for ensuring optimal IOL power calculations, ultimately enhancing the quality of cataract surgery and patient satisfaction. The use of intraoperative aberrometers, such as the ORA-VerifEye and other devices, is an exciting development that provides increased accuracy now and will likely continue to evolve using neural net and AI platforms to make 20/20 (6/6) vision an increasingly common and satisfying outcome for our future cataract surgery patients.

References

1. IOLMaster 700 – Swept Source OCT. Carl Zeiss Meditec. Available from: https://www.zeiss.com/meditec/en/products/optical-biometers/iolmaster-700-us.html

2. Portable Ultrasound Biometry. The handheld, multimodal ophthalmic biometer you need to take critical measurements from anywhere. Micro Medical Devices. Available from: https://micromedinc.com/portable-ophthalmic-ultrasound-biometry/
3. Pardianto G. What was known about biometry and IOL Power Calculation? In: Pardianto G, editor. The Intraocular Lens Power Calculation. Medan: Anak Sudarti Foundation; 2022. p. 11–23. ISBN 978-623-6763-50-6, e-ISBN 978-623-6763-51-3. Available from: https://bit.ly/TheIOLPowerCalculation
4. Jarstad JS. Cataract surgery 2020 and beyond: Pearls from my career. 2024. J Ophthal Res Pract. https://doi.org/10.25259/JORP_19_2024.
5. Labib KM, Ghumman H, Jain S, Jarstad JS. A review of the utility and limitations of artificial intelligence in ophthalmology: glaucoma, cornea and oculoplastics. Cureus. 2024;16(11):E73522. https://doi.org/10.7759/cureus.73522.
6. Jarstad JS, Mina H, Midathala G. Cataract surgery in challenging cases: a review. In: Pardianto G, Tassignon MJ, editors. Innovation in cataract surgery. Singapore: Springer; 2024. p. 153–9. https://doi.org/10.1007/978-981-97-5192-1_10.

Chapter 20
IOL Power Calculation for Toric IOLs and How to Battle Astigmatism

Muhammad Zidny Fahmi and Gede Pardianto

20.1 Introduction

Astigmatism, even at low levels (0.75 diopters (D) or more), can significantly affect postoperative uncorrected visual acuity and patient satisfaction. Toric intraocular lenses (IOLs) provide an effective solution when paired with accurate biometry, proper formula use, refined surgical planning, and attention to platform-specific nuances. This chapter reviews practical strategies to optimize toric outcomes in daily practice [1, 2].

20.2 Understanding Astigmatism

Astigmatism arises from irregular curvature of the cornea or crystalline lens. It is classified into:

Author declares no financial interest.
Table belongs to the author.

M. Z. Fahmi (✉)
JEC Java @ Surabaya, JEC Eye Hospitals & Clinics, Surabaya, Indonesia

G. Pardianto
Department of Ophthalmology and Vision Sciences, Universitas Prima Indonesia, Medan, Indonesia

Sabang Merauke Eye Center (SMEC), Medan, Indonesia

Prima Vision Eye Hospital, Medan, Indonesia

Star Premiere Eye Center (SPEC), Medan, Indonesia

G. Pardianto (ed.), *Intraocular Lens (IOL) Power Calculation*,
https://doi.org/10.1007/978-981-92-1223-1_20

- *Regular astigmatism*: Predictable axis, correctable with spectacles, contact lenses, or toric IOLs.
- *Irregular astigmatism*: Nonuniform curvature, often due to pathology (e.g., keratoconus, scarring).

Posterior corneal astigmatism (PCA) is critical to account for, especially in against-the-rule (ATR) patterns, where neglecting PCA often leads to undercorrection [3, 4].

20.3 IOL Power Calculation for Astigmatism Correction

20.3.1 Essential Biometric Parameter

Essential biometric parameters for reliable toric IOL calculations include:

- Axial length (AL) and anterior chamber depth (ACD)
- Keratometry (anterior &and posterior)
- Target refraction
- Surgically induced astigmatism (SIA)
- White to white (WTW)
- Central Corneal Thickness (CCT)

Swept-source optical coherence tomography or SS-OCT (e.g., IOLMaster 700 (Carl Zeiss Meditec, Dublin, CA)) and Scheimpflug (e.g., Pentacam AXL (Oculus Optikgeräte, Wetzlar, Germany)) devices allow better prediction of total corneal power.

20.3.2 Barrett and Kane Toric Formulas: Accuracy and Posterior Cornea Role

Modern toric IOL calculators significantly reduce residual astigmatism (RA). Barrett Toric estimates PCA and includes effective lens position (ELP) and SIA are among the most widely used modern calculators in routine eyes [1]. Kane Toric integrates artificial intelligence (AI) with theoretical optics, showing excellent performance in both normal and atypical eyes [2]. These formulas can detect the need for toric IOLs in borderline astigmatism (~0.75 D) and help guide precise alignment and lens power selection.

20.3.2.1 Studies Comparing Predicted Versus Measured PCA

Jung et al. (2022) suggested that measured PCA offered a slight benefit in high ATR eyes; otherwise, no major difference [3]. Yang et al. [4] evaluated the predictive accuracy of the Barrett Toric Calculator using measured posterior corneal astigmatism derived from swept-source OCT and Scheimpflug imaging. The authors reported that incorporation of measured PCA did not consistently improve refractive prediction accuracy compared with Barrett's predicted PCA model, supporting the continued use of predicted PCA for routine toric IOL calculations while reserving direct measurements for selected cases.[4]. Koch et al. [5] suggested that predicted PCA is sufficient for most, but measured PCA is advised in irregular corneas or postrefractive cases [5].

Clinical Tips Predicted PCA is reliable in most cases, but consider measured PCA in high-cylinder, oblique axes, or prior refractive surgery.

20.4 Choosing the Right IOL: Spherical Equivalent Versus Spherical Power

Most IOL platforms base selection on *spherical equivalent (SE)*:

$$SE = \text{Sphere} + \left(\text{Cylinder} \div 2\right)$$

However, *Zeiss toric IOLs* (e.g., AT Torbi, AT LISA tri toric) require *pure spherical input*:

$$\text{Zeiss } IOL \text{ formula : Spherical} = SE - \left(\text{Cylinder} \div 2\right)$$

Failing to apply this correction may lead to *myopic overcorrection* postoperatively (~−0.50 to −1.00 D) [1, 2].

Pearls Always check IOL platform conventions. Some calculators auto-adjust (e.g., Zeiss version of Barrett), while manual ordering via Callisto Eye (Carl Zeiss Meditec, Dublin, CA) requires surgeon input.

20.5 Refractive Targeting Strategy: Spherical and Astigmatic Considerations

20.5.1 Spherical Power Targeting

For most patients, the refractive goal is *emmetropia*. However, targeting slight *myopia (−0.25 to −0.50 D)* can be beneficial when:

- Patients prefer intermediate or near function without glasses.
- Eyes are long/short where IOL power accuracy is less predictable.
- Surgeon wants to avoid hyperopic surprises, especially postrefractive eyes [1, 2].

20.5.2 Toric IOL Residual Cylinder or RA Preference

When full cylinder correction is not possible due to toric step limitations, it is better to leave *low residual with-the-rule (WTR) astigmatism* than ATR or oblique.

- WTR is *better tolerated* due to lid anatomy and natural optical compensation.
- WTR tends to *decrease with age*, making it more self-neutralizing.
- ATR and oblique residuals are more visually symptomatic [1, 2, 6, 7].

Example:
Barrett offers two toric options:

(A) Residual −0.25 D at axis 90° (WTR)
(B) Residual −0.10 D at axis 180° (ATR)

Choose A, even though the cylinder is slightly higher.

20.6 Refining Incision Axis Planning

Shifting the incision axis from 25° to 35–40° may reduce the residual cylinder from >0.10 D to <0.10 D. Use calculators that simulate this (e.g., Barrett or Kane Toric) [7, 8].

20.7 Surgical and Postoperative Considerations

- Mark the axis using digital overlay systems such as the RoboMarker (Surgilum, Wilmington, NC) or manual ink marks at the slit lamp.
- Use consistent incision size and location to stabilize SIA.

Table 20.1 IOL axis evaluation: Days 1, 7, and 30 postoperatively [1, 2, 6, 7]

Timepoint	Goal	Tools
Day 1	Screen for major rotation (>10°)	Slit lamp + Mendez ring
Day 7	Check for mild drift (5–10°)	Pupil dilation + toric overlay/aberrometry
Day 30	Confirm rotational stability	Barrett Rx Check, iTrace Analyzer (Tracey Technologies, Houston, TX), OPDScan III (Nidek, Tokyo, Japan), iDesign (Johnson & Johnson Vision, New Brunswick, NJ)

- Maintaining an appropriately sized continuous curvilinear capsulorhexis (CCC) that will provide 360° complete overlap of the IOL's optic edge may improve centration and stability, as well as limit the IOL tilt.
- If performing femtosecond laser cataract surgery (FLACS), the laser system may assist with marking the axis of lens placement.
- Ensure complete removal of ophthalmic viscosurgical device (OVD) behind IOL to prevent early rotation.
- Postoperative IOL examination is compulsory to perform at days 1, 7, and 30 after surgery (Table 20.1) [1, 2, 6, 7].

Even if the anterior segment is clear and the OCT normal, *unexpected low uncorrected visual acuity (UCVA)* must raise suspicion of toric axis misalignment.

- 1° misalignment = ~3.3% loss of cylinder power
- 10° misalignment = ~33% loss
- 30° misalignment = complete loss of astigmatism correction
- 90° misalignment = the astigmatism will be doubled

Reposition toric IOL ideally within 1–2 weeks postoperative, if needed. The latest period is during 12 weeks postoperative. This will give enough time for the patient's refraction to stabilize but still allow for easy and safe rotation since fibrotic healing has not yet completed [7].

20.8 Clinical Recommendations

- Utilize Barrett Toric or Kane Toric formulas in all cataract surgery cases [1, 2].
- Aim for emmetropia or slight myopia (−0.25 to −0.50 D).
- Choose RA in WTR axis if full neutralization is not possible.
- Properly convert SE to Sph. when using Zeiss toric IOLs.
- Refine incision axis location to reduce RA.
- Recheck toric axis postoperatively at days 1, 7, and 30 [3, 4, 7].
- Consider measured PCA in high-risk corneas.
- Document and address RA >0.5 D with realignment or laser [3, 4].

20.9 Additional Recommendations

Haigis T, Abulafia-Koch Toric, Naeser-Savini, Hoffer QST (Kenneth J. Hoffer Q/Giacomo Savini/Leonardo Taroni), Hill-RBF (Radial Basis Function), and Holladay Toric Calculator are also the armaments to help surgeons to implant toric IOL and battle astigmatism [6, 7].

Some other formulas are favorable to battle the SIA and RA. The Holladay 2 formula includes correction for SIA. Surgeons could utilize Hill SIA calculator to calculate their personal SIA. Emmetropia Verifying Optical (EVO) 2.0 formula analyzes ELP and predicted PCA to calculate the total corneal power (TCP). The Barrett Rx formula is available through the American Society of Cataract and Refractive Surgery (ASCRS) website. It carefully combines the Barrett universal II (BUII) formula and Barrett Toric Calculator. This formula is able to suggest the IOL exchange and IOL rotation, as well as help the surgeons to determine if that IOL exchange or IOL rotation could improve the postoperative refractive results. Barret Rx can also be used to calculate the accurate power for a piggyback IOL in cases of refractive surprise [7, 8].

The Holladay 1 Consultant Program, the Alpins Statistical System for Ophthalmic Refractive Surgery Techniques (ASSORT) Toric Calculator from Dr. Noel Alpins, The Alcon Calculator, the Toric Results Analyzer Calculator or AstigmatismFix from Drs. John Berdahl and David Hardten, and the Baylor Nomogram are programmed to play a key role in the calculation of toric IOL power [7, 9, 10].

Guided systems for toric IOL alignments, such as Callisto Eye (Carl Zeiss Meditec, Dublin, CA), and the Alcon Verion Image Guided System (Alcon Laboratories, Inc., Fort Worth, TX) can be useful to battle postoperative astigmatism [9, 11]. Among other features, Callisto Eye allows the surgeon to bypass preoperative and intraoperative marking altogether [7].

Intraoperative (wavefront) aberrometry supports phaco to determine an axis adjustment for toric IOL power selection and manage its accurate placement [12]. Optiwave Refractive Analysis (ORA) System with Wavetec AnalyzOR (WaveTec Vision, Aliso Viejo, CA, now part of Alcon Laboratories, Inc., Fort Worth, TX) and Holos Intraop (Clarity Medical Systems, Inc., Houston, TX) are some of the intraoperative aberrometers in the market [9, 10]. ORA System employs Talbot-Moiré interferometry to take intraoperative wavefront measurements in aphakic conditions to guide IOL implantation against astigmatism [7].

Calculation for special situations or miscellaneous cases, as well as how to battle astigmatism, is crucial [7, 13]. Surgeons can also access online toric calculator formulas or online calculators from some toric IOL manufacturers [14, 15]. Recently, surgeons have been able to use some language-based AI chats (ChatGPT, DeepSeek, Gemini, etc.), as backup tools and means of verification, to determine whether their conventional calculations are correct (see Chap. 2).

20.10 Conclusion

The battle against astigmatism is won through meticulous attention to nuance—formula choice, posterior corneal modeling, incision axis refinement, appropriate refractive targeting, and vigilant postoperative review and monitoring. These practices empower ophthalmic surgeons to perform refractive cataract surgery with precision and confidence.

References

1. Connell BJ, Kane JX. Comparison of the Kane formula with existing formulas for intraocular lens power selection. BMJ Open Ophthalmol. 2019;4(1):e000251. https://doi.org/10.1136/bmjophth-2018-000251. PMID: 31179396; PMCID: PMC6528763.
2. Helaly HA, Said MH, Elnaggar OR, Elkhawaga MH. Accuracy of modern and traditional intraocular lens power calculation formulas in pediatric cataract surgery. Clin Ophthalmol. 2024;18:1761–9. Published 2024 Jun 20. https://doi.org/10.2147/OPTH.S468294.
3. Shammas HJ, Yu F, Shammas MC, Jivrajka R, Hakimeh C. Predicted vs measured posterior corneal astigmatism for toric intraocular lens calculations. J Cataract Refract Surg. 2022;48(6):690–6. https://doi.org/10.1097/j.jcrs.0000000000000819.
4. Yang X, Jiang Y, Lin S, et al. The predictive accuracy of Barrett toric calculator using measured posterior corneal astigmatism derived from swept source-OCT and Scheimpflug camera. Eye (Lond). 2024;38(1):132–7. https://doi.org/10.1038/s41433-023-02646-1.
5. Koch DD, Ali SF, Weikert MP, Shirayama M, Jenkins R, Wang L. Contribution of posterior corneal astigmatism to total corneal astigmatism. J Cataract Refract Surg. 2012;38(12):2080–7. https://doi.org/10.1016/j.jcrs.2012.08.036.
6. Savini G, Di Maita M, Hoffer KJ, et al. Comparison of 13 formulas for IOL power calculation with measurements from partial coherence interferometry. Br J Ophthalmol. 2021;105(4):484–9. https://doi.org/10.1136/bjophthalmol-2020-316193.
7. Kramer B. Toric IOL power calculation and managing residual astigmatism. In: Pardianto G, editor. The intraocular lens power calculation. Medan: Anak Sudarti Foundation; 2022. p. 75–84. ISBN 978-623-6763-50-6, e-ISBN 978-623-6763-51-3.
8. Krall EM, Arlt EM, Hohensinn M, et al. Vector analysis of astigmatism correction after toric intraocular lens implantation. J Cataract Refract Surg. 2015;41(4):790–9. https://doi.org/10.1016/j.jcrs.2014.07.038.
9. Gu X, Wang L, Breen M, Merchea M. IOL lens constant optimization. Alcon Medical Affairs; 2019. Available from: https://us.alconscience.com/sites/g/files/rbvwei1736/files/pdf/1906A277-US-ORA-19-E-1275-Lens-Constants-White-Paper.pdf.
10. Ferguson TJ, Kramer B, Berdahl JP. Cataract and lens surgery: how to battle astigmatism. In: Pardianto G, Tassignon MJ, editors. Innovation in cataract surgery. Singapore: Springer; 2024. p. 271–81. https://doi.org/10.1007/978-981-97-5192-1_18.
11. Berdahl J. Correcting residual astigmatism after the implantation of a Toric IOL: tips for determining whether to rotate the IOL or perform laser vision correction. Cataract Refract Surg Today. 2012;6:42–6.
12. Srinivas SP, Young AL, Behndig A, Chang DF, Dhubhghaill SN, Eom Y, Fan AH, Findl O, Gundersen KG, Khanna RC, Kohnen T, Mah FS, Miller KM, Nanavaty MA, Nuijts R, Oshika T, Pardianto G, Reus NJ, Ruit S, Sharma N, Venkatesh R, Zhang M, Zheng K, Rao SK, Alió JL. Controversies, consensuses and guidelines on modern cataract surgery by the Academy of Asia-Pacific Professors of Ophthalmology (AAPPO). Asia Pac J Ophthalmol (Phila). 2025:100224. https://doi.org/10.1016/j.apjo.2025.100224. PMID: 40628343

13. Goggin M. Toric intraocular lenses: evidence-based use. Clin Exp Ophthalmol. 2022;50(5):481–9. https://doi.org/10.1111/ceo.14106. Epub 2022 May 29. PMID: 35584257; PMCID: PMC9543206.
14. Ramsauer M, Luft N, Vounotrypidis E, Priglinger SG, Mayer WJ. Accuracy of toric intraocular lens power calculation depending on different keratometry values using a novel network based software platform. Front Med (Lausanne). 2024;11:1363286. https://doi.org/10.3389/fmed.2024.1363286. PMID: 38665295; PMCID: PMC11043607.
15. Liu C, Wang M, Long D, Zhang Y, Chen Y, Wu Q. Comparison of the accuracy of Toric intraocular lens formulas used by the online calculator of the European society of cataract and refractive surgeons. J Refract Surg. 2025;41(2):e120–30. https://doi.org/10.3928/1081597X-20241219-01. Epub 2025 Feb 1. PMID: 39937979.

Chapter 21
Power Calculation for Implantable Collamer Lenses and Piggyback IOLs

Tommy T. Atmaja and Gede Pardianto

21.1 Introduction

Refractive surgery has become increasingly common after cataract procedures, offering a spectrum of techniques designed to reduce dependence on corrective lenses. These procedures work by modifying the optical properties of the eye, allowing light to be focused accurately on the retina [1, 2].

Modern refractive surgery is broadly categorized into two major approaches:

1. Corneal-based procedures (keratorefractive surgery), which reshape the cornea to alter its refractive power. These include traditional incisional techniques such as radial keratotomy and arcuate keratotomy, as well as advanced laser vision correction techniques like photorefractive keratectomy (PRK), laser-assisted in situ keratomileusis (LASIK), and small-incision lenticule extraction (SMILE) or keratorefractive lenticule extraction (KLEx) [1, 2].
2. Lens-based procedures, which involve modifying the eye's refractive status by implanting or exchanging an intraocular lens. This category includes phakic

All authors declare no financial interest.
The table belongs to the authors.

T. T. Atmaja (✉)
Sabang-Merauke Eye Center (SMEC), Tanjung Pinang, Indonesia

G. Pardianto
Department of Ophthalmology and Vision Sciences, Universitas Prima Indonesia, Medan, Indonesia

Sabang Merauke Eye Center (SMEC), Medan, Indonesia

Prima Vision Eye Hospital, Medan, Indonesia

Star Premiere Eye Center (SPEC), Medan, Indonesia

G. Pardianto (ed.), *Intraocular Lens (IOL) Power Calculation*,
https://doi.org/10.1007/978-981-92-1223-1_21

intraocular lenses (phakic IOLs), such as the implantable collamer lens (ICL), and clear lens extraction or refractive lens exchange for specific cases [3, 4].

Among lens-based refractive approaches, the ICL and piggyback intraocular lenses (piggyback IOLs) are two important options used in different clinical scenarios. ICL implantation is indicated for patients with high refractive errors who are unsuitable candidates for corneal refractive surgery due to extreme ametropia, thin or irregular corneas, or other contraindications, and Piggyback IOLs are primarily used to manage residual refractive error following cataract surgery, especially when the initially implanted primary IOL fails to achieve the targeted postoperative refraction [4–6].

Both procedures demand precise preoperative power calculation to optimize visual outcomes. Accurate biometry and meticulous planning are critical to minimize the risks of undercorrection or overcorrection, which could significantly affect postoperative satisfaction and long-term success [7].

21.2 Principles of Biometry for ICL and Piggyback IOL

Biometry plays a critical role in the success of IOL surgery. Accurate measurements are essential not only to achieve the desired postoperative refractive outcome but also to ensure long-term ocular safety [8, 9]. In ICL surgery, biometry is performed to add refractive power without removing the natural crystalline lens [5, 10]. In contrast, for piggyback IOLs, an additional lens is implanted in an eye that already contains a primary IOL within the capsular bag to correct residual refractive errors [6].

These two procedures differ significantly in their biometric principles. For ICL implantation, the primary focus is on calculating the appropriate lens power and selecting the correct lens size (sizing) to achieve an ideal vault and avoid postoperative complications. On the other hand, piggyback IOL biometry primarily focuses on calculating the additional lens power required to correct postoperative residual refractive errors [6, 10]. This calculation is based on postoperative manifest refraction and standard biometric parameters, including axial length (AL) and keratometry (K) readings. Table 21.1 summarizes the key differences in principles and biometric parameters between ICL and piggyback IOL procedures. Understanding these differences is essential to minimize complications and achieve optimal visual outcomes.

Table 21.1 Comparison of biometric principles, power calculation, and clinical factors between ICL and piggyback IOL

Factor/parameter	ICL	Piggyback IOL
Location	Sulcus, in front of the natural crystalline lens	Sulcus, in front of the capsular bag IOL
Purpose	Add refractive power for correction of high myopia/hyperopia	Correction of residual refractive error after cataract surgery
Axial length (AL)	Determines ICL power, especially important for high myopia	Used to calculate additional power
Keratometri (K1, K2)	Important for toric ICL	Important for calculating refractive target
Anterior Chamber Depth (ACD)	Critical for sizing and safety (ideal >2,8 mm)	Not relevant
White-to-White (WTW)	Determine ICL diameter	Not relevant
Lens Thickness (LT)	Helps predict vault	Not relevant
Vault	Target 250–750 micron	Not relevant
Postop refraction data	Not required	*Mandatory* for piggyback IOL calculation
Power calculation principle	*Vergence formula* with vertex distance correction; data derived from manifest refraction. No need for effective lens position (ELP) prediction [11]	*Vergence formula* combine uses empirical methods formula such as Holladay or Barrett Rx [12]
Main complication	Abnormal vault can be risk for cataract and glaucoma	Iris chafing, interlenticular opacification

21.3 Power Calculation and Sizing or Vaulting of ICL

21.3.1 Power Calculation for ICL

The calculation of the ICL power differs fundamentally from the calculation of IOL power used in cataract surgery. In cataract surgery, the crystalline lens is removed and replaced with an artificial IOL, which requires advanced formulas to predict the effective lens position (ELP), such as Barrett Universal II (BUII), Holladay 2, or Sanders-Retzlaff-Kraff/Theoretical (SRK/T) [10, 11].

In contrast, during ICL implantation, the natural crystalline lens remains intact, and the ICL is positioned in the posterior chamber, specifically within the ciliary sulcus. Because the position of the ICL is relatively stable and predictable, there is no need to calculate or predict ELP. Instead, the primary objective of power calculation is to determine the refractive power required to shift the correction from the spectacle plane to the intraocular plane, using the vergence formula [12, 13].

The ICL functions like an "internal contact lens." Since the ICL is positioned much closer to the nodal point of the eye than spectacles, the lens power must be adjusted to account for this difference in location. This adjustment is done using a vertex distance conversion formula [9, 14]:

$$P_{ICL} = \frac{P_{\text{Spectacle}}}{1-\left(d\,P_{\text{Spectacle}}\right)}$$

Where:

- P_{ICL} = power of the ICL at the sulcus plane (diopters)
- P_{Spectacl}e = spectacle lens power (manifest refraction at the corneal plane)
- d = vertex distance in meters (usually 12 mm, or 0.012 m)

Example
If a patient has a manifest refraction of −12.00 D at the vertex distance of 12 mm:

$$\text{PICL} = \frac{-12.00}{1-\left(0.012\times-12.00\right)} = \frac{-12.00}{1+0.144} = -10.49\text{D}$$

The recommended ICL power would then be −10.5 D (diopter), which is matched to the closest available lens power provided by the manufacturer. For toric ICLs, both cylinder power and axis must be entered with high precision, as small errors can result in residual astigmatism or suboptimal outcomes. Modern clinical practice typically relies on the *STAAR Surgical Online Calculator*, which automates this calculation and provides recommendations for both lens power and sizing [15, 16].

21.3.2 Sizing and Vaulting of ICL

In addition to power calculation, one of the most critical factors for the success of ICL implantation is sizing, which refers to the accurate selection of lens length. Sizing determines the vault, defined as the vertical distance between the posterior surface of the ICL and the anterior surface of the crystalline lens. An ideal vault typically ranges between 250 and 750 μm, with approximately 500 μm considered optimal [1, 5, 6]. A vault that is too low may cause the ICL to touch the crystalline lens, increasing the risk of anterior subcapsular cataract formation. In contrast, a vault that is too high may push the iris forward, causing narrowing of the anterior chamber angle, a condition referred to as angle crowding, which can lead to elevated intraocular pressure and potentially progress to pupillary block or even acute angle-closure glaucoma [5, 6].

To accurately predict the appropriate ICL size, several key biometric parameters are utilized. These include anterior chamber depth (ACD), anterior chamber width (ACW) or angle-to-angle (ATA), white-to-white (WTW) corneal diameter, crystalline lens rises (CLR), sulcus-to-sulcus (STS) distance, and lens thickness (LT). Swept-source optical coherence tomography (SS-OCT) represents a major technological advancement in anterior segment imaging and forms the basis of modern anterior segment optical coherence tomography (AS-OCT) devices. Compared to earlier spectral-domain optical coherence tomography (SD-OCT), SS-OCT provides deeper tissue penetration, faster scanning speeds, and higher resolution images. These features allow for precise visualization of deep ocular structures, including the ciliary sulcus, scleral spur, and crystalline lens equator, which are essential for accurate measurement of parameters such as STS and CLR [17, 18]. Recent studies have demonstrated that SS-OCT-based imaging leads to more reliable and reproducible measurements, improving ICL sizing accuracy and reducing the incidence of complications like low or high vault [19].

These biometric parameters are now routinely measured using advanced SS-OCT–based AS-OCT systems, such as CASIA2 (Tomey Corporation, Nagoya, Japan) and ANTERION (Heidelberg Engineering, Heidelberg, Germany), which are widely adopted in clinical practice for ICL planning [20].

Over time, there has been considerable debate regarding the most accurate approach to determining ICL size. Traditional methods relying solely on WTW and ACD measurements have often proven inadequate, as they do not fully capture the internal anatomy relevant to ICL placement. Recent trends favor AS-OCT-based measurements, which provide comprehensive and more representative data regarding anterior segment structures [5, 21]. In addition, direct STS measurement using ultrasound biomicroscopy (UBM) or high-resolution AS-OCT has gained increasing popularity, as it allows for a more accurate estimation of the actual sulcus size [21]. Modern sizing techniques using these advanced imaging modalities have been shown to improve vault prediction and reduce the risk of complications associated with inaccurate sizing, such as excessively low or high vaults [19].

21.3.3 Current Formulas and Models for Predicting ICL Size and Vault

Advances in biometric measurement technologies and anterior segment imaging have significantly improved the methods used to predict the appropriate size and vault of the ICL. In earlier clinical practice, ICL sizing relied primarily on two parameters: WTW and ACD. However, these external measurements are limited because they only reflect the surface anatomy of the eye and often fail to represent the actual dimensions of the ciliary sulcus, the precise location where the ICL is placed [22, 23].

The introduction of SS-OCT-based AS-OCT devices, such as CASIA2 and ANTERION, has revolutionized the field by providing highly detailed imaging and accurate measurements. These devices allow for the evaluation of multiple parameters, including ACW, ATA, CLR, LT, and STS distance [24]. By incorporating these comprehensive measurements, clinicians can achieve more precise and individualized ICL sizing, thereby reducing the risk of complications such as low vault or high vault [18, 25].

21.3.3.1 Nakamura-Kamiya Formula

The Nakamura-Kamiya (NK-3) formula represents a modern approach to ICL sizing by leveraging the detailed biometric data provided by AS-OCT. This formula primarily uses ACW and CLR as its key parameters to predict the optimal ICL size [21, 22]. Larger ACW and CLR values generally indicate the need for a larger ICL size to maintain adequate spacing between the lens and the surrounding ocular structures, thus ensuring an optimal vault and maintaining safety margins. Once the formula provides a calculated result, this value is then mapped to one of the standardized ICL sizes available from the manufacturer [18, 22, 25].

The formula is expressed as follows:

$$\text{Optimal}\,ICL\,\text{Size}\,(\text{mm} = 5.307 + \left(0.0617 \times ACW\right) + \left(0.501 \times CLR\right)$$

For example, an eye with an ACW of 11.8 mm and a CLR of 0.4 mm would yield an optimal ICL size of approximately 12.4 mm, rounded to the closest available lens size. By aligning the calculated measurement with one of the four available ICL sizes, 12.1 mm, 12.6 mm, 13.2 mm, or 13.7 mm, surgeons can tailor the lens selection to match each patient's unique anterior segment anatomy, thereby improving vault predictability and postoperative outcomes [22].

21.3.3.2 Kojima-Shimizu (KS) Formulas

The KS formula, developed by Kojima and Shimizu, is one of the earliest and most widely used methods for determining the optimal size of an ICL. It primarily relies on WTW and ACD measurements to estimate lens size, with the aim of achieving a postoperative vault within the ideal range of 250–750 μm [26]. A larger WTW generally indicates the need for a longer lens, while greater ACD suggests more space in the anterior chamber, both of which influence vault and ICL positioning. Due to its simplicity and accessibility, the KS formula quickly became a standard tool in ICL sizing and remains popular worldwide, especially in settings without advanced imaging devices such as AS-OCT or SS-OCT. [18, 25]

However, the KS formula has limitations because it only considers external measurements and does not fully reflect the internal anatomy of the ciliary sulcus, where the ICL actually rests. This can lead to inaccurate predictions, sometimes resulting in excessively low or high vaults. Despite this, many surgeons continue to use the KS formula as a baseline calculation, often comparing it with modern formulas such as the NK-3 to improve accuracy [18]. This combined approach helps guide decision-making, particularly in borderline or complex cases, ensuring safer and more predictable surgical outcomes [24, 25].

21.3.3.3 Anterior-Based Multiple Regression Formula

Recent advances in AS-OCT technology have facilitated the development of multiple regression formulas that combine several biometric parameters into a single, more sophisticated model. One of the most notable innovations is an ANTERION-based regression formula, which integrates ACW, CLR, LT, and WTW data to provide a highly personalized prediction of the postoperative vault. The NK formula exhibited superior consistency and low predictive error compared to the KS formula in the 12.6 mm ICL group [26]. This multiparameter strategy is especially valuable for patients with complex or borderline anterior segment anatomy, where traditional formulas may be insufficient [18, 25].

21.3.3.4 STS-Based Approach

The STS distance directly represents the anatomical space where the ICL will be positioned. Historically, STS measurements were estimated indirectly using WTW or ACW values, but these external metrics could not reliably predict the true internal anatomy. With the advent of ultrasound biomicroscopy (UBM) and high-resolution AS-OCT, clinicians can now measure STS with much greater accuracy [22]. This direct approach provides a more physiological and precise method for ICL sizing. However, a unique challenge remains: manufacturers produce ICLs in only four discrete sizes 12.1 mm, 12.6 mm, 13.2 mm, and 13.7 mm [22].

As a result, continuous STS measurements must be mapped to one of these fixed sizes to determine the appropriate lens. For example, if the measured STS distance is 12.45 mm, the surgeon would typically select a 12.6 mm ICL, as it is closest to the actual measurement while ensuring safe vaulting. Conversely, if the STS distance is 13.4 mm, a 13.2 mm ICL would likely be chosen to avoid excessive vaulting. This mapping process is essential to prevent complications associated with inaccurate sizing, such as *low vault* due to undersizing or *high vault* caused by oversizing [27].

21.3.4 Power Calculation for Piggyback IOL

The calculation of power for a piggyback IOL follows the same basic principle as the ICL and does not require specialized formulas to predict the ELP, as is necessary in primary cataract IOL power calculations. The piggyback IOL is placed in the ciliary sulcus, positioned anterior to the primary IOL, and its primary purpose is to neutralize residual refractive errors following cataract surgery. This calculation focuses on the postoperative manifest refraction, supplemented with biometric data such as AL and K values to ensure accuracy [28].

In practice, the power of a piggyback IOL is commonly determined using the vergence formula, which converts the refractive correction from the spectacle plane to the intraocular plane where the piggyback IOL will be positioned. This adjustment ensures that the calculated lens power corresponds precisely to the lens location within the eye. Modern online calculators are now widely available and can integrate postoperative refractive data to generate highly accurate recommendations for piggyback IOL power [26, 28].

The selection of appropriate lens material and design, as well as thorough preoperative evaluation of ocular anatomy, is crucial to minimize complications. Lenses made from hydrophobic acrylic material with rounded, smooth edges are preferred, as they reduce friction and irritation to the iris. Choosing a piggyback lens with a slightly smaller optic diameter than the primary IOL also helps decrease the risk of mechanical complications caused by lens overlap or crowding [27, 28].

One of the most common complications associated with piggyback IOL implantation is interlenticular opacification (ILO). This occurs when protein and cellular debris accumulate in the narrow space between the primary IOL and the piggyback IOL, leading to a gradual reduction in visual quality. To prevent ILO, it is recommended that the two lenses be made from different materials, such as pairing a hydrophobic acrylic primary IOL with a hydrophilic acrylic piggyback lens. This material variation minimizes protein interaction and reduces the likelihood of opacification formation.

By carefully combining accurate power calculations with thoughtful selection of lens material, design, and size, piggyback IOL implantation can provide a safe and effective solution for correcting residual refractive errors, reducing the need for more invasive surgical interventions such as IOL exchange [28].

21.3.5 Modern Strategies for Calculating Piggyback IOL Power

In conventional clinical practice, the calculation of piggyback IOL power has primarily focused on residual refractive error measured after cataract surgery. This value is then converted from the spectacle plane to the intraocular plane using a basic vergence formula. Such an approach has been effective for many straightforward cases, particularly when the residual refractive error is mild to moderate. However, in cases of high ametropia, this traditional method often proves inadequate [26, 28].

Karjou et al. highlighted that secondary piggyback IOL implantation is an effective and safe technique for the correction of residual ametropia following cataract surgery. Three-piece IOLs can be safely placed as secondary piggyback IOLs in situations where specifically designed IOLs are not available [28, 29].

A modern piggyback IOL calculator can be adapted to integrate preoperative variables, including ACD, K reading, and details of the primary IOL, to enhance both the accuracy and consistency of postoperative refractive outcomes [28, 29]. One of the most widely used tools today is the Barrett Rx Piggyback IOL calculator, which allows clinicians to input postoperative refraction, primary IOL data, and multiple biometric parameters into a single platform [12].

This innovation represents a shift toward a more individualized and data-driven approach to piggyback IOL power calculation. Although these modern formulas and tools remain under active validation and refinement, preliminary results have demonstrated significant improvements in accuracy, thereby reducing the risks of undercorrection and overcorrection. Consequently, the integration of such calculators into routine clinical practice offers a practical and precise method for managing residual refractive error without resorting to invasive procedures such as primary IOL explantation [12, 15, 30].

21.3.6 Nowadays and Future of ICL and Piggyback IOL Power Calculation

Traditional formulas for IOL power calculation often face significant challenges, especially in complex cases such as ICL and piggyback IOLs. The emergence of artificial intelligence (AI) integration in IOL power calculation has brought revolutionary advancements to modern ophthalmology. AI algorithms can analyze massive datasets, including biometric data, anterior segment imaging, and postoperative outcomes, thereby providing a more precise and individualized power calculation process. This is particularly important for patients with unique anatomical variations or complex refractive needs [28, 29].

Several AI-based technologies have already been applied to IOL and piggyback IOL power calculations, offering improved accuracy and predictability [12, 15].

21.3.6.1 Barrett Rx Piggyback Calculator

The Barrett Rx Piggyback calculator, available through the Asia Pacific Association of Cataract and Refractive Surgery (APACRS) online platform, represents a modern predictive model that utilizes big data from thousands of cataracts and piggyback IOL surgical cases. This tool calculates piggyback IOL power based on postoperative residual refraction, the power of the primary IOL, and essential biometric parameters such as AL and K. By applying optimized algorithms, it provides more accurate results than traditional manual calculations [12, 31].

The performance of the Barrett Rx calculator has been especially promising in IOL exchange scenarios. In a study conducted by Kaiser et al., the formula demonstrated excellent accuracy, with 56% of eyes achieving results within ±0.25 D of the target refraction and 96% within ±0.50 D of the target [31]. However, clinical studies specifically evaluating the accuracy of Barrett Rx in the context of piggyback IOL implantation remain limited. Further research is needed to validate its role in secondary lens procedures.

21.3.6.2 AI-Based Predictive Analytics for ICL Sizing and Vaulting

In ICL implantation, AI has been utilized to predict vault height and select the appropriate ICL size with higher precision. These AI systems incorporate data from advanced biometric imaging modalities such as AS-OCT using devices such as CASIA2 or ANTERION. Key parameters include anterior chamber width ACW, ATA, CLR, and STS measurements [18, 25, 32].

Recent studies have demonstrated that machine learning models significantly reduce vault prediction errors compared to traditional sizing formulas such as KS and NK-3 [18, 24–26]. Improved prediction accuracy minimizes the risk of postoperative complications such as low vault, which may lead to cataract formation, or high vault, which can result in angle closure or elevated intraocular pressure [32, 33].

21.3.6.3 Ray-Tracing AI Modeling for Complex Piggyback IOL Cases

Ray-tracing technology simulates the path of light rays as they pass through the ocular structures, allowing for a detailed analysis of optical interactions between the primary IOL and the piggyback IOL. This advanced modeling predicts how the combination of lenses will affect visual quality, including aberrations, peripheral illumination, and overall retinal image clarity [28, 34].

Several research centers have incorporated AI-driven ray-tracing simulations to optimize piggyback IOL outcomes. These simulations enable surgeons to visualize how the piggyback IOL will interact with the preexisting primary IOL and predict the optimal power selection to correct residual refractive error without inducing additional optical aberrations. This approach is particularly beneficial in highly complex cases, such as those involving multifocal or toric lenses, where standard calculation methods may not adequately account for intricate optical interactions [28, 29, 35].

21.3.6.4 Intraoperative Aberrometry with AI Integration

The Optiwave Refractive Analysis (ORA) system (Alcon Laboratories, Inc., Fort Worth, TX) is a significant innovation in improving intraoperative aberrometry with IOL power calculation accuracy. ORA functions in real time, providing immediate feedback to surgeons about intraoperative refractive status, lens positioning, and required power adjustments. With AI integration, ORA can analyze intraoperative data rapidly and precisely, enabling more informed surgical decisions [36].

In the context of piggyback IOL implantation, ORA plays a crucial role by assessing the optical properties of the eye immediately after the primary IOL has been implanted. This direct measurement of residual refractive error allows for precise piggyback lens power determination without solely relying on preoperative data. The primary method involves calculating the aphakic spherical equivalent, measured when the eye is in an aphakic state before placing the secondary lens [37]. These data are then combined with biometric variables such as keratometry and the estimated ELP to optimize piggyback IOL selection.

21.4 Conclusion

The calculation of IOL power for both ICL and piggyback IOLs remains one of the most challenging aspects of modern refractive surgery. As surgical techniques evolve and patient expectations rise, the need for accuracy in lens power calculation becomes increasingly critical. This accuracy not only determines the success of the surgery in terms of achieving the desired refractive outcome but also plays a vital role in preventing postoperative complications that can arise from incorrect lens power selection.

Recent advancements, including AI-assisted calculations, advanced biometry devices, and intraoperative aberrometry tools such as ORA, represent a significant step forward in the field. These innovations allow for a more individualized and data-driven approach to lens implantation, shifting away from a "one-size-fits-all" model to one that accounts for each patient's unique anatomical and optical characteristics.

In conclusion, bridging the gap between traditional techniques and modern innovations is essential for improving outcomes in IOL power calculation. As this chapter has outlined, continuous research, clinical validation, and integration of new technologies into routine practice are vital for future progress. By embracing these developments, ophthalmologists can ensure safer surgeries, higher patient satisfaction, and more predictable visual outcomes, ultimately advancing the field of refractive lens surgery and improving the quality of care for patients worldwide.

References

1. Almutairi MN, Alshehri AM, Alhoumaily AY, Alnahdi O, Taha MA, Gangadharan S. Meta-analysis: clinical outcomes of laser-assisted in situ keratomileusis (LASIK) and photorefractive keratectomy (PRK) in hyperopia. BMC Ophthalmol. 2025;25(1):140. Published 2025 Mar 18. https://doi.org/10.1186/s12886-025-03956-6.
2. Reinstein DZ, Archer TJ, Vida RS, et al. Small Incision Lenticule Extraction (SMILE) for the correction of high myopia with astigmatism. J Refract Surg. 2022;38(5):262–71. https://doi.org/10.3928/1081597X-20220314-01.
3. Sanders DR, Vukich JA, Doney K, Gaston M, Implantable Contact Lens in Treatment of Myopia Study Group. U.S. Food and Drug Administration clinical trial of the Implantable Collamer Lens for moderate to high myopia. Ophthalmology. 2003;110(2):255–66. https://doi.org/10.1016/s0161-6420(02)01771-2.
4. Kamiya K, Shimizu K, Igarashi A, Kobashi H. Posterior chamber phakic intraocular lens implantation for the correction of myopia and myopic astigmatism: a review. J Cataract Refract Surg. 2018;44(6):725–39. https://doi.org/10.1136/bjophthalmol-2017-310164.
5. Packer M. The Implantable Collamer Lens with a central port: review of the literature. Clin Ophthalmol. 2018;12:2427–38. https://doi.org/10.2147/OPTH.S188785.
6. Fernández-Buenaga R, Alió JL, Pérez Ardoy AL, Quesada AL, Pinilla-Cortés L, Barraquer RI. Resolving refractive error after cataract surgery: IOL exchange, piggyback lens, or LASIK. J Refract Surg. 2013;29(10):676–83. https://doi.org/10.3928/1081597X-20130826-01.

7. Salouti R, Nazarpour-Servak M, Dehghani MM, et al. Implantable collamer lens sizing optimization based on the anterion AS-OCT biometric parameters. Eye (Lond). 2025;39(9):1730–6. https://doi.org/10.1038/s41433-025-03741-1.
8. Chen X, Chen F, Wang X, et al. Safety and anterior chamber structure of evolution implantable Collamer lens implantation with short white-to-white corneal diameters. Front Med (Lausanne). 2022;9:928245. Published 2022 Aug 17. https://doi.org/10.3389/fmed.2022.928245.
9. Kamiya K, Shimizu K, Ando W, Igarashi A, Iijima K, Koh A. Comparison of vault after implantation of posterior chamber phakic intraocular lens with and without a central hole. J Cataract Refract Surg. 2015;41(1):67–72. https://doi.org/10.1016/j.jcrs.2014.11.011.
10. Albo C, Nasser T, Szynkarski DT, Nguyen N, Mueller B, Libfraind L, et al. A comprehensive retrospective analysis of EVO/EVO+ implantable collamer lens: evaluating refractive outcomes in the largest single center study of ICL patients in the United States. Clin Ophthalmol. 2024;18:69–78. https://doi.org/10.2147/OPTH.
11. Holladay JT. Standardizing constants for ultrasonic biometry, keratometry, and intraocular lens power calculations. J Cataract Refract Surg. 1997;23(9):1356–70. https://doi.org/10.1016/s0886-3350(97)80115-0.
12. Barrett GD. Barrett Rx formula for piggyback IOL calculation. APACRS Online Tools. 2024; Available from: https://calc.apacrs.org/barrett_rx105/.
13. Reinstein DZ, Archer TJ, Srinivasan S, et al. Standard for reporting refractive outcomes of intraocular lens-based refractive surgery. J Cataract Refract Surg. 2017;43(4):435–9. https://doi.org/10.1016/j.jcrs.2017.04.005.
14. Kapoor G, Sharma VK, Singh P, et al. Objective and subjective outcomes following implantable collamer lens (ICL) implantation for the correction of myopia. Oman J Ophthalmol. 2025;18(2):187–92. Published 2025 Jun 24. https://doi.org/10.4103/ojo.ojo_171_24.
15. STAAR Surgical. ICL online calculator user guide. Monrovia: STAAR Surgical; 2024. Available from: https://evo-ocos.staarag.ch/Live/jsocoslive/calculator/dist/
16. Oshika T, Nakano S, Fujita Y, et al. Long-term outcomes of cataract surgery with toric intraocular lens implantation by the type of preoperative astigmatism. Sci Rep. 2022;12(1):8457. Published 2022 May 19. https://doi.org/10.1038/s41598-022-12426-8.
17. Dong J, Yao J, Chang S, Kanclerz P, Khoramnia R, Wang X. Evaluation of ocular diameter parameters using swept-source optical coherence tomography. Medicina (Kaunas). 2023;59(5):899. Published 2023 May 8. https://doi.org/10.3390/medicina59050899.
18. Nakamura T, Isogai N, Kojima T, Yoshida Y, Sugiyama Y. Implantable Collamer lens sizing method based on swept-source anterior segment optical coherence tomography. Am J Ophthalmol. 2018;187:99–107. https://doi.org/10.1016/j.ajo.2017.12.015.
19. Russo A, Filini O, Savini G, et al. Predictability of the vault after implantable collamer lens implantation using OCT and artificial intelligence in White patient eyes. J Cataract Refract Surg. 2023;49(7):724–31. https://doi.org/10.1097/j.jcrs.0000000000001182.
20. Dhawlikar NS, Dai YL, Hughes KV, Rao NK. IOL power calculation in special situations. In: Pardianto G, editor. The intraocular lens power calculation. Medan: Anak Sudarti Foundation; 2022. p. 43–73. ISBN 978-623-6763-50-6, e-ISBN 978-623-6763-51-3.
21. Zhang J, Shao J, Zheng L, Zhao X, Chen S. Implantable collamer lens sizing based on measurement of the sulcus-to-sulcus distance in ultrasound biomicroscopy video clips and ZZ ICL formula. BMC Ophthalmol. 2022;22(1):363. Published 2022 Sep 7. https://doi.org/10.1186/s12886-022-02583-9.
22. Thompson V, Cummings AB, Wang X. Implantable Collamer lens procedure planning: a review of global approaches. Clin Ophthalmol. 2024;18:1033–43. Published 2024 Apr 6. https://doi.org/10.2147/OPTH.S456397.
23. Xiong L, Wu J, Du H, Wang Z. Comparison of formulas in the implantable collamer lens vault prediction. Medicine (Baltimore). 2023;102(50):e36542. https://doi.org/10.1097/MD.0000000000036542.

24. Lei CS, Jiang X, Yang X, et al. Repeatability and reproducibility of anterior segment measurements with a new full-range SS-OCT and comparison with an AS-OCT. Photodiagn Photodyn Ther. 2025;55:104763. https://doi.org/10.1016/j.pdpdt.2025.104763.
25. Cerpa Manito S, Sánchez Trancón A, Torrado Sierra O, Baptista AM, Serra PM. Biometric and ICL-related risk factors associated to sub-optimal vaults in eyes implanted with implantable collamer lenses. Eye Vis (Lond). 2021;8(1):26. Published 2021 Jul 5. https://doi.org/10.1186/s40662-021-00250-6.
26. Zhong X, Li Y, Li Y, Wang G, Du Y, Zhang M. Comparison of predictability in vault using NK formula and KS formula for the implantable Collamer lens surgery. J Ophthalmol. 2024;2024:4256371. Published 2024 Jul 27. https://doi.org/10.1155/2024/4256371.
27. Lv M, Dai Y, Wu X. Quantitative analysis of iris-ciliary angle area to optimize ICL selection: a retrospective study. BMC Ophthalmol. 2025;25(1):488. Published 2025 Aug 27. https://doi.org/10.1186/s12886-025-04295-2.
28. Karjou Z, Haddad W, Saad E, Tabbara KF. A new formula for secondary piggyback intraocular lens power calculation in highly ametropic eyes. J Cataract Refract Surg. 2015;41(4):820–6.
29. Karjou Z, Jafarinasab MR, Seifi MH, Hassanpour K, Kheiri B. Secondary piggyback intraocular lens for management of residual Ametropia after cataract surgery. J Ophthalmic Vis Res. 2021;16(1):12–20. Published 2021 Jan 20. https://doi.org/10.18502/jovr.v16i1.8244.
30. Buonsanti D, Hoffer KJ, Coutinho CP, Savini G. The influence of anterior chamber depth on the calculation of piggyback intraocular lenses. Am J Ophthalmol. 2025;272:161–5. https://doi.org/10.1016/j.ajo.2025.01.013.
31. Kaiser KP, Jandewerth T, Wanten JC, et al. Barrett RX tool for intraocular lens power calculation in pseudophakic eyes undergoing intraocular lens exchange. J Cataract Refract Surg. 2025;51(11):972–8. https://doi.org/10.1097/j.jcrs.0000000000001732.
32. Zhang Q, Li Q, Yu Z, et al. Exploring machine learning models for vault safety in ICL implantation: a comparative analysis of regression and classification models. Ophthalmol Ther. 2025;14(8):1789–812. https://doi.org/10.1007/s40123-025-01173-4.
33. Yuan DQ, Tang FN, Wang Y, et al. Prediction of postoperative vault after implantable collamer lens implantation with deep learning. Int J Ophthalmol. 2025;18(7):1197–204. Published 2025 Jul 18. https://doi.org/10.18240/ijo.2025.07.02.
34. Hassan AH, Sayed KM, ElAgooz M, Elhawary AM. Refractive results: safety and efficacy of secondary piggyback Sensar™ AR40 intraocular lens implantation to correct Pseudophakic refractive error. J Ophthalmol. 2016;2016:4505812. https://doi.org/10.1155/2016/4505812.
35. Li T, Reddy A, Stein JD, Nallasamy N. Ray tracing intraocular lens calculation performance improved by AI-powered postoperative lens position prediction. Br J Ophthalmol. 2023;107(4):483–7. https://doi.org/10.1136/bjophthalmol-2021-320283.
36. Otani A. Accuracy of intraoperative Aberrometry-based prediction of postoperative refraction and astigmatism after novel Toric intraocular lens implantation. Clin Ophthalmol. 2025;19:2681–9. Published 2025 Aug 11. https://doi.org/10.2147/OPTH.S534932.
37. Greenwood MD, Hutchison JW, Gorham RA, Kramer BA. The use of intraoperative Aberrometry in normal eyes: an analysis of intraocular lens selection in scenarios of disagreement. J Refract Surg. 2022;38(5):304–9. https://doi.org/10.3928/1081597X-20220331-01.

Chapter 22
Integrated Artificial Intelligence and Chat Program for Intraocular Lens Power Calculation

Ferdian Ramadhan, Evelyn Komaratih, and Gede Pardianto

22.1 Introduction

Phacoemulsification is the most performed ophthalmological surgical procedure, specifically in cataract management. Over time, patients' expectation for correct sight after cataract surgery has been rising [1]. Postoperative vision depends on many factors, and one of the most important among them is accuracy of the intraocular lens (IOL) power implanted [2].

The prediction of refractive outcomes after cataract surgery has steadily improved, with more recent IOL power formulas generally outperforming those of prior generations. There is still considerable debate about which formula provides the most accurate refractive prediction. No single formula has been shown to be highly accurate across a range of eye characteristics; some authors have suggested that cataract surgeons should use different formulas for eyes of varied ocular dimensions [2, 3].

Recent studies have found that 70–80% of eyes obtained a postoperative refraction within ±0.50 D of the predicted value. A few sources reported that the

All authors declare no financial interest.

F. Ramadhan (✉)
Klinik Utama Sumenep, Sumenep, Indonesia

E. Komaratih
Department of Ophthalmology, Universitas Airlangga, Surabaya, Indonesia

G. Pardianto
Department of Ophthalmology and Vision Sciences, Universitas Prima Indonesia, Medan, Indonesia

Sabang Merauke Eye Center (SMEC), Medan, Indonesia

Prima Vision Eye Hospital, Medan, Indonesia

Star Premiere Eye Center (SPEC), Medan, Indonesia

G. Pardianto (ed.), *Intraocular Lens (IOL) Power Calculation*,
https://doi.org/10.1007/978-981-92-1223-1_22

percentage of the prediction error within ±0.5 D after cataract surgery was 73.7% [4, 5]. The most widely used IOL power formulas are Sanders-Retzlaff-Kraff/Theoretical (SRK/T), Hoffer Q, Holladay 1, and Haigis. These formulas are estimating the effective lens position (ELP) using different parameters, for example, axial length (AL), keratometry (K), anterior chamber depth (ACD), white to white (WTW) distance, and lens thickness (LT) [6].

Artificial intelligence (AI) was introduced in the 1950s by John McCarthy. Alan Turing is assumed to be the father of theoretical computer science and AI. In 1948, he presented many of the main concepts of AI [7]. Ophthalmology quickly adopted AI technologies in many areas, such as visual fields, fundus photography, and optical coherence tomography, obtaining excellent classification performances in the detection of retinopathy [8]. AI refers to techniques for machines that mimic human behavior; machine learning is a subset of AI whereby machines can improve without explicit programming, and deep learning is a subset of machine learning whereby machines can self-train to perform tasks using extensive data sets fed into multilayered neural networks [9]. However, the advent of AI has begun to transform the landscape of IOL power calculation, offering new methodologies that can enhance precision and predictability.

22.2 AI for IOL Power Calculation in General

The integration of AI into IOL power calculation is a significant advancement in the field of ophthalmology, particularly in cataract surgery. Understanding this integration is crucial for several reasons:

1. Enhanced accuracy: Traditional methods of IOL power calculation often rely on empirical formulas that may not account for individual variations in patient anatomy. AI algorithms can analyze vast datasets, including biometric measurements, to provide more accurate predictions of ELP and postoperative refractive outcomes. Studies have shown that AI-driven models can reduce mean absolute errors compared to conventional formulas, resulting in better visual outcomes for patients [10].
2. Personalized medicine: AI can facilitate a personalized approach to IOL power calculation by taking into account individual patient characteristics, such as age, corneal topography, and previous ocular surgeries. This adaptability is particularly beneficial in complex cases, such as those involving high myopia or astigmatism, where standard formulas may fall short. Personalized calculations can lead to improved patient satisfaction and reduced rates of postoperative refractive surprises [10, 11].
3. Real-time adjustments: The use of AI in conjunction with advanced imaging technologies, such as swept-source optical coherence tomography (SS-OCT) and intraoperative aberrometry, allows for real-time adjustments during surgery. This capability ensures that any intraoperative changes in ocular parameters can

be immediately addressed, enhancing the accuracy of IOL power calculations and improving surgical outcomes [10, 12].

4. Backup to conventional methods: AI can serve as a valuable backup to conventional IOL power calculation methods. By providing a second opinion or confirming calculations made using traditional formulas, AI can enhance decision-making and reduce the risk of errors. This dual approach can be particularly useful in complex cases or when dealing with atypical ocular anatomies [10, 13].
5. Continuous learning and improvement: AI systems can continuously learn from new data and outcomes, allowing for ongoing refinement of IOL power calculation methods. As more data become available, AI algorithms can be updated to improve their predictive capabilities, ensuring that practitioners have access to the most effective tools for patient care [10, 14].
6. Training and adaptation: Understanding AI in IOL power calculation prepares ophthalmologists for the future of surgical practice. As AI tools become more prevalent, practitioners must be equipped to utilize these technologies effectively. Training in AI applications can enhance surgical skills and improve patient outcomes, positioning ophthalmologists at the forefront of innovation in eye care [10, 11].

The importance of understanding IOL power calculation with AI lies in its potential to enhance accuracy, personalize treatment, enable real-time adjustments, and serve as a reliable backup to traditional methods. As the field of ophthalmology continues to evolve, embracing AI technologies will be essential for improving patient care and outcomes in cataract surgery [10–12].

The application of AI in IOL power calculation encompasses both fundamental principles and cutting-edge innovations. Traditional formulas, such as SRK/T and Hoffer Q, have been the foundation of IOL power calculations for decades. These formulas utilize biometric data to predict postoperative refractive outcomes, often relying on assumptions regarding ELP that may not hold true for all patients. In contrast, AI-driven methods leverage large datasets and machine learning algorithms to refine these calculations, potentially leading to more accurate predictions. For example, studies have demonstrated that machine learning techniques, such as eXtreme Gradient Boosting (XGBoost) and support vector regression, can yield lower mean absolute error (MAE) compared to traditional formulas [10, 12].

22.3 Intraocular Lens Calculation Formulas Based on AI

The FullMonte method, the first AI-based IOL power calculation formula, was introduced by Gerald Clarke. As a hybrid formula, in addition to optical components, it used a Monte Carlo Markov Chain simulator to improve its refractive predictions [15]. recently, some newer formulas have appeared with promising results. They used the latest methodologies, including AI, and a large number of preoperative eye parameters to calculate the postrefractive error [15, 16]. We can divide them into methods applying AI only and hybrids, that is, formulas that are based on an optical approach or ray tracing and that use AI to refine them. In addition, there are universal algorithms utilizing AI to improve the trueness of existing formulas (Table 22.1) [16].

IOL formula calculation is based on a simple scheme, shown in Fig. 22.1. And this scheme is much more complete when using the AI formula (Fig. 22.2) [17]. There are two AI-based formula structures: in the first AI methods can be designed to either predict postoperative spherical equivalent (SE) for a known IOL power, and the second can predict the IOL power engrafted given the postoperative SE and biometric data [18].

First, they are created using large datasets. Second, they use advanced machine learning algorithms that are excellent at creating predictive models. Third, they can be updated and improved as postoperative refractive data become available. Examples of publicly available AI formulas include the Radial Basis Function (RBF) 2.0, Emmetropia Verifying Optical Formula (EVO) 2.0, Kane, Postoperative spherical Equivalent prediction using ARtificial intelligence and Linear algorithms by Guillaume Debellemanière, Damien Gatinel, and Alain Saad (PEARL-DGS), Hoffer Q Savini/Taroni (Hoffer QST), and Ladas Super Formula 2.0 [19].

The Kane formula was introduced in 2017 and developed using several large data sets from selected high-volume surgeons. It used about 30.000 eyes. This formula is a combination of theoretical optics, thin lens formulas, and big data techniques to make its predictions. The Kane formula requires A-constant (ACD-constant), AL, K, ACD, and sex or gender as variables. A-constant formula is similar to SRK/T formula; LT and central corneal thickness (CCT) will improves predictions, therefore there were optional [20].

Table 22.1 Variables used in the formula based on hybrid and AI

Formula		Logic approach classification	Variables utilized								
			AL	K	KmA	KmP	ACD	LT	CCT	WTW	G
FullMonte		Hybrid	C				C	C			
Ladas		Hybrid	C	C			C				
Hill-RBF	1.0	AI	C	C			C				
	2.0		C	C			C				
	3.0		C	C			C	O	O	O	O
PEARL-DGS		Hybrid	C	C			C	C	C	C	
Kane		Hybrid	C	C			C	O	O		C
Karmona		AI	C		C	O	C	O		C	C
Hoffer QST		Hybrid	C	C			C				C
Nallasamy		AI	C	C			C	C	O	C	

AL axial length, *K* keratometry, *KmA* keratometry-mean anterior, *KmP* keratometry-mean posterior, *ACD* anterior chamber depth, *LT* lens thickness, *CCT* central corneal thickness, *WTW* white to white, *G* gender, *Hill-RBF* Hill-radial basis function, *PEARL-DGS* Postoperative spherical equivalent prediction using ARtificial intelligence and Linear algorithms by Guillaume Debellemanière, Damien Gatinel, and Alain Saad, *Hoffer QST* Hoffer Q, Savini, Taroni, *C* compulsory, *O* optional, *AI* artificial intelligence

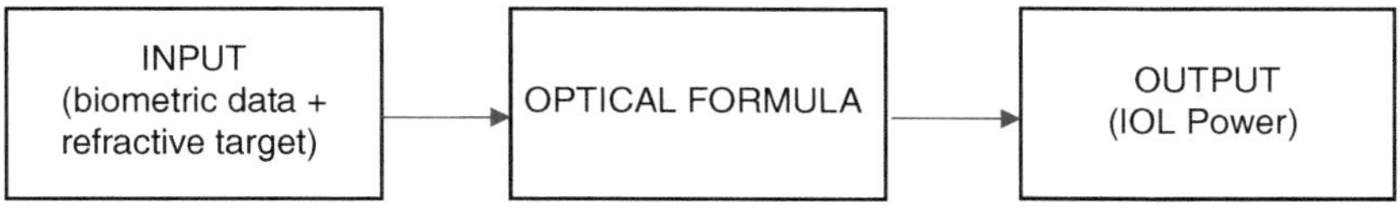

Fig. 22.1 The classic scheme of IOL power calculation using a classic optical formula

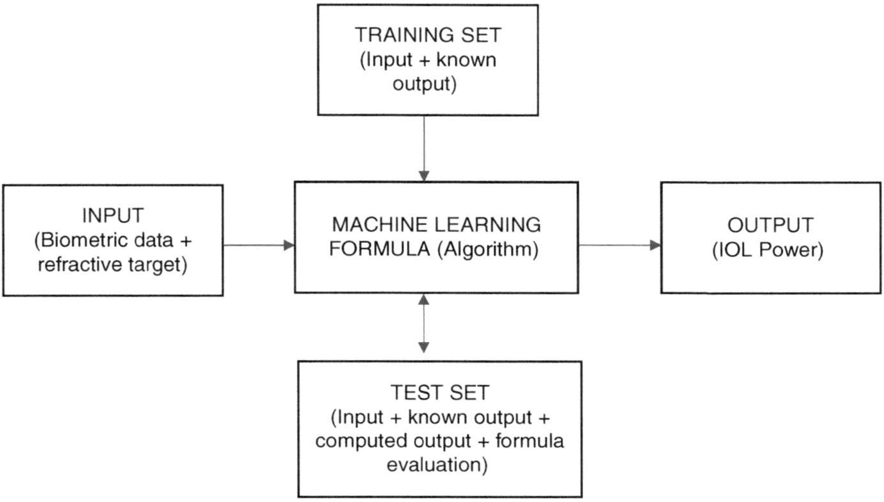

Fig. 22.2 IOL power calculation using an artificial intelligence formula

PEARL-DGS was developed by Guillaume Debellemanière, Damien Gatinel, and Alain Saad in 2017 using optical biometry and a machine learning model. This is a thick lens formula based on the prediction of the theoretical internal lens position (TILP), a distance from the posterior corneal surface to the anterior IOL surface. TILP is calculated by different machine learning algorithms, for examples, neural networks, gradient boosted trees, and support vector regression. This formula uses AL, K, ACD, LT, WTW, and CCT. Output linearization, adjustable IOL constant, and no retraining for new models are typical of the PEARL-DGS method [21].

The Ladas Super Formula AI was developed in 2015 by John G. Ladas, Uday Devgan, Albert Jun, and Aazim Siddiqui. The formula is based on the idea of super formula IOL. It predicts the refractive outcome by using one of five third-generation formulas (Holladay 1, Hoffer Q, Holladay 1, SRK/T) and fourth-generation formulas (Haigis). This formula was developed using mathematical equations with the potential to be graphed on the x, y, and z axes and elaborated them in three dimensions, which will provide the framework to analyze the formulas in three dimensions. Using this observation, the super-surface IOL formula was constructed [22]. I mean, depending on most of literatures especially [23], Ladas Super Formula AI is the most accurate formula in combining AL and K.

The Hill-RBF uses deep learning from a large data set to predict refractive outcomes (a pure AI regression method). This formula, introduced in 2016 by Warren E. Hill, MD, adds a validating boundary model by which it refuses to provide a refractive prediction as it is more likely to be inaccurate. This is a pure data-driven IOL power calculation method and uses pattern recognition developed by MATLAB and a refined form of data interpolation. The Hill-RBF online calculator adjusted for used with LENSTAR LS 900 (Haag-Streit, Köniz, Switzerland) optical biometer in combination with the Alcon SN60WF (Alcon Laboratories, Fortworth, TX, USA). Hill-RBF 3.0 formula uses AL, K, ACD, LT, WTW, CCT, and gender as variables [24].

The Karmona formula is the newest IOL power calculation formula, designed by David Carmona G between 2018 and 2021. This formula is the result of pure AI without Gaussian theoretical components. It is based on two combined models of machine learning, called a regularized Bayesian neural network and a Cubist decision tree. The data variables include AL, ACD, K, WTW, and corneal anterior surface central radius. Karmona is optimized for anterior keratometry with IOL Master® 700 (Carl Zeiss Meditec, Dublin, CA) and for posterior keratometry with Pentacam® (Oculus Optikgeräte GmbH, Wetzlar, Germany). However, this formula is continuously improving [25].

Hoffer QST is an evolution of the Hoffer Q formula to improve its accuracy by utilizing AI. The founder tried to increase the accuracy of Hoffer Q in long eyes by improving the prediction of ELP. The variables used for this formula are K, AL, ACD, corneal radius, and gender. The formula is calculated for IOL power by using linear machine and integrating with AI adjustment [26].

The Nallasamy formula, announced in 2022 by Li, Stein, and Nallasamy, is based on an ensemble machine-learning model that has recently been introduced. This formula is based on a data set of 5016 eyes, obtained by Lenstar LS 900 optical biometers (Haag-Streit USA; EyeSuite software V.i9.1.0.0) at the University of Michigan's Kellogg Eye Center. The formula uses six compulsory variables such AL; K; ACD; WTW; LT; and CCT. This formula utilizes an ensemble machine learning model consisting of two layers. The first layer is preoperative data and IOL power as input data and the postoperative refraction as the target value. The second layer includes a meta-model, and the output is the final predicted refraction [27].

22.4 Comparison of AI IOL Formulas

Many IOL formulas have been developed over the years, with the aim to achieve the most accurate refractive outcome. Recent formulas, based on AI, have been launched with complex parameters, resulting in greater accuracy. Many studies compared the accuracy of AI IOL formulas with refraction target $< \pm 0.5$ D SE and lower MAE as parameters. Lower MAE values indicate higher accuracy in predicting the correct IOL power [17].

Stopyra et al., in 2023, compared the twelve intraocular lens power calculation formulas for eyes smaller than 22.0 mm in terms of absolute error (AE), percentage of postoperative emmetropia, by using Holladay 1, SRK/T, Hoffer Q, Holladay 2, Haigis, Barrett Universal II (BUII), Hill-RBF, Ladas, Kane, EVO, Pearl-DGS, and K6 formulas. Three months after phacoemulsification, refraction was measured, and the mean AE was calculated. Results showed Kane and Hill-RBF obtained the lowest agreement interval, by mean Kane formula is recommended for intarocular lens power calculation for eyeballs with the axial length smaller than 22.0 mm [28].

Voytsekhivskyy et al., analyzing 24 intraocular lens formula(s) accuracy; BUII, Castrop, EVO 2.0, Haigis, Hoffer Q, Hoffer QST, Holladay 1, Holladay 2, Holladay 2 (AL Adjusted), K6 (Cooke), Kane, Karmona, LSF AI, Naeser 2, OKULIX, Olsen (OLCR), Olsen (standalone), Panacea, PEARL-DGS, RBF 3.0, SRK/T, T2, Voytsekhivskyy Regression Function (VRF), and VRF-G (gender). The IOL Master 700 was used for biometric measurements with optimized lens constants, the mean PE and its standard deviation (SD), the median absolute error (MedAE), the MAE. The result showed that Kane, Hoffer QST, and BUII were more accurate than the older formulas, yielding the highest percentage of refractive accuracy [29].

The latest research of Stopyra et al. [16] concluded that among AI-based formulas, Kane seems to be the most accurate. It achieves the lowest MAE and the highest percentage of eyes within ±0.5 D [17].

22.5 AI Chat Programs

Nowadays, AI chat programs have become useful tools for confirming the accuracy of calculations made by IOL calculation machines, ranging from the most conventional to the most advanced, including the IOLMaster 700. In cases where AL and K-readings are too extreme, or in eyes with abnormalities, or eyes that have undergone certain previous surgeries, such as keratorefractive surgery, vitrectomy, scleral buckle, etc., AI chat programs can be utilized to confirm the results of machine calculations.

To date, calculations using machines such as the IOLMaster 700 remain the gold standard in IOL power calculation. Internet-based IOL power calculation tools or online calculators, as presented by various professional organizations and many IOL manufacturers, as well as calculations using AI-based formulas such as Kane, Ladas Super Formula, Hill-RBF, PEARL-DGS, etc., can also be relied upon as first-line calculation tools. However, AI chat programs cannot yet be fully relied upon as first-line calculation tools. Nevertheless, AI chat programs can be used to confirm IOL power calculations in cases that are questionable and require additional attention.

Currently, there are various AI chat programs, including ChatGPT, DeepSeek, Claude, Llama, Gemini, Bard, Replika, Jasper, Perplexity, Tidio, ManyChat, Landbot, and others. Each has its own utility based on the initial programming intentions of its service providers. Please study them carefully to determine which is most reliable in helping to confirm IOL calculations with conventional machines, online calculators, or AI-based formulas.

If we perform cataract surgery in any area with only basic biometry tools and limited data available, as long as the internet is accessible, we can optimize the IOL power calculations and confirm their various calculations using AI chat programs.

22.6 How to Use AI Chat Programs to Confirm any IOL Power Calculations

Using ChatGPT as one of the AI chat programs, for example, to assist with IOL power calculations can be a valuable way out for ophthalmologists and eye care professionals. However, it's important to note that ChatGPT itself does not perform calculations directly. Instead, it can guide you through the process, provide information on relevant formulas, and help you interpret the results. Here's how to effectively use ChatGPT for IOL power calculations:

22.7 Step-by-Step Guide to Using ChatGPT for IOL Power Calculation

1. *Gather patient data*: Before using ChatGPT, collect all necessary biometric measurements for the patient, including:
   - AL, K1, K2, ACD, WTW, LT, CCT, etc.
   - Any previous surgical history (if applicable)
   - IOL data, A-constant, material (hydrophobic, hydrophilic), multifocal, toric, etc.
2. *Choose the formula*: AI will guide you to a specific IOL calculation. However, we can propose certain formulas. Determine which IOL power calculation formula you want to use. Common formulas include:
   - SRK/T
   - Hoffer Q
   - BUII
   - Kane Formula
   - Others based on the specific situation
3. *Ask for guidance*: You can ask ChatGPT-specific questions related to the formula you are using. For example:
   - "What is the SRK/T formula for calculating IOL power?"
   - "How do I calculate ELP using the BUII formula?"

4. *Input data*: Provide the necessary patient data to ChatGPT. For example:
   - "Using the SRK/T formula, if the axial length is 25 mm, the keratometry is 44.00 D, and the ACD is 3.0 mm, what is the IOL power?"
5. *Calculate manually or use a calculator*: Based on the guidance provided by ChatGPT, you may need to perform the calculations manually or use a scientific calculator. If you need assistance with the calculations, you can ask:
   - "Can you help me understand how to calculate the effective lens position for the given measurements?"
6. *Interpret results*: Once you have the calculated IOL power, you can ask ChatGPT for help in interpreting the results. For example:
   - "What does an IOL power of +22.00 D suggest for this patient?"
7. *Double-check*: Always verify the calculations with established medical software or tools specifically designed for IOL power calculations, as ChatGPT is not a substitute for clinical judgment or specialized software.

22.8 Example Interaction

Here's an example of how you might interact with ChatGPT for IOL power calculation:

User: "What is the formula for calculating IOL power using the SRK/T method?"
ChatGPT: "The SRK/T formula is given by:

$$P = A - 0.9 \times K - 2.5 \times AL$$

Where:

- P = IOL power
- A = A-constant of the IOL
- K = Keratometry reading
- AL = Axial length in mm."

User: "If the A-constant is 118, K is 43.00 D (diopter), and AL is 25 mm, what is the IOL power?"
ChatGPT: "You can calculate it as follows:

$$P = 118 - 0.9 \times 43 - 2.5 \times 25$$

This simplifies to:

$$P = 118 - 38.7 - 62.5 = 16.8$$

Thus, the IOL power is approximately +16.8 D."

We can repeat our calculations using various prompts and keywords until we gain confidence in the IOL power value that is closest to the most accurate value.

22.9 Conclusion

The integration of AI into IOL power calculation represents a significant advancement in cataract surgery. IOL power calculation formula based on AI has the potential to achieve the most accurate postoperative refractions after cataract surgery. By leveraging machine learning algorithms and advanced biometric measurements, ophthalmologists can enhance the accuracy of IOL power predictions, ultimately improving patient outcomes. As the field continues to evolve, ongoing research and collaboration will be essential to fully realize the potential of AI in optimizing IOL power calculations and addressing the complexities of individual patient care.

AI chat programs cannot yet be fully relied upon as first-line calculation tools. Nevertheless, AI chat programs can be used to confirm IOL power calculations in cases that are questionable and require more meticulous attention.

Using ChatGPT as one of the AI chat programs can enhance your understanding and support your decision-making process in IOL power calculations. We expected the future improvements to this AI-based formula and the application could contribute to better outcomes for every patient. However, it is still very crucial to combine this assistance with clinical expertise and validated tools to ensure the best outcomes.

References

1. Aristodemou P, Sparrow JM, Kaye S. Evaluating refractive outcomes after cataract surgery. Ophthalmology. 2019;126:13–8. https://doi.org/10.1016/j.ophtha.2018.07.009.
2. Melles RB, Holladay JT, Chang WJ. Accuracy of Intraocular Lens calculation Formulas. Ophthalmology. 2018;125:169–78. https://doi.org/10.1016/j.ophtha.2017.08.027. (Aristodemou P, Knox Cartwright NE, Sparrow JM, Johnston RL. Formula choice: Hoffer Q, Holladay 1, or SRK/T and refractive outcomes in 8108 eyes after cataract surgery with biometry by partial coherence interferometry). J Cataract Refract Surg 2011; 37(1): 63–71. 10.1016/j.jcrs.2010.07.032).
3. Lee AC, Quazi MA, Pepose JS. Biometry and intraocular lens power calculation. Curr Opin Ophthalmol. 2008;19:13–7. https://doi.org/10.1097/ICU.0b013e3282f1c5ad.
4. Nemeth G, Modis L Jr. Accuracy of the Hill-radial basis function method and the Barrett Universal II formula. Eur J Ophthalmol. 2021;31:566–71. https://doi.org/10.1177/1120672120902952.
5. Norrby S. Sources of error in intraocular lens power calculation. J Cataract Refract Surg. 2008;34:368–76. https://doi.org/10.1016/j.jcrs.2007.10.031.
6. Grzybowski A. Artificial intelligence in ophthalmology. Cham: Springer Nature; 2021. p. 1–286. https://doi.org/10.1007/978-3-031-83756-2.

7. Schmidt-Erfurth U, Sadeghipour A, Gerendas BS, Waldstein SM, Bogunović H. Artificial intelligence in retina. Prog Retin Eye Res. 2018;67:1–29. https://doi.org/10.1016/j.preteyeres.2018.07.004.
8. Ramessur R, Raja L, Kilduff CL, Kang S, Li JPO, Thomas PB, Sim DA. Impact and challenges of integrating artificial intelligence and telemedicine into clinical ophthalmology. Asia-Pac J Ophthalmol. 2021;10:317–27. https://doi.org/10.1097/APO.0000000000000406.
9. Zhu L, et al. The Zhu-Lu formula: a machine learning-based intraocular lens power calculation formula for highly myopic eyes. BMC Ophthalmol. 2023;23(1):1–9. https://doi.org/10.1186/s12886-023-00442-5.
10. Wang Y, et al. A study on repeatability and agreement of keratometry & refractive prediction between Verion and IOL Master. J Pak Med Assoc. 2021;71(2):1–9. https://doi.org/10.47391/jpma.3842.
11. Kim JH, Park SH. Investigation of the myopic outcomes of the newer intraocular lens power calculation formulas in Korean patients with long eyes. Sci Rep. 2023;13(1):1–8. https://doi.org/10.1038/s41598-024-63334-y.
12. Hoffer KJ, et al. Predictive accuracy of Barrett TK toric calculator compared to measured posterior corneal astigmatism using Pentacam in toric IOL power calculation. Indian J Ophthalmol. 2023;71(6):1–7. https://doi.org/10.4103/ijo.ijo_1386_23.
13. Ahuja AS, Paredes Iii AA, Eisel MLS, et al. Applications of artificial intelligence in cataract surgery: a review. Clin Ophthalmol. 2024;18:2969–75. Published 2024 Oct 17. https://doi.org/10.2147/OPTH.S489054.
14. Clarke GP, Burmeister J. Comparison of intraocular lens computations using a neural network versus the Holladay formula. J Cataract Refract Surg. 1997;23(10):1585–9. https://doi.org/10.1016/s0886-3350(97)80034-x.
15. Hipólito-Fernandes D, Luís ME, Serras-Pereira R, Gil P, Maduro V, Feijão J, Alves N. Anterior chamber depth, lens thickness and intraocular lens calculation formula accuracy: nine formulas comparison. Br J Ophthalmol. 2022;106:349–55. https://doi.org/10.1136/bjophthalmol-2020-317822.
16. Stopyra W, Cooke DL, Grzybowski A. A review of intraocular lens power calculation formulas based on Artificial intelligence. J Clin Med. 2024;13(2):498. https://doi.org/10.3390/jcm13020498.
17. Stopyra W, Voytsekhivskyy O, Grzybowski A. Accuracy of 7 artificial intelligence-based intraocular lens power calculation formulas in medium-long eyes: 2-center study. Can J Ophthalmol. 2025;60(4):200–7. https://doi.org/10.1016/j.jcjo.2025.01.020.
18. Rojas JD, Ladas J. AI models for IOL calculation. In: Cataract & refractive surgery today; 2023.
19. Kane J. Kane Calculator. Available online: https://iolformula.com.
20. Debellemanière G, Dubois M, Gauvin M, Wallerstein A, Brenner LF, Rampat R, Saad A, Gatinel D. The PEARL-DGS formula: the development of an Open-source machine Learning-based thick IOL calculation formula. Am J Ophthalmol. 2021;232:58–69. https://doi.org/10.1016/j.ajo.2021.05.004.
21. Siddiqui AA, Juthani V, Kang J, Chuck RS. The future of intraocular lens calculations: Ladas super formula. Ann Eye Sci. 2019;4:19. https://doi.org/10.21037/aes.2019.04.02.
22. Ladas JG, Siddiqui AA, Devgan U, Jun AS. A 3-D "Super Surface" Combining Intraocular Lens Formulas to Generate a "Super Formula" and Maximize Accuracy. JAMA Ophthalmol. 2015;133:1431–6. https://doi.org/10.1001/jamaophthalmol.2015.3832.
23. Hill W. Hill-RBF Calculator. Available online: https://rbfcalculator.com.
24. Carmona-González D, Palomino-Bautista C. Accuracy of a new intraocular lens power calculation method based on artificial intelligence. Eye. 2021;35:517–22. https://doi.org/10.1038/s41433-020-0883-3.
25. Taroni L, Hoffer KJM, Pellegrini M, Lupardi E, Savini G. Comparison of the New Hoffer QST with 4 Modern Accurate Formulas. J Cataract Refract Surg. 2023;49:378–84. https://doi.org/10.1097/j.jcrs.0000000000001126.

26. Li T, Stein J, Nallasamy N. Evaluation of the Nallasamy formula: a stacking ensemble machine learning method for refraction prediction in cataract surgery. Br J Ophthalmol. 2023;107:1066–71. https://doi.org/10.1136/bjophthalmol-2021-320599.
27. Stopyra W. The accuracy of intraocular lens power calculation formulas for eyes longer than 25.00 mm and the correlation between method accuracy and eye axial length. Klin Ocz. 2021;123:129–33. https://doi.org/10.5114/ko.2021.107849.
28. Stopyra W. Analysis of accuracy of twelve intraocular lens power calculation formulas for eyes with axial hyperopia. Saudi J Ophthalmol. 2023;37:125–30. https://doi.org/10.4103/sjopt.sjopt_64_22.
29. Voytsekhivskyy OV, Hoffer KJ, Tutchenko L, Cooke DL, Savini G. Accuracy of 24 IOL power calculation methods. J Refract Surg. 2023;39:249–56. https://doi.org/10.3928/1081597X-20230131-01.

Index

G. Pardianto (ed.), *Intraocular Lens (IOL) Power Calculation*,
https://doi.org/10.1007/978-981-92-1223-1

GPSR Compliance

The European Union's (EU) General Product Safety Regulation (GPSR) is a set of rules that requires consumer products to be safe and our obligations to ensure this.

If you have any concerns about our products, you can contact us on ProductSafety@springernature.com

In case Publisher is established outside the EU, the EU authorized representative is:

Springer Nature Customer Service Center GmbH
Europaplatz 3
69115 Heidelberg, Germany

Batch number: 10732090

Printed by Printforce, the Netherlands